# *Intrusive Interventions*

# Rochester Studies in Medical History

Senior Editor: Theodore M. Brown
Professor of History and Preventive Medicine
University of Rochester

Additional Titles of Interest

*Barefoot Doctors and Western Medicine in China*
Xiaoping Fang

*Beriberi in Modern Japan: The Making of a National Disease*
Alexander R. Bay

*The Lobotomy Letters*
Mical Raz

*Plague and Public Health in Early Modern Seville*
Kristy Wilson Bowers

*Medicine and the Workhouse*
Edited by Jonathan Reinarz and Leonard Schwarz

*Stress, Shock, and Adaptation in the Twentieth Century*
Edited by David Cantor and Edmund Ramsden

*Female Circumcision and Clitoridectomy in the United States: A History of a Medical Treatment*
Sarah B. Rodriguez

*The Spanish Influenza Pandemic of 1918–1919: Perspectives from the Iberian Peninsula and the Americas*
Edited by María-Isabel Porras-Gallo and Ryan A. Davis

*Infections, Chronic Disease, and the Epidemiological Transition: A New Perspective*
Alexander Mercer

*Save the Babies: American Public Health Reform and the Prevention of Infant Mortality, 1850–1929*
Richard A. Meckel

A complete list of titles in the Rochester Studies in Medical History series may be found on our website, www.urpress.com.

# *Intrusive Interventions*

## *Public Health, Domestic Space, and Infectious Disease Surveillance in England, 1840–1914*

Graham Mooney

University of Rochester Press

First published 2015

University of Rochester Press
668 Mt. Hope Avenue, Rochester, NY 14620, USA
www.urpress.com
and Boydell & Brewer Limited
PO Box 9, Woodbridge, Suffolk IP12 3DF, UK
www.boydellandbrewer.com

ISBN-13: 978-1-58046-527-4
ISSN: 1526-2715

**Library of Congress Cataloging-in-Publication Data**

Mooney, Graham.
Intrusive interventions : public health, domestic space, and infectious disease surveillance in England, 1840–1914 / Graham Mooney.
pages cm. — (Rochester studies in medical history : ISSN 1526-2715 ; v. 33)
Includes bibliographical references and index.
ISBN 978-1-58046-527-4 (hardcover : alk. paper) 1. Communicable diseases—History—England—19th century. 2. Epidemiology—History—England—19th century. 3. Medicine, Preventive—History—19th century. 4. Public health—England. I. Title.
RA643.M66 2015
362.10942—dc23 2015016147

A catalogue record for this title is available from the British Library.

This publication is printed on acid-free paper.
Printed in the United States of America.

To the memory of my grandmother
Florence Taylor (née Schofield), 1901–97

# Contents

Acknowledgments ix

Abbreviations xiii

Introduction 1

## Part One: Making Infectious Disease Surveillance

1 Finding Disease in the Victorian City 19

2 "These Bastard Laws": Infectious Disease, Liberty, and Localism 40

## Part Two: Spaces of Risk and Opportunity

3 Sequestration and Permeability: Isolation Hospitals 69

4 "Combustible Material": Classrooms, Contact Tracing, and Following-Up 93

5 Disinfection, Domestic Space, and the Laboratory 121

6 Rules for Home Living: Tuberculosis and the Consumption of Self-Help 154

Conclusion 179

Notes 183

Bibliography 233

Index 265

# Acknowledgments

I have to disagree with Friedrich Nietzsche, who once wrote that "all truly great thoughts are conceived while walking." Really? For me, it's while on public transport. Sit me on a bus or a train and the idea mill just starts churning. So, my first acknowledgment has to go to the public transport system in Cagliari, Sardinia, on which the idea to write a book on infectious disease surveillance was hatched. Even though it has taken the better part of two decades to get my stuff together, I don't regret that particular thought. I have thoroughly enjoyed researching and writing this book, and it gives me great pleasure to express my gratitude to the many wonderful people and organizations that have sustained and supported me.

I have had many scholarly mentors over the years, but none were more inspirational and generous than my PhD supervisors in the Department of Geography at Liverpool University, Gerry Kearns and the late Bob Woods. What a great team they made—outstanding examples of collegiality, inquisitiveness, and rigorous high standards. The kernel of this book can be found in my PhD dissertation, so it is to them that I owe my longest-term debt. I'm deeply sorry that Bob is not around to read this book, though I know there aren't enough graphs in it for him!

Three other colleagues have also been instrumental. Anne Hardy showed faith in the project from an early stage and has shepherded me through my career in various ways since then. I was extremely fortunate to work with Bill Luckin for a large chunk of the 1990s as I was trying to find my way at the intersections of public health, geography, and history. As many others have discovered, Bill is an avid supporter of junior scholars' work. He is also a living, breathing, editorial red pen. He kindly read drafts of chapters and made helpful suggestions at a crucial stage. My office at the Institute of the History of Medicine at Johns Hopkins University happened to be next door to that of the late Harry Marks—and what a remarkable stroke of spatial luck that was. Harry took me under his wing, shared his vast store of knowledge, and continually provoked me to think harder (frequently indicated by nothing more than a raised eyebrow). If nothing else, I trust that some of the long footnotes in this book do justice to his cherished memory.

Other colleagues have also played important roles. At the Institute, Mary Fissell, Randy Packard, Gianna Pomata, and Dan Todes all read draft chapters and encouraged me to find a distinctive voice. I have done my best to take their advice to heart. I am lucky to have them all as colleagues, but I am truly grateful to Mary and Randy who have been particularly supportive in a whole host of other ways. Vicky Blake, Nadja Durbach, Chris Hamlin, Matthew Newsom Kerr, Jonathan Reinarz, Simon Szreter, Andrea Tanner, and Rebecca Whyte have either read various bits of the book or pointed me in the direction of primary sources. My graduate students Eli Anders (at Johns Hopkins) and Anne Clark and Sue Smith (at the Open University) always took a keen interest in the progress of the book, and have taught me more than they probably realize. My apologies to those people I have left out.

Another example of spatial luck has been to have departmental digs next to the lovely people in the Rare Book Room in the Institute library. Their ability to uncover readings, find obscure references, and smile all the while is a constant source of amazement to me. Thank you, Linda Bright, Eliza Hill, and most of all Christine Ruggere, who is not only the best book curator and primary source locator but a good friend. Meanwhile, the administrative support of Coraleeze Thompson at the institute has got me out of a hole on many occasions.

Archives scattered across provincial England provided access to much of the content I have used. I am profoundly grateful to the indefatigable staff of city and county archives and various libraries and collections in Birmingham, Leicester, Liverpool, Manchester, Nottingham, Salford, Sheffield, and Newcastle. In London, I spent time in the British Library, the British Medical Association Archives, the Fawcett Library, the London Metropolitan Archives, the Parliamentary Archives, and the Wellcome Library.

This book would not have been possible without very generous funding from the Wellcome Trust in the form of a postdoctoral fellowship. I was also a visiting fellow at the University of Nottingham's Institute for the Study of Genetics, Biorisks and Society in 2003, where I was able to conduct archival research in Nottingham and strike up a friendship with Patrick Wallis, who was extremely generous during my stay there. Ted Brown and Sonia Kane at the University of Rochester Press have been very patient, encouraging, and helpful.

Friends and family have, of course, sustained me throughout the writing of this book. Ian Callaghan and Amelia Foster in Oxford, and Mark and Julie Arnull in Birmingham, put me up on numerous occasions and have been great friends during some difficult times. My mum, Margery Mooney; my late dad, Gerard Mooney; as well as Margaret Mooney, Paul and Gel Mooney, Violetta Hionidou, and Mary Alice Ernish have all supported me in myriad ways. Thank you. I'm incredibly lucky to have two wonderful children, Ilia and Yuri, who never fail to keep me going with their great senses of humor and love. You two are the best. Finally, this book is dedicated to the memory of my maternal grandmother, Florence Taylor. It took me many years to realize it, but it is to her that I owe my love of history.

I wish to thank the publishers of the following articles for their permission to reproduce here revised sections from these articles: "The Material Consumptive: Domesticating the Tuberculosis Patient in Edwardian England," *Journal of*

*Historical Geography* 42, no. 1 (2013): 152–66, © 2013 by Elsevier; "Infection and Citizenship: (Not) Visiting Isolation Hospitals in Mid-Victorian Britain," in *Permeable Walls: Historical Perspectives on Hospital and Asylum Visiting*, ed. Graham Mooney and Jonathan Reinarz (Amsterdam: Clio Medica/Rodopi, 2009), 147–74; "Public Health versus Private Practice: The Contested Development of Compulsory Notification of Infectious Disease in Late-Nineteenth-Century Britain," *Bulletin of the History of Medicine* 73, no. 2 (1999): 238–67, © 1999 by the Johns Hopkins University Press; and "The Prevention and Control of Infectious Childhood Diseases in Late-Nineteenth- and Early-Twentieth-Century London: The Case of Diphtheria and Measles," in *Questioni Di Popolazione in Europa: Una Prospettiva Geografica*, ed. Russell King and Marie-Luisa Gentileschi (Bologna: Patron Editore, 1996), 255–71.

# Abbreviations

| | |
|---|---|
| AO | attendance officer (school board) |
| BMA | British Medical Association |
| CLH | Common Lodging Houses |
| CMO | chief medical officer (Board of Education) |
| GP | general practitioner |
| GRO | General Register Office |
| LCC | London County Council |
| LGB | Local Government Board |
| LMI | Liverpool Medical Institution |
| LMS | Leicester Medical Society |
| LSB | London School Board |
| MAB | Metropolitan Asylums Board |
| MOH | medical officer of health |
| MSSA | Manchester and Salford Sanitary Association |
| NDMS | Northumberland and Durham Medical Society |
| PLB | Poor Law Board |
| PLMO | Poor Law medical officer |
| RSC | Royal Sanitary Commission |
| SCPSR | Select Committee on Police and Sanitary Regulations |
| SMO | school medical officer |
| SMOH | Society of Medical Officers of Health |
| SMS | School Medical Service |
| VADPR | Vigilance Association for the Defence of Personal Rights |

# Introduction

In an 1876 address that was reported in both the medical and popular press, the newly inaugurated president of the Society of Medical Officers of Health, Dr. George Buchanan, spoke to his colleagues about "Citizenship in Sanitary Work."[1] As one of the first medical officers of health in London—appointed in 1856 at the parish of St. Giles in the Fields—and at the time an assistant medical officer to the Local Government Board, Buchanan had been steeped in the public health problems of English urban life for two decades.[2] Despite this wealth of experience—or more likely because of it—that October Friday night Buchanan drew inspiration from the American state of Massachusetts. He pointed to the great strides in sanitation since the formation of the Massachusetts State Board of Health in 1869. Buchanan recounted at length the part played by the board in the recent establishment of an abattoir in the neighborhood of Brighton, which had lately been annexed by the city of Boston.[3] The board's attempt at nuisance control had met with predictable resistance from local butchers, but by 1876 the city had an exemplary facility that, remarkably, found favor with the butchers and was ready to be administered by the city of Boston itself.

So what did Buchanan want his metropolitan audience of medical officers to take from this transatlantic story? Certainly he made no attempt whatsoever at comparison with the regulation of the meat trade in Britain.[4] Rather, his message concerned the broader philosophical issues of compulsion and citizen participation in public health matters. It was, Buchanan observed, through the careful formulation and implementation of compulsory legislation that the Massachusetts Board of Health was able to intervene against slaughterhouses. The board was encouraged by petitions lodged by Brighton's inhabitants, who were fed up with blood running in the streets and the offensive stench of offal. In the very same spirit of commonweal, Bostonians had lobbied successfully for the creation of a local board of health for the city in 1872.[5]

"I have told the story of Massachusetts' sanitary progress very badly," Buchanan said, "if there is any need to point its moral for ourselves."[6] Of course, he spent the rest of his speech doing exactly that. And the moral was this: the need to educate ignorant and careless people in the individual and community-wide benefits of sanitary reform. As Buchanan saw it, Britain's problem was that general national laws did not cover all the aspects of public health that concerned a local community. Local bylaws, meanwhile, only dealt with a limited range of topics. So, the key to filling this vacuum in Britain's efforts to solve urban health problems was to raise the sanitary consciousness of the public, with the intention that the community would take a more vocal and active role in its own government.[7]

Buchanan sketched out how a diligent medical officer of health (MOH) should communicate knowledge by writing reports in an accessible manner and by participating at public meetings. Health officers might also help organize local societies that promoted public awareness of sanitary subjects through lectures and pamphleteering. How to get scientific knowledge across to the lay public was a knotty problem for Buchanan and his colleagues, but he was excited about the potential to do so. According to him, greater public interest in hygienic matters would make for a robust political culture of citizenship because "people will understand better their rights as well as their duties in local self-government."[8]

To illustrate the importance of community participation in sanitary matters, Buchanan concluded his address with the matter of infectious disease notification:

> A community wants to take all possible precautions against scarlet fever, and to begin by making a municipal law that every householder shall inform the sanitary officers of the existence of the disease. Why should it not be able to order this, and to take any like action that it considers suitable to its circumstances? And why should it have to wait, for its proper security, until Parliament has come to the conclusion that it may exceptionally be endowed with the required authority, or until Parliament is pleased to consider such course of action fit for enforcement everywhere throughout England? The direct right of a local community, while subject to general law, to make for itself what additional law it considers necessary for its sanitary welfare, is at present but imperfectly acknowledged. . . . Without such a right, admitted and acted on, a city arranged by Hygeia herself would presently fall short of the ideal of the goddess.[9]

Did Buchanan pluck this example randomly from thin air? Hardly. In that same year, 1876, the Yorkshire town of Huddersfield had introduced the first local legislation for infectious disease notification. Meanwhile, other towns—Bolton in England, Greenock in Scotland—were preparing to take local improvement bills to Parliament in 1877 that also incorporated the measure. These pioneering forays into the systematic reporting of infected people to local authorities were copied by many other localities in the 1880s and 1890s to the point where a nationwide mandate was eventually passed into law in 1899. For the likes of Buchanan, local interest in infectious disease notification was a victory for a "participatory" public health that championed the rights of householders across the country. Buchanan spoke of citizenship as the right of a local community to protect itself, adding that members of a community had a responsibility to report cases of infectious disease. This should not surprise us; after all, what is the politics of public health in modern democracies about if not the balance between rights and responsibilities, and between the competing interests of individuals and communities?[10]

But citizenship is not a static concept. It is subject to perpetual negotiation. Political conflict over citizenship was particularly intense in the lead-up to the 1867 Reform Act, just at the time when public health, as an organized response to the challenges posed by urbanization and industrialization, was becoming embedded as a state practice.[11] Historian Keith McClelland has quite rightly ring-fenced the preeminence of political considerations as the respectable workingman's portal of entry into citizenship, but he does nevertheless reiterate that

> a much fuller account of working-class politics and the relationship of it to the wider patterns of political and social formation . . . would need to say something about how this figure [the citizen] came to be defined not only by some social and economic forces and by his own manner of self-presentation, but also by other agencies . . . [and would need] . . . to examine the impulses from civil society that differentiated the sober, respectable and desirable male figure and his family from others and that situated him as a suitable object for social inclusion and even celebration.[12]

McClelland's own brief list of "impulses from civil society" includes the Temperance Movement, the New Poor Law (since it punished the able-bodied man who did not, or would not, work), sanitary reform, and the regulation of prostitution through the Contagious Diseases Acts. There are, of course, many other "impulses": from the realm of public health I would readily add the campaign against compulsory infant smallpox vaccination in which antivaccinationists argued for their rights as parents to withhold their children from vaccination, whereas provaccinationists saw vaccination as a form of community participation that granted entry into the national polity.[13]

Rather than thinking of citizenship as the political expression of an individual's relationship to the nation-state, McClelland and Sonya Rose hint that it is much more productive to frame it "as a language by means of which people can make claims on the political community concerning rights and duties, political and moral or ethical practices, and criteria for membership."[14] This notion—that questions of citizenship need to be seen through a variety of nonpolitical lenses—has been reiterated for the mid-Victorian period by Martin Pugh, who argues that legislation in the post-1868 Gladstone era was very much concerned with removing barriers to individual development for those who paid rates and taxes, respected the law, and actively sought to help themselves.[15] These three criteria are helpful in thinking about citizenship as related to matters of public health because they were tangled up with it: property taxes (i.e., rates) funded the expansion of public health activity; laws (some of which were contested, as we shall see) enabled and circumscribed public health and people's relation to it; and self-help was both assisted and challenged by public health.

The sort of disease reporting Buchanan wanted was imbued with the question of citizenship because the interventions it facilitated reconfigured hygienic and sanitary norms.[16] It did this in a number of ways: a physician's hitherto confidential diagnosis of infectious disease was made public property; the movements of infected and uninfected people across space were circumscribed;

infectious patients were removed to hospital using force;[17] the behavior of those patients and their visitors was regulated; and parents were held accountable for the prevention of infectious disease in their offspring and its transmission to other children. The rights and freedoms of citizens became conditional on their responsible conduct in the face of infectious disease. What sort of freedoms are these? Eugenio Biagini has questioned the assumption "that classical liberals followed Thomas Hobbes in believing that 'liberty is the absence of restraint.' . . . *Popular* liberals held quite a different concept of liberty—one characterized by an emphasis on 'civic virtue' and participation and indistinguishable from what is commonly described as the 'republican tradition.'"[18] One of the key themes of *Intrusive Interventions,* then, is that public health mediates liberty and government on multiple levels of civic virtue and participation. In other words, "freedom" means the freedom of the local state to govern autonomously,[19] and the freedom of individuals to live without interference from the state.

Historians of Victorian liberal governmentality have used the insights of Michel Foucault to study the rationalities and technologies of nineteenth-century urban government, of which public health was an important part.[20] However, in a simultaneously trenchant and sympathetic critique of this approach, Simon Gunn has argued that the focus on the exercise of rule through freedom has operated at such a level of abstraction that it leaves "unanswered the question of how historical change occurs and who or what contributes to it."[21] I agree with these sentiments (though it has to be said that studies of liberal governmentality are *very* much concerned with the "how"), so the approaches of pioneering social and political historians of the British urban local state, such as Peter Hennock, are no less relevant to how I want to tell the story of infectious disease surveillance than are those of historians adopting a Foucauldian framework.[22]

Moving toward the particularities of public health in this way also represents a response to the recent observation made by Michael Worboys that historians need to think more about the *practices* of science in the history of medicine. Referring to the agenda for his groundbreaking book *Spreading Germs,* Worboys says:

> I focused on new procedures such as antisepsis, disinfection, and isolation, which were targeted at the ways germs passed between and into bodies. In charting how approaches to prevention and treatment moved from being inclusive and multifactorial to being exclusive and focused on single factors, I gave relatively little attention to the techniques, methods, and operation of germ management in the clinic, laboratory, and field. . . . I now know that I missed a trick with regard to all of my themes: I could, and should, have said more about the performative aspects of the germ practices—that is, the techniques, materials, and methods of germ management.[23]

Part 1 of *Intrusive Interventions,* "Making Infectious Disease Surveillance," chronicles the administrative-bureaucratic interest in the creation of a system of sickness registration that eventually morphed into infectious disease notification. Part 2, "Spaces of Risk and Opportunity," constitutes the "doing" of infectious disease surveillance and deals with the "performative aspects of the germ practices" that Worboys feels escaped him (with the qualification, of course, that such practices were not necessarily thought of as germ based).

One advantage of contemplating practice is that it draws us more fully into the messy world of social relations. Take the questions of coercion and resistance; or, in the language of governmentality: "counter-conducts," the protests and struggles "against the processes implemented for conducting others."[24] These have been relatively underplayed in histories of Victorian British public health, apart from the somewhat exceptional and well-documented examples of compulsory infant smallpox vaccination and the Contagious Diseases Acts.[25] Indeed, in contrast to these high-profile campaigns, historians have suggested that people accepted disease reporting and compulsory sequestration in late Victorian Britain as part and parcel of a new public health rationality that trimmed their traditional freedom to be left alone, sick or not.[26] Eugenio Biagini has asserted that, in more general terms, the "task of reconciling liberty and community, individual rights and social control turned out to be simpler in Britain than anywhere else in Europe, with the exception of Switzerland and the Scandinavian countries."[27] *Intrusive Interventions* attempts to refine this somewhat sanguine historical picture by tracing the contentious debate that centered on infectious disease surveillance's articulation of state coercion and its interference with the moral character of family life. There was substantial pushback against its attack on traditional modes of domiciliary patient care (an approach that was partially reversed in the early twentieth century in the case of tuberculosis, as outlined in chapter 6). In sum, the piecing together of infectious disease surveillance—which in the mid-Victorian period was by no means a given and had no identifiable end point—put liberal subjectivity at stake.

Documenting practice also allows me to address historical scholarship that has suggested bacteriological knowledge solidified existing public health activities and somehow made them more palatable to the general public. I want to pose an alternative to this form of technoscientific determinism. Bacteriology notwithstanding, infectious disease surveillance had to be continuously reshaped in order to negate the political fallout of coercion and interference. This was done through minimizing the impact of intrusion, maximizing the mobility and portability of public health technologies, embracing mechanical autonomy, and creating optimal conditions for the regulation of self-governing individuals.

## Infectious Disease Surveillance

*Intrusive Interventions* explores how and why infectious disease notification came about. It documents the transition of notification from a locally determined measure to a full-blown law that was compulsorily enforced across the country. It also examines how the practices of isolation, disinfection, and contact tracing were assembled around notification. Despite their piecemeal implementation, patchy uptake, and partial origins in port authority control, these measures taken together were recognizably characteristic of a national approach to infectious disease prevention that came to be known as the "English System."[28] This book investigates how these techniques help us to think about a much broader set of issues related to the ideology and practice of public health and urban government, particularly to do with the freedoms, rights, and responsibilities of individuals living under the auspices of Victorian liberal democracy.

Sitting between the great age of sanitary engineering in the mid-nineteenth century and a supposed "new" public health in the early twentieth, the final decades of the 1800s were a transitional period in the history of British public health. Until relatively recently, the familiar version of events has been that a unified germ theory challenged and overturned some long-held beliefs and practices in public health. Obviously, the remediation of the public environment was never abandoned; but there was a shift away from the preoccupations of the sanitary movement toward the medical management of biologically dangerous individuals, a transformation that was wrought by a knowledge of germs produced in the laboratories of the bacteriological revolution.[29] This narrative of scientifically propelled progress has not gone undisputed. For example, Worboys's study of the interaction between scientific knowledge and medical practice demonstrates that it is no longer acceptable to speak of a germ "theory" of disease, or even of a bacteriological "revolution" in Victorian medicine. Worboys dates the move toward person-centered policies to the early and mid-1870s, at least concurrent with, and in some cases preceding, the landmark discoveries of Louis Pasteur and Robert Koch.[30] At this time, influential sanitarians were advocating interventions such as disinfection and isolation that relied on the identification of individual cases—George Buchanan's promotion of infectious disease notification in 1876 is a good example—through clinical observation, not bacteriological investigation (even though the language of intervention was sometimes infused with the embryonic language of germs).[31]

While the disinfection of people and their belongings and the sequestration of pathologically dangerous patients both have a history that stretches back centuries, the formalization of infectious disease reporting in the towns and cities of Britain that began in the 1870s facilitated these interventions on a scale that was historically unprecedented, at least outside of epidemic crises. Without infectious disease notification, public health authorities would have disinfected far fewer houses and would have had far fewer patients in their isolation hospitals. But disease reporting did not in itself create new forms of public health regulation; rather, it allowed for the more comprehensive implementation of laws that already existed.[32] The compulsory removal of patients to hospital, the temporary closure of businesses thought to be sources of disease, and domestic visitations by the local sanitary police were all pretty much part and parcel of urban life before infectious disease notification came along.[33] Reporting diseases simply allowed more of these interventions to happen more frequently. In so doing, it justified an expansion of the local state's budget on public health activities—why bother adopting notification legislation to identify even more diseased people if there were no hospitals to send them to.

This bundle of public health intrusions—notification, disinfection, and isolation—has been referred to as "exclusive" by Worboys, who contrasts them with the "inclusive" sanitary reforms of earlier in the century. Peter Baldwin calls them "neo-quarantine," a neat expression that encapsulates the way in which a "traditional" form of sequestration was applied to the "modern" management of diseased individuals. Meanwhile, in his book on hygiene and public health in nineteenth-century France, David Barnes coins the phrase "sanitary-bacteriological synthesis" to characterize much the same set of ideas and techniques.[34]

In a paper published in 1999 I broadly concurred with Worboys, Baldwin, and Barnes in saying, "Notification was *the* crucial policy development in the move toward the individualization of public health strategies in the late nineteenth century. Indeed the scientific therapies and bacteriological examinations that were adopted on a large scale would not have been possible without it."[35] My own thinking on this, however, has changed over the years. While it is true to say that these policies certainly were more tightly focused on individuals with disease and the individual causal factors of disease, this did not mean that their object was as narrowly defined and "exclusive" as we have assumed. Here, I hope to provide a more nuanced reading that demonstrates how infectious disease surveillance opened up the multifaceted world of individuals to the intrusive scrutiny of public health. Nondiseased family members and friends of patients became the objects of education and supervision; domestic space was transformed into a specific focus of intervention; and the school came to be seen as a place of pathogenic exchange through which infectious disease was transferred between people, and from one part of a city to another.

Under these circumstances, to term such efforts that sought to break the cycle of disease transmission as having an "exclusive" focus on the infected individual does them something of a disservice. Baldwin's invoking of "quarantine" (as in "neo-quarantine") also seems restrictive and carries with it an implicit assumption about what quarantine itself was. Consequently, "surveillance" seems to be a more appropriate moniker; it conveys the far-reaching scope of public health that went way beyond the individualization of policies designed to prevent the spread of infectious disease. Surveillance is also more fitting than "neo-quarantine" because of our current understanding of it as the "ongoing systematic collection, analysis, and interpretation of health-related data for use in the planning, implementation, and evaluation of public health practice, closely integrated with the timely dissemination of these data to those who need to know. The final link in the surveillance chain is the application of these data to prevention and control."[36] The volume and type of information used in surveillance today is, of course, extensive, and it is no longer confined to infectious disease.[37] However, the procedures referred to in contemporary disease surveillance systems were first developed and realized in the Victorian period, when a recognizably modern form of "surveillance" began to integrate clinical, epidemiological, and bacteriological intelligence in the service of interventions that traversed all aspects of social life.

Before mandatory national legislation for infectious disease notification in the late 1890s, surveillance constituted a set of measures that were adopted and implemented locally, made possible by "bastard laws," as the title of chapter 2 indicates. Although notification did extend to the vast majority of the urban population by that point, the experience of isolation and disinfection was not uniform across the country. If the uneven uptake of notification is anything to go by, the idea that municipal authorities were eager for a comprehensive system of surveillance seems questionable. Such geographical inconsistencies do indeed point to the importance of local political sensitivities in the determination of urban public health interventions. However, in her comparative study of Birmingham and Gothenburg, Marjaana Niemi came to the conclusion that public health policies were insulated "from political contention and conflict" by the authority of scientific knowledge.[38] Niemi argues that it was mainly because of a lack of citizen interest in the late nineteenth and early twentieth centuries that the field of public health was left to the devices of elected politicians (city councilors) and appointed officials (such as health officers and hospital superintendents) who set great store by expert knowledge.

Such an interpretation is only a partial version of events. I attempt to flesh this out by using archival evidence from a selection of English cities—Liverpool and Manchester in the northwest; Birmingham, Nottingham, and Leicester in the Midlands; and London—that reflect a variety of experiences with infectious disease surveillance. This evidence reveals, first, that the basic tools of surveillance were put in place well before their bacteriological logic was "scientifically" proven: disinfecting apparatus was mobilized, isolation hospitals were built, and schools were temporarily closed in the absence of anything like positive "scientific" confirmation that closure actually staved off infectious disease in the community.

Second, council chambers from one city to the next constantly reverberated to the sound of animated arguments about many areas of public health policy, and infectious disease surveillance was no different. Neither councilors nor MOHs can be said to represent undifferentiated constituencies. They each varied in the production, reproduction, and deployment of popular and expert knowledge about diseases and interventions. These forms of knowledge themselves varied widely in quality and, to use a more recent phrase, transferability. One might wonder why, *if* scientific knowledge *was* so obviously persuasive, elected and appointed public health officials across the country met with such varying degrees of success when trying to convince their fellow citizens of the benefits of infectious disease surveillance. The answer is that in a number of places counterarguments were made about how surveillance impinged on the interests of one group or another, or encroached on the rights and freedoms of ordinary people; sometimes, these groups and people were listened to and interventions were limited accordingly or abandoned altogether.

Third, the amount of political work that had to be done to create a viable space for scientific knowledge to operate should not be underestimated. In this respect, Chris Otter's formulation of "inspectability" in *The Victorian Eye* suggests a valuable framework for understanding infectious disease surveillance. According to Otter, urban technologies became inspectable through the principles of legibility, accessibility, portability, and agglomeration. Though I would define some of these in a slightly different way, and though I am concerned as much with the human-centered materiality of surveillance as I am with the nonhuman material aspects of it, Otter's principles do characterize rather well some of the tactics of infectious disease surveillance.

Otter defines *legibility* quite literally: for example, information about food and drink had to be clearly written and conspicuously displayed. These and other signs and labels made all sorts of inspection possible to both government inspectors and the general public. In the case of infectious disease, family practitioners authorized that the patient's body was sick. This legibility was expressed in the form of a named disease on a notification certificate that became the property of the state; but the causes and modes of transmission of many of these named conditions were open to dispute, and notification often forced this naming exercise on GPs when they would have preferred to avoid it.

*Accessibility* to subterranean and hard-to-reach sanitary hardware was increasingly built in to utility networks via inspection plates and chambers (manholes). For infectious disease, notification was equivalent to the manhole cover because it granted access to the hidden confines of domestic space and the family. For inspectors of infrastructural systems, mobile instruments of measurement and record were not confined to specialist devices, but included everyday items like feathers, balloons, pencils, and notebooks. Disease surveillance generated its own forms of *portability*. Ambulances specifically designed to convey infected patients to isolation hospitals are one example. Special carts for the transport of infected personal property are another. Other technologies of disinfection, such as pump sprayers, also had to be mobile to guarantee their effectiveness in domestic spaces (and, indeed, to enable them to pass easily through doorways and up narrow staircases). Municipal disinfecting teams also devised a handy paper system of documenting disinfection practice that could be taken on the road.

Finally, *agglomeration*. Otter develops this idea in relation to the inspectability of abattoirs, but it is striking that he uses a medical example to introduce it. By bringing patients together in a single space, he says, it "became possible to discern medical identities and differences that remained below the threshold of visibility when the sick remained isolated in the home or small hospitals."[39] This was certainly the case for isolation hospitals, as shown in chapter 3. In addition, agglomeration can be applied to the type of thinking about population that characterized liberal governmentality. As a leading public health figure, Arthur Newsholme stated in Baconian terms, "Knowledge was always power, and it was self-evident that any local authority using the information given it by notification, was in better position to adopt early preventive measures against the spread of disease."[40] But such information was more subtly instrumental than this. Within the hospital setting itself, the agglomeration of data from lots of patients allowed for interrogation of the natural history of infectious diseases that otherwise eluded the collective efforts of medical practitioners elsewhere.[41] Furthermore, with increased knowledge of disease incidence in the community, the calculation of case fatality rates became more reliable. These rates might be broken down by age and sex and compared and contrasted to death rates. In addition, localities with ongoing vulnerability to disease outbreaks could be identified even when case fatality rates were falling (as in the case of scarlet fever). In other words, the agglomeration of numbers calculated and recalculated the geographies of life, sickness, and death.

## Spaces of Risk and Opportunity

Note how Otter's formulation is inherently spatial: accessibility, portability, and agglomeration are all geographical frames.[42] In an essay review of Otter's *Victorian Eye*, historian Iwan Morus argued that if we want "to understand the cultures of Victorian surveillance and spectacle we need to understand their spaces and to understand those spaces we need to get to grips with their specific peculiarities and the particular regimes of production and consumption that sustained them."[43] It can hardly be doubted that infectious disease surveillance broadened the state's penchant for interfering in everyday life and interrupting channels of biological risk.[44] At the same time, it created, opened up, and shaped specific spaces to ideas about how freedom from infection, and the possibilities of life, could be achieved. As many spatial theorists have remarked, a deeper appreciation of the complexity of space is crucial in order to comprehend this exercise of power and the potentialities of freedom.

In an observation that is particularly salient to many of the themes addressed in this book, geographer David Harvey notes that "state apparatuses obsessed with identities, control, and surveillance turn again and again to the absolute conceptions of space and time as central to their mission of effective governance and control."[45] This understanding of space as *absolute*—that is, immovable, fixed, and mapped—is the means of pinpointing individual persons, things, and processes.[46] Yet, as Harvey argues, an absolute conception of space submerges much of what is, or could be, relative and relational. With *relative* space, the preexisting and bounded absolute spaces that are vital for individuation and governance—hospitals and schools, for example—do not go away, but they are conditioned by phenomena and processes within a space-time framework; they are historically spatial and spatially historical.[47] Spaces only exist in relation to other spaces, giving them multiple, not singular, geometries, depending on the location and circumstances of the observer and the observed. *Relational* space, meanwhile, is a means of thinking about the potentiality of space, focusing on processes that produce their own space and time in which identities are "open, fluid, multiple, and indeterminate . . . [which] is how we live day by day."[48]

If we are to understand the meaning of a disinfection laboratory, an isolation hospital, or a school classroom of nonimmune children (at least for a particular slice of time), then we need to grasp the "relational politics of the spatial." "What if," geographer Doreen Massey has asked, "space is the sphere not of a discrete multiplicity of inert *things* . . . [but of] . . . a heterogeneity of practices and *processes?* . . . Then it will be not an already-interconnected whole but an ongoing product of interconnections and not." Conceived in this way, space "will always be unfinished and open."[49] The multiple forms of sociospatial relations can be expressed along dimensions that incorporate scale,[50] place,[51] and networks that do not necessarily privilege any one of these over the other.[52]

I call isolation hospitals, disinfecting stations, laboratories, schools, and homes "spaces of risk and opportunity," because while they were marked out as biologically threatening, at the same time they were also spaces where potential citizens were educated in the management and regulation of their behaviors and social relations.[53] The simultaneity of risk and opportunity draws attention to the potentiality of *uncertainty*, which is precisely what gives these processes of regulation and management their power.[54] As Massey notes, it is not so much the openness or closure of spaces such as laboratories and homes (two kinds of spaces that she herself has studied) that should be the sociopolitical question; rather, it is the terms on which uncertainty is established. How are the range and nature of social relations constructed? What geometries of power are exercised? What trajectories of experience and knowledge are accessed and denied? What connections are made with and to other spaces? In other words—and it is something to which I aspire in my understanding of infectious disease surveillance—the absolute, relative, and relational spaces that public health works through need to be held in dialectic tension.

Health care is a spatialized enterprise. The vast majority of people in the mid-nineteenth century sought remedies for their illnesses from long-standing and intimate sources: the first resort for most ailments was the dispensary or apothecary, the general practitioner, the Friendly Society physician, the street vendor, or friends and relations.[55] Nevertheless, multiple sites existed for the consumption of health care. General and specialist hospitals and workhouses proliferated and continued to multiply in the Victorian city, and individuals' experience of ill health and health care doubtless became increasingly institutionalized. Chapter 1 reveals how, as part of a wider argument about the ways in which vital statistics could be used to govern urban populations, a bureaucratic process of sickness registration in the late 1860s and early 1870s culminated in the realization that the financial costs and biological risks of outdoor poor relief for infected people was unsustainable. This realization was very much predicated on the construction of a kind of environmental absolute space as a means of managing "vital geographies."[56] Just as large infrastructural projects of urban environmental and sanitary reform gathered pace, a parallel rationale emerged that poor and working-class people with an infectious or contagious disease should be documented, so that the wider community would benefit from having them cleansed, isolated, monitored, and returned to health.

Simultaneously, urban public health administrations were beginning to take concrete form across most of the country. The professionalizing cadre of public health professionals (appointment of an MOH was compulsory from 1875, but many towns and cities had one before that date) claimed a stake in this epidemic territory. Hospital superintendence and management materialized as a significant public health activity and a legitimate route of career advancement for public health doctors. The number of isolation hospitals exploded, from a sprinkling of privately run fever and smallpox hospitals in the early years of the century to more than 700 just before World War I. These newer hospitals were built (or adapted from previous uses) by local authorities, often with the help of low-interest financing from the central government. The repayment of government loans and ongoing running costs came out of local property taxes (rates). As such, institutionalized health care became politicized in new ways.

The scale of routine aggregation of the infected was unprecedented. Certainly, people with infectious diseases had been hospitalized in the distant and not-too-distant past. Pest houses during plague epidemics in the fourteenth century, venereal disease hospitals in the early modern period, and cholera hospitals in the early nineteenth century are three obvious examples. With the exception of lock hospitals, which concentrated on a small, though historically important section of the population, these institutions tended to be only temporary structures and placed transient demands on local government. Once infectious disease notification began to reveal the whereabouts of scores of diseased bodies that had hitherto remained beyond the reach (if not gaze) of public health, many local authorities began to exercise their powers of removal, and isolation hospitals became massive-scale, year-round repositories of biological risk. For example, the first four years of notification in Birmingham, 1890–93, witnessed as many scarlet fever hospital admissions (6,220) as there had been in the previous fifteen (6,236). Between 1890 and 1910, the percentage of notified scarlet fever cases admitted to hospital in Birmingham fell below 80 percent on only one occasion.[57] In the first full year of infectious disease notification in Salford in 1883, 26 percent of all scarlet fever cases were hospitalized. Within three years, this proportion had risen to almost 50 percent.[58] Curiously, given that thousands of people were admitted to isolation hospitals every year, relatively little is known about what went on in these hospitals, certainly compared to general voluntary hospitals, other specialist hospitals, and workhouses (though one could say that Poor Law medical wards are another historical blind spot).[59]

Chapter 3 sets out how institutionalization of infected patients became routinized, the diseases that were targeted, and the identity of the populations most liable to be sequestered. The extent of hospital isolation varied across England, but from the early 1870s hundreds of thousands of young children suffering from scarlet fever, diphtheria, enteric fever, and smallpox were isolated for weeks on end. Isolation was very much a test case for liberalism because its focus predominantly was on children whose citizenship status was ambiguous. It had political valence through its association with coercive removal, the role of infection rituals for patients and staff within the hospital, and the tight regulation of visiting.[60] Coexisting with these indications of anxiety was the opportunity to inculcate norms of infection avoidance in patients and their families. These processes gave form and identity to isolation hospitals.

Notification recalibrated the power of the state to interfere with everyday life, but by no means did its long arm reach across the full landscape of disease.

Highly infectious and sometimes fatal common ailments such as measles and whooping cough were not included on the schedule of compulsorily notifiable diseases. Therefore, schools played a crucial role in the control of what came to be known as "nonnotifiable diseases." Elementary public education from the 1870s meant that schools were used as an important source of information about the existence of infectious disease in the community. Schools were reconceptualized as spaces of extreme biological risk. Education was only one purpose for the space of the classroom: schools were also used as quasi-public health laboratories, in which attempts were made to plot the progress of an epidemic among pupils in the same class, between classrooms, and between the school and home. Chapter 4 juxtaposes initial scientific uncertainties about modes of disease transmission and herd immunity with a somewhat less ambiguous set of normative assumptions regarding the social relational behaviors of pupils and their siblings in the classroom, in school, on the street, and at home. I argue that the micromapping of student infections created room for a debate about policies that balanced the demands of political and social efficiency, community protection, and science. The expansion of mass education on the one hand, and the refinement of the spatio-epidemiological technique of contact tracing on the other, offered the state another route of entry into the domestic sphere, which brought home (figuratively and literally) to parents the duties and responsibilities they were expected to bear in the name of a healthy community.

Notions about the inviolability of domestic space and the protective sheath of domesticity were central to British national identity in the Victorian period. The home was both a canonical and contentious space. Infectious disease surveillance provided not only unparalleled access to the homes of the poor, but also a set of tools to destroy and neutralize the biological threat posed by the intimacy of domestic space. Disinfection cleared domestic space of biological dangers, so understanding how disinfection was transformed over the period offers an important perspective on the meaning of Victorian domesticity and contributes to the recent historiography that challenges its supposed conceptual stability.[61] In chapter 5, I depart from other historians' explanations about the apparent widespread acceptance of disinfection, which have emphasized the benefits of public education for medical science and the consequent public acceptance of disinfection's intrusiveness.[62] Rather, I argue that in order to be widely accepted, the municipal disinfection of homes and material belongings was transformed into a mobile, technologically sophisticated, and less obtrusive practice. I explore the adoption and integration of steam disinfection as a safe and easily managed technology that maximized the obliteration of germs but minimized the ruin of material possessions. House disinfection with chemical spraying became a portable, rapid, and directed intervention capable of destroying germs in the darkest corners of the home. I also analyze in some detail the creation, in Manchester's public health laboratory, of an experimental room that was designed to replicate the conditions of domestic space. This domestic laboratory, I argue, was a spatial expression of the uncertainty of science and the deeply contingent nature of laboratory research.

Chapter 6 builds on chapter 5 by demonstrating that municipal disinfection capacity was *the* vital criterion that persuaded central government in 1906 to grant Sheffield the power to make the notification of respiratory tuberculosis compulsory. As such, a fresh narrative of tuberculosis reporting is provided. Here, the focus on domestic space as an arena of liberal governmentality intensifies, since the fundamental rationale of tuberculosis notification clearly was the configuration of self-governing individuals. The making of the domiciled tuberculosis patient has been virtually ignored by historians, who have preferred to concentrate on the characteristics of sanatorium treatment. This is remarkable given that more than 90 percent of tuberculosis sufferers never saw the inside of a sanatorium. I argue that medical professionals sought to create the autonomous patient through a therapeutic approach that collapsed the spaces of the sanatorium and the home. Self-help manuals guided domiciled patients in the practices of auto-quantification and appropriate ways of living. Such technologies of the self were complemented by the marketing of commodities to homebound tuberculosis patients—baths, reclining chairs, bed rests, reading stands, heating devices, and so on—in a way that imbued these objects with scientific knowledge about hygienic and moral therapy, and incorporated tubercular patients into the realm of late-Victorian mass consumerism. In all, I call these market-centered activities the "preventive therapy" of the home.

While the (often coercive) management of individual behaviors was seen as the route to controlling epidemics, the social relations of the family were the agency through which self-governance was most effectively realized. As the final section of this introduction discusses, accessing domestic space, and neutralize it not only as a harbor of infection but also as a site of deficient family rearing, became a key endeavor of public health by the turn of the twentieth century.

## Public Health, Domestic Space, and the Family

Speaking on the subject of "Domestic Health" to the 1881 meeting of the Sanitary Institute in Brighton, public health activist Alfred Carpenter made the claim that "there is scarcely a house in the kingdom in which excreta are not to some extent retained." By "excreta" Carpenter meant all forms of seepage from the body. Skeptical that bacteriology would ever deliver a knockout punch to cholera, diphtheria, and other infectious diseases in the way that vaccination seemed to be doing to smallpox, Carpenter argued that the key to prevention lay in

> removing from our persons and from our habitations those debris which arise from the act of living. . . . The most civilised and luxurious home is, in some cases, carefully prepared for the cultivation of disease-germs or factors, if they come into our midst: carpets, curtains, and comforts of all kinds retain the *débris* from our skins and our pulmonary membranes; the excreta from our sweat-glands are allowed to settle upon our uncleaned windows, out-of-the-way cornices, useless ledges, and so-called architectural or upholstering ornaments.[63]

There are multiple layers of meaning in this short quote. The first is the stark materialization of infection; Carpenter's language is suffused with the proto-terminology of germ specificity that would not have been acceptable, or even comprehensible, to his audience just a few years earlier. The second relates to how Carpenter represents the sources of risk: skin falling away, emanations of the respiratory system, and the outpourings of the sweat glands were now just as threatening as expulsions from the bowels and the urinary tract (for which, of course, technologies of removal existed). This is not simply the debris of illness, of disease, or of malfunction: *normal life* is dangerous; Carpenter is saying that we are all dangerous. Third, and most crucial, this debris was not necessarily dangerous in and of itself: rather, it was rendered dangerous—*cultivated*, in fact—by the form and content of the modern Victorian home. Indeed, some considered the subdivided middle-class single-family dwelling to be no less of a dirt-laden threat than the much vilified lodging house.[64]

At around the time that I began the research for this book, I picked up a copy of *The Family Story: Blood, Contract and Intimacy, 1830–1960*, published in 1999. I read that, apart from a few exceptions, the "home has never been of direct interest to academics or intellectuals."[65] This observation was somewhat misleading; it overlooked, for example, pivotal works by influential thinkers such as Gaston Bachelard and Mary Douglas, not to mention humanistic geographers such as Yi-Fu Tuan, who saw "home" as central to their explanatory worlds.[66] It is fair to say, however, that the home had escaped *sustained* historical attention because of its seemingly mundane role in everyday life. The blossoming of cross-disciplinary work on domestic space over the past decade or so will have gladdened the authors of *The Family Story*. This research, reflected in the proliferation of new journals, collections of papers, textbooks, readers, and active networks of scholars, has started to take apart what we thought we knew, and what scholars had rarely looked for, in domestic space.[67]

It will become apparent throughout this book that of particular interest to me are questions of how "domestic" is produced as a geographical scale and how the "home" was managed as a site of risk and opportunity, both of which reveal much about the structure and exercise of power through the family.[68] While these concepts and spaces are, of course, continually under negotiation and dispute, there are good reasons to think that the period after 1780 was transformative.[69] First, "family" became more associated with the nuclear family, rather than with a household comprising an assortment of family members, servants, borders, or others. Second, the home was increasingly perceived as more private and more feminine than it had been before.[70] Recognizing that these changes took place is not meant to indicate unqualified support for the existence of separate "public" and "private" spheres, a position laid out by Leonore Davidoff and Catherine Hall in 1987. Rather, it is to understand the need to challenge and reformulate the notion of separate spheres, as many authors have done.[71]

Sensitivity to the production of the domestic scale, the site of the home, and the concept of family helps disclose the underlying scope of regulation.[72] For example, many historians have shown that the "sanitary revolution" of the early

Victorian period was as much about altering the appalling conditions of domestic space as it was concerned with improving the physical urban environment.[73] *Intrusive Interventions* follows this idea through to the early twentieth century, demonstrating how infectious disease surveillance governed through the agency of family and through the concept of domesticity—domesticity being that which makes the building a dwelling, the house a home—the responsibility for which primarily fell to women.[74]

The practices signaled by the hospital (isolation of people), the school (contact tracing), and the disinfection chamber (destruction and neutralization of biological threats) involved the production and reproduction of space in ways that both disrupted and reinforced the centrality of the family and domesticity in Victorian culture.[75] One of the crucial questions for liberal democracies has been how the state relates to the private family in shaping duties, responsibilities, rights, and needs.[76] Ready access to domestic space retrained the attention of public health officials onto the everyday behavior of families and the child-rearing abilities of parents, for whom, as Siân Pooley notes, "child health was a central concern, and at times an all-consuming priority."[77] Along these lines, many studies have examined domestic visiting, the infant welfare movement, child protection, and school welfare. What I try to show—particularly in chapters 5 and 6 when discussing disinfection and tuberculosis preventive therapy—is how the national and local state came to share the regulatory site of the home with alternate, but complementary, bureaucracies of power. Some experts outside formal government were armed with medical knowledge and hygienic ideas; others deployed marketing strategies, advertising skills, and the language of selling.

It is important not to lose sight of nineteenth-century gender roles here. There are obvious striations between and within class lines, and according to local cultural, economic, and social conditions, but it is fair to say that for the majority of working-class nuclear families, houses—or just as likely rooms within houses—were made into homes by women, as wives and mothers; family life and parenting responsibilities centered on the woman, even if she was engaged in paid work (which in many cases was home based, as with child-care, lodging, sewing, or laundry).[78] A little of the same could be said of the middle classes that dominated professional life and shaped many of the public health practices that appear in this book. The middle classes were highly attuned to the role that family played in maintaining respectability and building moral character.[79] There were, of course, important changes to these prevalent family forms, the situation of men vis-à-vis the home and domesticity, ways of parenting, and what "family" actually meant. *Intrusive Interventions* suggests that infectious disease surveillance assumed a role in these changes that was perhaps less obvious than, say, the infant welfare movement and domestic visiting, but no less powerful. Forced hospitalization, the cleansing of homes and property, and tracing the microgeographies of children within and between schools and homes are as good examples as any of how the state sought to govern through the family and domestic space.[80]

*Part One*

# Making Infectious Disease Surveillance

# Chapter One

# *Finding Disease in the Victorian City*

The English System of infectious disease surveillance crystalized in the latter part of the nineteenth century, when preventive interventions such as hospitalization and disinfection blended with scientific discoveries in aseptic surgery and bacteriology. Legislatively speaking, the fulcrum for this was the Infectious Disease (Notification) Acts of 1889 and 1899. These acts forced general practitioners to report cases of infectious disease to the local sanitary authority, which then pursued existing public health laws to isolate patients in hospital, disinfect property and belongings, suspend schooling, and temporarily close businesses.[1]

Most accounts of public health ideology and practice in the late nineteenth century accept that infectious disease surveillance was a "modern" response to age-old biological threats. This is reflected in the terms that historians use to depict the triad of notification, isolation, and disinfection. Peter Baldwin's "neo-quarantinist techniques" indicate that, to some extent, the English System was new wine in old bottles: quarantine and fumigation were refined and repackaged as isolation and disinfection. Expanding on ideas put forward by Margaret Pelling, Michael Worboys's "exclusive" public health stresses how bacteriology put the focus of intervention onto individuals and their behaviors, in contrast to the "inclusive" approach of environmental sanitation that prevailed earlier in the century. There are shades of this in David Barnes's phrase the "sanitary-bacteriological synthesis," in which "the commonsense cultural appeal and broad applicability of the old knowledge (for example, that foul-smelling substances are bad for one's heath) . . . [were brought] into harmony with the specificity and scientific mastery inherent in the new knowledge of microbes."[2]

The discovery of infected individuals and the management of their behavior was, however, something more than just a rejuvenated preventive apparatus that held up a mirror to medical science. It was a public health policy that expressed modern liberal government. Victorians sought to impose some sort of order on their increasingly complex and sprawling cities.[3] Information about rapidly growing populations enabled government to tax, plan, and regulate. Historians' interest in these aspects of modern urban life is echoed in the proliferation of "governmentality" studies of censuses, maps, surveys, and the collection of data. By no means was the "information state" unique to the nineteenth century, but its breadth and depth certainly was widened and intensified during the Victorian period. As James Scott notes in *Seeing like a State,* "The idea that one of the central purposes of the state was the improvement of all members of society—their health, skills and education, longevity, productivity, morals, and family life—was quite novel" in the nineteenth century.[4]

The bureaucratic point of this improvement was the perfectible city, the creation of a "diagram" in which autonomous individuals would regulate themselves, pursue their own interests without harming others, and take responsibility for their actions.[5] Mary Poovey called the predominantly urban environmentalist view of this diagram the "social body." Modern liberal society, she writes, "assumed that semi-autonomous realms like the economy or population would govern themselves as long as society was organised to conform to specific natural laws."[6] In the perfectible city, bodies and spaces, and bodies *in* spaces, were the focus of attention: "the spatial relation of citizen to habitat was turned into one that can and should be governed."[7] The morals, habits, and conduct of the poor in their urban environment were subjected to inquiry, enumeration, and surveillance.

As cities were constantly remade and took on new forms, these bureaucratic tools of information became central to a biopolitical logic of governmentality that cycled through observation, judgment, and regulation.[8] Through this prism, complex urban space was rendered visible. Though these techniques were implemented unevenly and rarely fully realized, knowledge of urban territory and awareness of the things that cities contained could be used by self-governing individuals to behave rationally. The need to know was fundamental to the management of urban life and the government of populations by experts "at a distance."[9] Ian Hacking neatly summarizes this with the term "making up people." This has particular resonance for historical studies of medicine and public health, because the projects of observation, categorization, classification, and calculation undertaken by the Victorian state sought to reconfigure the scope of life itself, since they aspired to redefine the "possibilities for personhood."[10] Thomas Osborne and Nikolas Rose have characterized this as "benign panopticism" in which "gazes and visibilities are diffused, local, reciprocal, and towards which the end is not contrition and reform but happiness, mutuality, solidarity."[11]

But where, and how, does a history of infectious disease surveillance fit into all of this? In the realm of infectious disease surveillance, how did the techniques and sites of infectious disease surveillance relate to this nexus of knowledge and power?[12] Benjamin Ward Richardson's 1875 utopian urban vision, *Hygeia,* provides an excellent starting point, even if it has been mined by historians countless times already.[13] The titular city Hygeia's one hundred thousand residents enjoyed a mortality rate of no more than five per thousand.[14] Its wide boulevards, subterranean transport links, and low-rise housing set a premium on light, ventilation, and quiet. Hygeia was a cityscape that achieved health through the spatial separation of human beings from their own waste and the wastes of industry. Sewers and water pipes were underground. Urban utilities—sewage treatment plants, pumping stations, gas works, and so on—were located symbolically beyond the city boundary. So, too, were pollutant-spewing factories. Hygeia was the archetypal liberal eudemonic diagram, and it provided direct inspiration for Ebenezer Howard's "garden city" movement, which "invoked the idea of the city as a space of transparency and perfect administration."[15] While historians have commented on the idealism of Richardson's plan, they have also observed that many aspects of Hygeia, from the structure of its sanitary administration to its material technologies, were already being assembled in Britain's industrialized cityscapes. Chris Otter has argued that Richardson's plan "showed how the city's problems with sanitation and government could almost be reduced to problems of perception, which were, in turn, soluble through careful attention to the material form of the city: its streets, pavements, subways, and walls."[16]

While the mastery of material form and technology certainly was a means to govern through freedom, it cannot be reduced to infrastructure alone, for the control and management of pathogenic risk in Hygeia required a panoptic vision. All medical men practicing in Hygeia had to notify the sanitary office of their patients' illnesses, so that "every death, every disease of the living world in the district, and every assumable cause of disease, comes to light and is subjected, if need be, to inquiry."[17] Such inquiries were made by Hygeia's medically qualified health officer and his well-staffed team of inspectors. Infected patients were isolated in one of the city's twenty hospitals, each of which served an average of five thousand people and which were placed at equidistant intervals along the main streets.[18]

Richardson himself acknowledged that, for the most part, Hygeia was not far removed from the mid-Victorian reality.[19] Though patchily implemented across the country, many features of Hygeia's public health administration either had been in place for some time or had been created by the Public Health Acts of 1872 and 1875. Local health authorities already possessed the power to disinfect homes and remove the infected to hospital. An impressive corps of officers was employed across the country to inspect and abate sanitary nuisances. And some things that were not yet part of the public health landscape had been raised as *possible* by the Royal Sanitary Commission (RSC) in its 1871 report and provided the basis for the public health legislation of the 1870s. One of these possibilities was the comprehensive system of sickness registration of which Richardson had dreamt.

Both Richardson and the RSC toyed with a vision of complete sickness registration that transformed private practitioners into the eyes and ears of the sanitary department. This is understandable. GPs were invariably on call twenty-four hours a day. Many of them owned the means of rapid mobility across the city. All had potential access to every domestic space. They possessed diagnostic expertise that sanitary inspectors, for all their experience and powers, simply could not claim. The GP's gaze was unequivocally diffuse and yet intensely microscopic.

The RSC recognized the potential epistemic and practical value of sickness registration. In Britain, vital statistics was a profoundly instrumental discipline compared to practices in other nation-states.[20] In the hands of statistical and medical experts, sickness registration could be a tool through which the state would know and, as Hacking would have it, remake its subjects. Vital statisticians and public health administrators wanted to construct an "index of sickness" to demonstrate the relationship between health and the urban environment. In Henry Wyldbore Rumsey's words, "It is the amount and duration of sickness, rather than the mortality, that tell on the prosperity of a community; and the sanitary condition of a State cannot be adequately predicated from a simple enumeration of deaths."[21]

Ultimately, however, the registration of sickness by GPs was frozen out as a realistic proposition by the RSC, which recommended instead the collation of data based on returns from Poor Law practice.[22] This chapter explores why this happened. For a variety of practical and intellectual reasons, physicians in the mid-nineteenth century were suspicious of attempts to collect their clinical observations together. Furthermore, three schemes—in London, Manchester and Salford, and Newcastle—demonstrated that information on illnesses from Poor Law practice and charitable institutions that did not depend on GPs and focused specifically on poor people was useful for anticipating epidemics and locating infected people.

Although the conclusions derived from data about sickness were fragmentary, partial, and sometimes at odds with each other, they nevertheless made a noteworthy contribution to the configuration of infectious disease surveillance in ways that have been overlooked by historians. Data on sickness produced a map of disease incidence among the poor that facilitated a shift in the technique of public health governance. By finding out where infected people lived, sickness registration meant that intensive and expensive house-to-house searches for ill people could be abandoned and replaced with cheaper and more immanent (though not necessarily more effective) techniques of persuasion, such as pamphleteering and lecturing. These latter practices buttressed the liberal rhetoric of self-help that demonized the unhygienic habits of the poor and identified the home as the key space of infectious risk in the Victorian city. Furthermore, the registration of Poor Law sickness revealed the huge number of paupers who were infectious. They were biologically dangerous and, in the case of those on outdoor relief—that is, people receiving help from the parish but not admitted to the workhouse—financially burdensome. It made both medical and economic sense to take as many poor people as possible out of their homes and sequestrate them in hospitals. These findings were implicitly acknowledged by the RSC when it argued that sickness registration might stay the toll of epidemics by providing medical officers with early information about the incidence of infectious disease in poor people. This claim unlocked the full prophylactic potential of the English System and summarized the public health case for a narrower form of sickness registration: infectious disease notification by GPs, the fraught establishment of which is dealt with in the next chapter. The importance of sickness registration for establishing the principle of infectious disease notification is explored below.

## The Royal Sanitary Commission and Sickness Registration

An impressive cabal of medical, public health, and statistical luminaries testified to the importance of sickness registration at the RSC in the late 1860s including

John Simon, William Farr, Henry Rumsey, Major George Graham, and William Burke (superintendent of the Statistical Department, GRO, Dublin) and Robert Druitt (then president of the MOH Association).[23] Curiously for an inquiry that produced landmark public health legislation in the 1870s, the RSC itself has received little attention from historians. It was prompted by a memorial in May 1868 from a joint committee of the Social Science Association and British Medical Association that requested investigation into a number of key areas in medicine and public health, including coroners' inquests, the role of medical and scientific advice, sanitary organization and medical officers, and the consolidation of sanitary laws.[24] The first request, however, was for an exploration of the "manner in which the cases and causes of sickness and of death are and should be inquired to and recorded."[25]

Three years later, the RSC concluded that a national register of sickness was desirable on as many as seven grounds. First, the emergence of epidemics could be more closely monitored. Second, the amount of poverty and grief caused by disease that did not lead to death could only be guessed at. In fact, the RSC noted that death represented an economically efficient outcome of illness for a variety of reasons: the cost of burial could be a trifling amount compared to the financial hardship brought about by a long period of sickness and convalescence; the long-term health consequences of a bout of epidemic sickness—diseases of the ears, bones, joints, glands, for example—hampered the productivity and earning potential of the afflicted and their caregivers well into the future; economic losses associated with illnesses such as ague, scrofula, rheumatism, and bronchitis were probably much greater than those of epidemic outbreaks. Sickness registration would allow these disease-related economic burdens to be estimated with precision.[26] Third, sickness registration would help illuminate the connections between occupations, social habits, and health in order to guide legislation. The commission observed that the investigations of the Medical Department of the Privy Council had taken some steps in this direction.[27] Expectations were high that sickness registration would uncover whether or not "social vices and vicious habits of life" were in fact sources of "sickness, poverty and decay." If they were not, then "considerable expenditure of money and of executive force" on these social vices could hardly be justified.[28]

Fourth, the geography of disease would be more accurately ascertained, since sickness would be registered according to place of residence. It was well known that deaths in a hospital were credited to the district in which the hospital was located. This seriously compromised the integrity of ecological interpretations of spatial mortality variation.[29] Fifth, many people who had a protracted illness that exacted an economic premium ultimately died from a completely unrelated condition. Insanity was a case in point: it was costly and wasteful but did not quite destroy life itself and often did not appear on death certificates, even as a secondary cause of death. Institutional efficiency was a sixth reason for sickness registration, particularly given the dangerousness of cross-infection in hospitals. While hospitals recorded deaths by cause, they failed to clarify whether illnesses such as fever and erysipelas were acquired in hospital by patients admitted for other ailments. Finally, the collation and analysis of statistics on sickness might reveal not only susceptibility to disease by locality and occupational class, but also immunity. Why were brass workers resistant to cholera? Why were country dwellers less prone to blood infections following injuries than city residents? "And," argued the commissioners, "if these are facts, it is not likely that they are the only facts of the kind; there must be many more, which a registration of sickness must help to detect."[30]

The case for sickness registration seemed incontestable. The main sticking point was whether GPs could or would relinquish information on patients. Provided that the information was given to a trusted public official and kept confidential, William Farr thought they might.[31] Of all the witnesses to the RSC, on this issue Farr was in a minority of one.[32] However, it is worth spending some time exploring why Farr went out on a limb here, even directly opposing his superior at the General Register Office.

## William Farr, the Army, and Sickness

Much of William Farr's work was characterized by attempts to reveal general and reproducible regularities in the structure of mortality. One might point to his early work on the relationship between the incidence of cholera and elevation above sea level. Another example is his application of actuarial methods to the construction of a life table, the "biometer" of health. Earlier work by Thomas Rowe Edmonds on the "Laws of Vitality" argued that there was a fixed relationship between the age-profiles of morbidity and mortality.[33] Edmonds used data prepared by Farr from the London Hospital and benefit societies that appeared in an edition of the *British Medical Almanack* for 1836, edited by Farr.[34]

Farr's understanding that mortality only revealed the tip of an epidemiological iceberg was prompted by his professional interactions with Edmonds in the 1830s.[35] Farr developed these concerns when he was invited to become a member of a three-man committee to devise proposals for the statistical branch of the Army Medical Department.[36] This committee's recommendations were published in 1861 and formed the basis of Farr's opinions on sickness registration in the general population that he later expressed to the RSC and elsewhere.

The committee planned an impressive level of medical surveillance for each soldier, the foundation of which would be a dense and portable set of documentary technologies. Every sickness episode from recruitment to discharge (or death) would be recorded in the medical history for each soldier. All the individual medical histories would be kept together in a Medical Histories Book held at the regiment level, but if a soldier was to be transferred his medical history sheet would accompany him. An annual Admissions and Discharges Book would contain the particulars of every regimental death, both on and off the battlefield. The committee also intended that the regimental surgeon would keep a Medical Case Book to record all those cases that were "considered important in an etiological, a pathological, or a therapeutical point of view."[37]

Farr was already in the process of creating a biopolitical geography of mortality at the GRO, based on the aggregation and classification of individual deaths at the district level. Similarly, he sought to map the ecology of sickness across the army, regiment by regiment. Just as a national death rate concealed local variations in mortality, so did a statistical report for the whole army hide differences in the sanitary condition of particular regiments: "the most deplorable state of a single suffering regiment might be swamped in a general return."[38] While the composition of each regiment might not differ as widely as, say, the population of a London district, information on new cases of illness presented regiment by regiment might yet point to the influence of "foul air, defective sewerage, want of cleanliness, and intemperance."[39] The committee sought a temporal layering as well as a spatial one. The existing practice of monthly regimental returns was not frequent enough, since the mean duration of diseases encountered in the army was no more than two weeks: a crisis could come and go before the central administration knew what was happening on the ground. For centuries the London bills of mortality had demonstrated the sanitary value of a weekly return, and it was urged that the same be applied to the military population.[40]

The ecological and temporal dialogue between the practiced analysis of mortality in the general population and the projected analysis of morbidity in the army was given concrete form by a pilot study in February 1858. Returns were taken from the First and Second battalions of the Grenadier Guards, all twenty-four regiments at Aldershot, the Royal Engineers, the East India Company Engineers, and three depot battalions at Chatham. In just one week there were 606 new cases of sickness among 22,000 men. Diagnoses were arranged under Farr's nosology from the Sixteenth Annual Report of the Registrar-General, and a set of weekly, quarterly, and annual pro forma returns were mocked up. The GRO provided staff to see the pilot through to press, replicating its operation for London's weekly return.[41]

The study revealed a high number of "ineffective" soldiers. The committee calculated that over the course of a year, the army might expect a rate of 135 cases of sickness for every one hundred men.[42] One extrapolation demonstrated that a minimum of 13,000 soldiers were in hospital at any given time, a not insubstantial fraction of a force of some 200,000.[43] A regular weekly return would help to diminish the amount of individual suffering and also underline the potential economic losses caused by disease. A bigger spatiotemporal picture would also work through the army's medical officers, who could graft the evidence of illnesses in individuals onto the wider topography:

> The medical officers of the army will learn from the reports the prevailing diseases against which they have to guard. They will be able to compare the cases occurring in their own and in other regiments. By observing the development of pathological phenomena, in bodies of men under every variety of circumstances, they will accumulate materials for induction, and will teach us to distinguish causes from coincidences. In stating principles and in giving

> opinions, they will have at hand tangible proofs and clear illustrations. . . . They have masses of men similarly constituted constantly under observation; and see them exposed to every variety of circumstances, so that the effect of physical causes on health must be striking. . . . Under the system which we propose, medical officers will be able to record their observation with increased accuracy, to classify phenomena, and to discuss the relations of every order of facts. A good system of army reports will enable the Army Medical Department to develop all its energies, and to distinguish itself by sanitary discoveries, which will increase the efficiency of Her Majesty's army, advance science, and be beneficial to mankind.[44]

Phrases such as "distinguish causes from coincidences," "stating principles," "tangible proofs," and "the relations of every order of facts" remind us of the search for regularities in data that characterized so much of Farr's work on mortality. But we also begin to see the basis of the RSC's sympathy for a national sickness register, particularly its role in epidemic prevention, in revealing the economic burden of morbidity, and in making connections between geographical phenomena and disease. In the army, details relating to all episodes of sickness were potentially available from the regimental surgeons. The only way that such a system could be replicated in civilian life was to have both public and private practitioners report all cases of disease that they discovered.

Two years later, this is exactly what Farr called for at the Fourth International Statistical Congress in London in July 1860. His ambitious set of national information requirements included an impressive array of potential measures of morbidity, not to mention anthropological data and records of environmental conditions.[45] While reaffirming his faith in mortality rates and life tables for distinguishing between healthy and unhealthy districts, Farr further recommended that the census should collect information on "the numbers suffering from the chief infirmities." Infirmity and sickness, he noted, "are far from expressing ideas so definite as death; the sense in which they are used should, therefore, be defined."[46] He favored enumerating the blind, deaf, dumb, idiotic, insane, and lame. In addition to disability, Farr advocated that the census should make a record of diseases in individuals as had been carried out and analyzed in the Irish census from 1841.[47] With such records, and with Friendly Society returns, it would be possible to "determine the amount of that kind of sickness which disables the working classes from following their usual occupations."[48]

Farr also called for the registration of all diseases and injuries that fell under the observation of medical men. Such a register could be tallied on an annual basis to show, by age, the annual number of attacks of disease, their duration, and the ensuing mortality. "The medical profession alone," Farr insisted, "can carry out such a great work in entire populations."[49] In drawing attention to how certain diseases "furnish unusually valuable indications of the sanitary state of the people," Farr cast GPs in the role of information providers in the service of statistics.

## The Statistics of Private Practice

Ten years later, the RSC was unmoved by Farr's lonely voice. While the commissioners accepted his estimate that 13 million or more annual cases of sickness prevented work or required medical assistance, it countered that the cost of registering such a vast number of illnesses was beyond the financial wherewithal of any government department. The RSC's bald, unqualified statement that "it would be impossible to register all cases in private houses" seemingly brooked no argument.[50]

Perhaps more than any other witness save John Simon, it was Farr's immediate superior, Registrar-General Major George Graham, who steered the RSC's attention away from GPs. In both his oral evidence and a written memorandum, Graham resisted the idea of a system of national sickness registration. He did not "expect to see the day that I should be called to appear before a Royal Commission and asked to register all the complaints which do not kill but only annoy and afflict the 22,000,000 of inhabitants of England and Wales."[51] He gave three examples designed to make the whole enterprise seem impractical, if not faintly ridiculous. Would the commission, he wondered, seriously expect the GRO to record every sniffle, headache, and indigestion of the 800,000 babies born every year? Registering the long list of complaints suffered by the old and infirm—from gout to gravel, deafness to dyspepsia—would be no less daunting. Finally, what about adults' most sensitive ailments? Need private practitioners inquire of their male patients whether their case of syphilis was a primary or secondary infection? Could female cases of hysteralgia, chlorosis, or dysmenorrhea be registered without making annoying inquiries?[52] The exasperation in his voice is palpable when he complained: "I do not know where I am to begin or where I am to end."[53]

Graham felt the GRO could deal with the potential demands of handling sickness records from public institutions, but its resources would be defeated by a more widespread collection:

> There are no statistics in the world that we cannot get, if you give us the money. I have taken two censuses, and I think if we could get a census of the whole population of England all in one day, by bringing out 36,000 men as I did, and sending out waggons along the Strand conveying 50 tons weight of paper, *there is nothing that we cannot collect in the way of statistics if you give us the money, excepting the diseases of the public.*[54]

He later wrote that if the commission really was going to advocate the registration of all sickness episodes, then it had better be done by the Medical Department of the Privy Council and not the Registrar-General's office. Fixed in his belief, Graham's dismissive parting shot was that such proposals were "undesirable, Utopian, and unattainable."[55] Graham was an astute manager of his staff, an adroit administrator, and possessed a deep understanding of the GRO's operations, both centrally and in the localities.[56] Clearly, he couched his objections to sickness registration as an operational issue for his office, but he also understood that GPs would not welcome the additional burden involved in reporting every minor case of illness that they came across.

While other witnesses to the RSC provided no direct evidence of this—that private physicians would not tolerate such an imposition seems to have been taken for granted—many indications of such resistance had been accumulating since the 1850s. That decade witnessed two attempts to persuade GPs to register the illnesses of their patients. Weekly tables of disease and meteorological observations were published by the Provincial Medical and Surgical Association between 1853 and 1855. Doctors in eight different locations provided daily recordings of air pressure, temperature, humidity, wind direction and force, ozone, the amount and class of cloud, precipitation, and diseases and deaths.[57] These so-called "medico-meteorological observations" were supplied by interested private practitioners, and there was no restriction placed on the type and class of disease reported. In any event, the use of these observations for determining the relationship between local conditions and disease was limited because an insufficient number of observations were made overall. Later in the century, Charles Paget reckoned that the scheme was overly "scientific" and that the majority of private practitioners were too busy to fill in the necessary forms.[58]

Richardson himself developed a scheme for sickness registration along similar lines, but with a focus on epidemic disease. At one point he had as many as fifty-five practitioners in forty-four locations reporting cases of disease on a quarterly basis, from the Shetlands in the north of Scotland to the Isles of Scilly off the southwest coast of England.[59] Richardson supplied observers with forms to tick off whether scarlet fever, smallpox, measles, whooping cough, croup, catarrh, influenza, erysipelas, cholera, ague, remittent fever, diarrhea, dysentery, typhus, puerperal fever, or carbuncle (probably in its anthrax form) were present in their area each week. Reports were returned to him on the first day of March, June, September, and December. He published the results in the *Journal of Public Health and Sanitary Review*, the first journal devoted to public health and of which Richardson was editor.[60]

This project lasted from 1855 to 1859. Richardson's own account of it appears in an essay entitled "The Registration of Disease," but it would be completely wrong to imply that his scheme was anything other than an attempt to indicate local disease presence, since observers were not required to report every single case.[61] Ultimately, it was too expensive and time-consuming for Richardson to continue single-handedly, but the experience led him to argue two points: first, the perfection of such a registration system, even if only over a period of ten or fifteen years, would bring about the "entire comprehension of the laws by which epidemics, at least, are governed"; and second, at the end of the day, his scheme was the victim of its own success, a consequence of the physicians' boundless energy and enthusiasm.[62]

We can only speculate that the energy and enthusiasm of Richardson's correspondents may have waned had he ventured to ask them to report *every* case of illness rather than just epidemic cases. Indeed, pressure of time on GPs was one of the reasons the BMA's later push for Collective Investigation failed so miserably in the 1880s. As Harry Marks has shown, Collective Investigation—the centralized collation of clinical histories of specific conditions in order to ascertain common patterns in the natural history of disease, relationships between different symptoms, and the effectiveness of therapeutic remedies—highlighted the division between the scientific demands of consultant physicians trained in morbid anatomy and the harsh realities of market-based general practice.[63] The problems of Collective Investigation were foreseen in the early 1860s by one of its main proponents, Manchester's Arthur Ransome. Ransome suggested some form of collective medical inquiry to the BMA as early as 1864, premised on his involvement with the system of disease registration initiated by the Manchester and Salford Sanitary Association (MSSA) four years earlier (this scheme is discussed below). Ransome proposed broadening a system of sickness reports from Poor Law institutions and voluntary hospitals to cover as many medical practitioners as possible, though for a limited number of diseases. He anticipated that objections to his scheme would arise from the medical profession's suspicion of statistical inquiries and the difficulty of obtaining the required information from doctors who were already very busy.[64] Ransome hoped the latter problem would be overcome if GPs trusted those responsible for administering the inquiries and that "the public spirit and self-denying energy of our profession" would win out. As Harry Marks demonstrates, two decades later the BMA's Collective Investigation Committee found that it did not win out at all.

## Enumerating Pauper Disease

Given that these attempts to prize diagnostic information from GPs failed, it was unsurprising that the RSC sidelined Farr's opinion that medical practitioners would readily give up their observations. It rejected the possibility of reporting all cases of sickness by GPs—"I think and hope that by no legislative enactment could you get physicians to give such information," said Irish registrar-general William Burke—and narrowed the focus to public institutions.[65] Poor law sickness registration, it was thought, could be had for relatively little additional effort and expense, since Poor Law medical officers (PLMOs) could easily send in a form containing the pauper's name, age, residence, and occupation; the disease, the date symptoms began; and the final outcome of the illness.[66]

Some suggested that similar reports could also be submitted from charitable institutions, voluntary hospitals, asylums, dispensaries, and from club doctors. Charles Dickens believed that the secretaries of friendly and benefit societies and dispensaries might be financially induced to fill in forms of sickness episodes, under the condition of anonymity for the patient. These would give up information not about the most impoverished, but about the respectable and comparatively healthy working class.[67] Dickens sided with those who argued that statistics of sickness provided a more sensitive gauge of sanitary science than mortality. In what stands as a classic statement of liberal governmentality and the potential reconfiguration of personhood itself, Dickens anticipated the implications for individual citizens:

> It is most true that we have never studied, are still neglecting to study, with any accuracy, the statistics of sickness and health, to which the statistics of death, even if they were perfect, would afford no clue. So far as care of the body goes, it concerns a man more to know his risks of the fifty illnesses that may throw him on his back, than the possible date of one death that must come, and of which the time is to him personally—in spite of libraries full of statistics—utterly unknown and uncertain.[68]

A deputation of the Medical Society of London, the Association of Medical Officers of Health, the St. Andrews Medical Graduates' Association, and, significantly, the PLMOs Association made the same arguments to the Poor Law Board in November 1869.[69] George Graham agreed that the GRO could indeed tabulate and publish pauper sickness returns if required.[70]

This kind of data collection already had multiple local histories that were somewhat troubled. In the late 1840s, both William Henry Duncan in Liverpool and John Simon in the City of London encouraged PLMOs to communicate with them whenever a case of disease occurred in their practice. They met with varying degrees of success. Simon, who took up his post as MOH in October 1848, blithely recounted that "before I had long been in office, the eleven Poor Law Medical Officers of the City voluntarily took upon themselves the trouble of each sending me a weekly return (often with additional notes) to acquaint me of any new cases of fever which had arisen in their respective districts."[71] Simon's biographer, Royston Lambert, painted a rather less sanguine picture. Initially the overworked PLMOs flatly refused to provide the necessary reports unless they were each paid an additional £50 per annum and granted the title District Medical Officer. These proposals eventually fell into abeyance until the cholera panic of 1849, upon which the PLMOs relented, albeit amid a continuing atmosphere of distrust and animosity.[72]

Duncan was similarly successful during Liverpool's fever epidemics, but at other times he lamented the lack of systematic reports.[73] In part, this reflected the legislative framework in Liverpool at the time. Under the Nuisances Removal Act of 1846, the Select Vestry of the Parish administered medical relief and was responsible for public health activity during epidemics; the Liverpool Sanatory [*sic*] Act of the same year, meanwhile, handed preventive duties to the borough.[74] Given these duplicitous circumstances, Duncan's achievement in securing any of the PLMOs' cooperation is noteworthy, yet it is perhaps understandable that "the Select Vestry was nervous about the use Duncan might make of 'their' data."[75] A similar sentiment was expressed by the PLMOs in London: not only was Simon's request for a weekly return designed to swell his recent appointment, they said it was also borne of "mere idle and inquisitive questions." To underline just how idle and inquisitive they believed Simon's demand to be, the PLMOs listed the MOH's deficient oversight of water and gas supply, scavenging, and domestic sewerage. Unless these problems were tackled, "no reports of ours can possibly be made available to public safety or benefit."[76]

Subsequent developments in London, Manchester and Salford, and Newcastle proved that collecting this sort of data was both viable and useful. These local schemes depended in large part on the goodwill and motivation of a small number of activists, many of whom were already in public service and belonged to an organized local body, such as the MSSA, the Northumberland and Durham Medical Society (NDMS), or the Association of Metropolitan Medical Officers of Health. Professional associations and societies—however divergent in constitution, aims, and working methods—smoothed the way for disease reporting by PLMOs and other physicians serving in institutions. Such societies provided ready access to the full range of local medical professionals in all their guises. The NDMS, for example, had nearly one hundred members in the early 1860s. They brought together under one roof the demand (i.e., the MOH) and supply side (i.e., the PLMO and Workhouse Infirmary surgeons) of sickness registration.[77] And they used subscription income to fund the publication of morbidity statistics as instruments of knowledge about local disease incidence.

In April 1857 the Association of Metropolitan Medical Officers of Health collated reports of cases of illness in London that occurred in nineteen workhouses, twenty-four Poor Law practices (outdoor cases and infirmaries), seven general hospitals, twenty-four dispensaries, four lunatic asylums, a prison, and two military and naval hospitals.[78] The returns were printed and circulated by the General Board of Health on a weekly and quarterly basis, along with observations gathered by the association's meteorological committee.[79] They soon expanded to include reports on twenty-two separate diseases from as many as 80 of the 180 metropolitan PLMOs, while 50 of the 109 metropolitan hospitals and dispensaries proffered information. Although this scheme was short lived, a victim of voluntarism and expense,[80] disease registration was continued in a number of metropolitan districts, including St. George's Hanover Square, St. Giles-in-the-Fields, St. Marylebone, Islington, and Whitechapel.[81]

Very few accounts of these schemes survive other than in MOH reports. One analysis was by Islington MOH Edward Ballard, who collected data from the parish workhouse, the infant poorhouse, eight outdoor medical relief officers, and two local dispensaries. Ballard related annual, quarterly, and monthly rates of sickness to broad climatic conditions.[82] He also tabulated comparisons of sickness among Islington's paupers with the mortality of the wider population according to the percentage contributions made by each disease to the total. Thus, respiratory diseases claimed the greatest percentages of mortality and morbidity in paupers and all people. Ballard's choice of analytic comparisons was instrumentally limited. The data did not allow him to compare like with like: sickness only from paupers, deaths from the whole population of Islington.[83] His use of proportionate rates did not account for differences in the age- and sex-structures of the two populations; Poor Law patients invariably were older than the general population. In addition, it was difficult to judge how his results were influenced by an increase in the district's population from little more than 95,000 in 1851 to about 200,000 in 1868.[84]

The best-known system of disease reporting, and certainly the most durable, was operated by the Manchester and Salford Sanitary Association from September 1860. Proponents frequently lauded the epistemic and instrumental purposes of sickness registration. But the immediate reason it started in Manchester was more prosaic. The MSSA was in a parlous financial state and needed to reduce the exorbitant costs of house-to-house visits. These visits were used to uncover infection and reveal technological deficiencies in housing construction and sanitation. The MSSA advocated a Chadwick-inflected, holistic vision of a technologically complete sanitary city and consistently harried the town council to provide one.[85] However, by the late 1850s the visitors "seldom found that unsanitary conditions of the districts" could be blamed on the "want of attention or diligence, on the part of the municipal bodies of either Manchester or Salford."[86] Martin Hewitt argues that such visits only ever reached a small proportion of the population anyway.[87]

As early as 1854 the MSSA had urged the Home Secretary Viscount Palmerston to make all boards of guardians provide, within sixty days of the end of each quarter, a list to the sanitary authority of the houses where deaths and cases of cholera, diarrhea, scarlatina, or any other disease had occurred. The intention was to investigate the localization of disease and its causes.[88] In the continuing absence of such returns, in September 1860 the MSSA began to collect and publish the weekly number of all cases under treatment in various public institutions. The system, modeled directly on the London scheme described above, lasted until 1880.[89] Arthur Ransome helped set up the MSSA's Subcommittee for the Registration of Disease and personally canvassed institutional physicians and medical officers to secure their voluntary returns.[90] It was doubtless an advantage that the MSSA counted a number of local PLMOs among its ranks and that the subcommittee normally included at least one PLMO or workhouse surgeon.[91] While the MSSA now had a means to compare the relative healthiness of different districts within the city and provide a spatially defined focus for sanitary and charitable work, the returns also provided real-time information on epidemic outbreaks.[92]

The returns served other purposes as well. By using sickness returns to locate disease, monies were freed up from house visits that could be channeled toward educational activities that promoted working-class self-help. The MSSA's version of public health citizenship emphasized the right of the poor to complain but also their duty to behave responsibly. Resources were devoted to lectures and pamphlets that aimed to reform working-class habits through liberalism's favored modus operandi of "moral suasion."[93] In Manchester (and elsewhere, of course), "the values of thrift, frugality, sobriety, industriousness, and above all, self-help . . . ," writes Martin Hewitt, "comprised a constantly reiterated canon of middle-class behavioural morality."[94] The MSSA never abandoned its mission to remind the city of its sanitary obligations, nor did it stop house inspections altogether, but it also reminded residents that it was "their duty to complain to the constituted authorities, whenever such interference is necessary."[95]

The Lancashire Cotton Famine of the early 1860s offered a swift opportunity for the sickness returns to reinforce the MSSA's belief that high rates of mortality and morbidity were due to working-class behaviors. The MSSA used its disease incidence data to reject the notion that destitution in the city produced increased mortality from typhus fever. It argued that the surge in mortality in the first six months of 1862 was not due to causes influenced by distress or starvation. The sickness returns indicated an upturn from whooping cough and measles caused by parents exposing their children to infection, rather than by any adverse impact of destitution.[96] George Buchanan's report for the Privy Council disputed this interpretation. He also consulted the MSSA's weekly sickness returns during his visit to Manchester and ultimately contended that whooping cough and measles *were* associated with malnutrition. Poverty and distress were making inroads into the health of the unemployed mill workers, and this was also reflected in a typhus epidemic.[97]

The MSSA challenged Buchanan's claims and countered that there were no more typhus deaths in the second half of 1862 than there had been in the first, and that the records of the fever wards at the Manchester Infirmary showed only fourteen cases in the last six months of 1862.[98] The *Times* reflected that "actual want" did not directly account for very many deaths, but that "there has been a general descent from ample and health-sustaining food to an insufficient diet," which was enough to excite some diseases and predispose to others. Buchanan's report demonstrated that typhus had to be "fed out" and that the minimum allowance granted to applicants for public assistance during the Cotton Famine had to be raised.[99] This was a touchy subject for Manchester's social and political elite. By using the sickness records to deny that typhus and malnutrition had gained a hold in the city, the MSSA defended the generosity of middle-class parochial and charitable relief efforts. It even went so far as to say that because of these efforts there had been no deterioration of health or strength among the operatives, something that should be applauded given the one-third increase in the number of paupers over the previous year.[100] In promoting the effectiveness of the relief operation during the Cotton Famine, the MSSA lauded the forced changes in working-class habits that scarcity had brought about, arguing that "causes will also have been in operation—such as the greater sobriety of the working classes—from inability to procure stimulants, the larger amount of outdoor employment, and the more constant care which the mothers have been able to bestow on their children."[101]

The only other provincial scheme of note was set up in Newcastle. In late 1863 Dr. George Philipson prompted the Northumberland and Durham Medical Society to collect information from private physicians along the lines adopted by Richardson in the mid-1850s. Philipson, the physician to Newcastle's Dispensary and Fever Hospital, anticipated potential objections and noted that while the procedure might "engross the time of the often overworked practitioner," the benefits, even if only to pathology, would make the exercise worthwhile.[102] The NDMS covered the expense of publishing tables that showed for zymotic diseases new cases, recoveries, and deaths broken down by age and sex.

Philipson reported to the society on a monthly basis, but his limited project was replaced in 1867 by the registration of diseases occurring in public institutions, based on the more ambitious Manchester and Salford operation. The "Health and Meteorology of Newcastle and Gateshead" listed new cases of twenty-five separate diseases drawn from twenty-four different sources—including Poor Law districts, infirmaries, workhouses, hospitals, dispensaries, and the jail—alongside deaths.[103]

One feature of the Newcastle system was the efficient and close cooperation of the board of guardians and the city authorities.[104] The PLMOs were in weekly contact with the sanitary committee, provided information on disease outbreaks from the weekly reports, and granted the committee access to their books on the sources of disease.[105] In this sense, then, the weekly returns of the NDMS formalized activities between the board of guardians and the city that had developed over the course of the previous decades. This is in striking contrast to what had happened during W. H. Duncan's time in Liverpool in the 1840s and what was happening in Manchester, where the city council very nearly had full control of sanitary matters and expressed little sense of need for reliance on the cooperation of the board of guardians.[106]

In his evidence to the RSC in 1870, Manchester's town clerk, Joseph Heron, appeared to be unaware that the MSSA had been collecting Poor Law data on the incidence of pauper sickness for the better part of a decade.[107] Heron's oversight would be less remarkable were it not for the fact that his own MOH recently had used the MSSA's disease incidence data to criticize the city's hospital accommodations. In 1869 Manchester's MOH John Leigh drew attention to the fact that while there had been about 16,000 infectious disease deaths in the whole of the 1850s (Manchester and Chorlton registration districts), there had been more than 31,000 cases of infectious disease in public practice in the seven years 1861–67. Leigh was scathing in his assessment of hospital provision for infectious diseases, and the publication of his report prompted a public meeting in the town hall on the subject.[108] The council subsequently opened a fever hospital with 128 beds at Monsall and a Children's Hospital in Pendlebury. According to one of the MSSA's honorary secretaries, isolation of the infected in these hospitals meant that "a constant and methodological supervision must be had over all parts of the city." As with Hygeia, this supervision could only be exercised through the notification of infectious diseases by private practitioners.[109]

## Infectious Paupers

In the early 1860s, Gavin Milroy reckoned that the PLMOs treated more than 1 million paupers every year.[110] Rumsey put the figure above 1.5 million. Another estimate reckoned the average annual number of cases treated by 3,200 PLMOs was 3.5 million.[111] The "truth" of these estimates matters less (indeed, they may all have been "true" in any given year) than the political impact this sort of knowledge had. The amount of "medical" support given under the Poor Law was staggering, but the detail of these sicknesses remained a mystery. Yet, while the GRO was willing to bear the cost of recording and sifting the records of these treatments, the analytic benefit of analyzing them was unclear. First, the medical relief list compiled by the PLMO was intended as a tool of economic and not sanitary surveillance: it allowed the board of guardians to keep an eye on the medical supplies ordered by the PLMO for enumerated cases of sickness.[112] The Local Government Board (LGB) itself did not ask for any returns of cases treated as indoor or outdoor relief, and there was no obligation on the medical superintendents of workhouse infirmaries to keep notes on their patients.[113] More often than not the lists of medical relief, laughed at as "beef tea and brandy lists" by some, ended up in the wastepaper basket.[114]

The lists were useless for comparative statistical purposes because they were carelessly or incompletely filled out, being low on the list of priorities for the underpaid PLMOs, who were "diligent workers in the medical hive, whose lives are distinguished by much toil and little pay."[115] It is readily understandable why PLMOs should take such a dismal view of record-keeping. Valuable therapeutic time was otherwise taken up with accounting for the "extras," classifying paupers for work and dietary purposes, and determining their fitness to withstand punishment.[116]

Simon mooted in 1868 that a quarterly return on the incidence and prevalence of pauper sickness would have some preventive value.[117] Edward Smith, the principal medical officer of the Poor Law Board (PLB), who had been Simon's "inspired" choice as a dietary inspector during the Lancashire Cotton Famine, was skeptical. Smith himself carried out an examination of the Poor Law sickness returns.[118] In the 1860s the PLB began to patch together information on the numbers of sick paupers, especially in London, but sickness never featured much in its annual reports.[119] So, in a one-off exercise, Smith secured a list from PLMOs across the country of all indoor and outdoor paupers who received medical treatment on December 18, 1869. Smith's inquiry was initiated to "give the public as clear an idea as possible of the actual physical condition of the great multitude of paupers." Smith was wise to restrict his survey to one day, since an incredible 153,245 sick paupers left an imprint on the return. Smith's analysis was unprecedented in its detail: it was national; it dealt with outdoor and indoor claimants; and it considered age, sex, and disease together.[120]

Writing in 1870, Smith was well aware of the RSC's recommendation for the registration of pauper sickness, which the BMA and Poor Law Medical Officers' Association reaffirmed in October with yet another deputation to the PLB.[121] But in producing a prototype of morbidity analysis envisioned by the RSC, he drew attention to its many limitations. A number of outdoor paupers were given medical advice without a formal order and were not added to the books of the PLMO. Not only were cases missed; they were duplicated (even though the survey was supposed to be de facto). The age classifications used for Poor Law administrative purposes (e.g., nine to sixteen years for children) were not comparable to the quinquennial groupings commonly used elsewhere. Individual

PLMOs varied greatly in their application of medical and surgical classifications. The GRO's nosology was not generally used. PLMOs found the demarcation between "acute" and "chronic" problematic and faced difficulty naming diseases, especially for vague classifications such as "debility." In sum, "there is a degree of laxity in making these records which is undesirable, and detracts from their value."[122] Add to this the fact that the production of a report for just one day in the life of Poor Law medical relief had been something of a mammoth task, and the prospect of piling on the workload of the PLMOs to generate an annual account became unthinkable. The advantage gained would be insufficient compensation for the "increased labour and imperfection involved."[123]

Smith's grids of sex and age were straightforward calculations. There were trivial differences in the level of sickness between men and women—the hazards of industrial labor for men were balanced by anxiety, privation, and other diseases for women. He confirmed that the sick pauper population was heavily skewed toward the elderly, especially for the indoor poor. The spatial analytic was much more complicated. With such a large number of observations at his disposal, Smith resisted the temptation to drill down to the 4,000 or so unions and parishes as he would have liked to have done (data for unions was printed; the tabular sections of the report ran to more than 400 pages).[124] But even the large county divisions showed that rural counties of the south and east had the highest proportions of sick paupers. Not surprisingly for the man who rapidly was becoming "the greatest living authority on matters of nutriment,"[125] Smith concluded that this geographical difference was "associated with a low state of health in the labouring classes generally, due to deficiency of food," compared to "the well paid and well fed labourers of the northern counties."[126]

Interesting though these findings were, the single most significant fact was that around 70 percent of all pauper illnesses—more than 100,000 cases in all—were treated at home. For Smith, the remarkable extent of outdoor medical relief was "perhaps the most important question in Poor Law administration."[127] Outdoor sick cases cost more to maintain than indoor ones. Economically speaking, it made sense that sick paupers, and especially those with infectious disease, should be treated in "well-arranged" hospitals. Furthermore, the probability of therapeutic success was higher in hospitals than in the homes of the poor, which were "not only ill-adapted to their cure, but particularly fitted for the spread of those diseases."[128]

Smith's data on the overreaching scope of outdoor medical relief found resonance in the LGB's subsequent "crusade" to trim expenditure and reduce the financial demands outdoor relief placed on the Poor Law.[129] Furthermore, Smith was an influential participant in the concurrent debate about the condition and efficiency of metropolitan workhouse infirmaries. The mid-1860s witnessed intense public discussion about the adequacy and operation of the metropolitan workhouse system.[130] The *Lancet* made a highly critical survey of London's workhouse infirmaries in 1865, and the PLB's response was to dispatch Smith to study conditions in metropolitan and provincial workhouses in 1866.[131] A further inquisition by Thomas Watson, president of the Royal

College of Physicians, recommended that sick paupers be treated in separate buildings.[132] The culmination of these assorted inquiries was the creation of the Metropolitan Asylums Board (MAB), in which London's Poor Law unions combined to provide hospital accommodations for the infectious sick.[133] Thus, Smith's pertinent comment in 1870 about "well-arranged" hospitals was a politically loaded one. Not coincidentally, his recommendation about the isolation of infectious patients came just as the MAB was opening the doors of its fever hospitals. This sparked a long-running argument about pauperization and isolation of the infectious that lasted for almost two decades, and which I will discuss in chapter 3.

Historians who have sought to explain the rise of infectious disease surveillance in Victorian Britain have not paid attention to the importance of sickness registration. Sickness registration was a multivalent tool with layered meaning, and this makes its relevance difficult to tease out. Several constituencies wanted to make use of sickness registration. Government ministers, vital statisticians, local sanitary authorities, Poor Law guardians, institutional physicians, moral guardians, and social reformers all expressed an interest in what it had to offer: a complex and diverse array of epistemic and utilitarian possibilities.

Debates about nutrition and disease during the Lancashire Cotton Famine, the massive provision of outdoor medical relief across the country, the localized sources of epidemics, and hospitalization of the infected demonstrate how sickness registration assumed contested biopolitical significance. It offered fresh ways of interpreting and reconfiguring urban life, and not just in the abstract sense of providing fodder for reams of blue book tables that represented the diseased poor in a new statistical light.[134]

For all their limitations, early schemes of sickness registration became embedded in the practice and discourse of Victorian modes of urban governance. Between the 1850s and the late 1870s, local health departments, sanitary and medical societies, charitable agencies, voluntary organizations, and other bodies used sickness registration to locate disease in the Victorian city. This in turn provided a cost-effective framework to critique (as in Manchester) and enhance (as in London and Newcastle) public health activity, justify middle-class charitable efforts toward improving the lot of the urban poor, and refine liberal techniques of persuasion and self-help.

It is worth recalling Patrick Joyce's remarks about the liberal state's information equilibrium, which "depended on reaching a balance which involved not only knowing the governed but *not* knowing them as well . . . knowing enough not to have to know more. What it knew, or sought to know, was vital to it, but of equal importance was securing the trust of citizens by not attempting to know too much."[135] The question of sickness registration illustrates the ambiguities of knowledge gathering rather well. As the RSC's deliberations made clear, the landscape of pauper sickness really *was* something that government "sought to know." But Smith's report exposed the limits to Poor Law sickness registration as a means to understanding for central government. It was hard to obtain the data, and the quality of that data was fundamentally unreliable. Smith's investigation demonstrated the potential to indicate some very broad trends, spatial variations, and differences between pauper subpopulations that had important policy implications. But there was little chance that a regular and systematic scrutiny of pauper sickness would ever do all the work that the RSC wanted it to. S. W. North, president of the Yorkshire Association of Medical Officers of Health, told his audience in 1878 that sickness registration had limited scientific value from a medical perspective and was too expensive to administer. "The registration of disease," he argued, "will answer no useful purpose, and . . . would necessitate an army of clerks for its proper tabulation. . . . The cost . . . would be something enormous, and such as no community would endure."[136] As Ballard's local study of Islington had demonstrated, without comparable information on morbidity in the general population, sickness registration drawn only from pauper and charitable voluntary institutions would, by definition, only ever reveal the condition of the poorest of the poor.

Gathering information about sickness among the poor was not discarded as a workable national long-term project because government feared losing the trust of its citizens by wanting to know too much about paupers, as Joyce suggests. Rather, the cost was prohibitive and the detailed results were unreliable, which, taken together, rendered its analytic utility questionable. Expense was also a factor in rejecting the even larger project of comprehensive sickness registration by GPs that the likes of Richardson, Farr, Rumsey, and Ransome wanted. Here, the question of trust *was* significant in two ways that were related to the medical profession. First, the demands of comprehensive sickness registration would strain relations between government and the medical profession. Physicians did not have the time, energy, or inclination to perform the tasks required—something that became obvious through the failed schemes in the 1850s and the BMA's doomed venture into Collective Investigation. Second, inquiries into the sensitive nature of certain illnesses represented an intolerable intrusion into the privacy of individual citizens. In the name of knowledge gathering alone, these were two steps too far. By the end of the 1870s, even Richardson conceded the impracticality of collecting information on all cases of sickness via private physicians and thought it best to confine the effort to epidemic disease.[137] Here is MOH S. W. North again: "If we meddle with social arrangements, interfere with business, encroach on household privacy, or run counter to the prejudices of society, we must have reason and practical utility on our side, or we shall fail to justify our proceedings; for this purpose, we must not ask for information unless we are prepared to show that we can make it useful in promoting the goals of the community."[138] This heavy emphasis on instrumentality was a characteristic feature of British vital statistics more generally. What North was saying was that sickness registration had to be about more than the acquisition of knowledge; it must be *useful* to the community.

In his book about social investigation and the culture of government blue books, Oz Frankel makes the point that the "state could not exercise full mastery over the process of inquiry . . . or the fate of its printed reports once they were issued and promiscuously published."[139] Thus it was that Smith's report, which was primarily designed to investigate the "actual condition of the great multitude of paupers," took on greater significance when it was inserted into the wider political debate about isolating the infectious sick. Similarly, sickness registration data became more than just a cartographic device to map the urban geography of infection. In the hands of Manchester's MOH John Leigh, for example, the burden of infectious diseases borne by the poor was transformed into an immutable case for building a proper isolation hospital in the city. Clearly, *some* form of registration was needed if these hospitals were to be peopled by patients, thereby giving value for ratepayers' money.

So it was that, as Arthur Newsholme reflected in 1896, "gradually, the idea of compulsory notification of infectious diseases, as the most urgent branch of a national system of registration of diseases, came to the front."[140] Some of the reasons why infectious disease notification "came to the front" were to do with what it was *not*: it was not the blanket registration of all sicknesses; and it was not concerned with socially sensitive diseases such as syphilis. This left the door ajar for systems of notification by all physicians, not just those employed by public or voluntary institutions. But notification also became "urgent" once it was realized that although existing public health laws already provided the ends to improve health—isolation, disinfection, suspension of businesses—the means were limited. Notification constituted the means.

Chapter Two

# "These Bastard Laws"

## Infectious Disease, Liberty, and Localism

In February 1882, Nottingham's MOH Edward Seaton outlined the benefits of infectious disease notification:

> I have urged the adoption of a system of notification because by this means we should undoubtedly be in a better position to control the spread of disease. I have urged it in the case of smallpox, because we may thus get patients thoroughly well isolated and by getting the persons who are likely to be exposed to the infection vaccinated, we may stop the course of this highly infectious and terrible disease; I have urged it in the case of scarlet fever because we should be thus enabled to limit its spread by preventing children who are in an infectious state attending school, by preventing the carrying on of lace and hosiery work in the very same rooms as those in which the sick person lies, and, speaking generally by preventing other heedless and unnecessary exposure of infected persons or things; I have urged it in the case of enteric (typhoid) fever, and also diphtheria, because it would enable us to make a more searching examination of the houses and premises in which cases occur, with a view to discovering unhealthy conditions than is otherwise possible, and also because we could thus secure the efficient disinfection of those particular emanations by which the disease is known to be propagated, most frequently through the recognised channels, water, milk, or sewer gas.[1]

In the absence of a national register of sickness, salaried public health officials up and down the country pressured their employers to legislate for infectious disease notification by GPs, which might bring all infected individuals—regardless of their economic means or occupation—under the gaze of the local sanitary department.[2] The key words of Seaton's advocacy are "control" and "enable." Notification afforded unprecedented accessibility to the infected and their households. Such access promised control of the diseased and the nondiseased because it facilitated the swift implementation of existing public health laws. No longer would an MOH be reliant on inconsistent and unreliable sources of information. A daily list of infectious cases in the community provided by competent medical attendants promised to trim the fat from onerous and speculative house-to-house inspections. The inspectorial staff in the public health office would be able to visit patients as soon as they became known to them, in order to better direct municipal resources and apply legislation that gave them the power to remove the infected to hospital, disinfect belongings and homes, and suspend business operations.

Compulsory infectious disease notification first appeared on the national statute books as an optional measure in 1889 and then as a mandatory law in 1899. Historians have focused mainly on the introduction of this national legislation as an indication of the interventionist tendencies of the British state.[3] For Dorothy and Roy Porter, the acts represented "a striking infringement of the traditional freedom to be sick, and to spread one's sickness, with impunity." Despite this, they argue, notification aroused little public opposition because "by the last quarter of the nineteenth century the public was becoming acclimated to a new medical rationality that might involve the trimming of its liberties."[4] Yet the 1889 act only came about after experiments with local legislation in fifty provincial towns and cities that had adopted some form of notification through a local act of Parliament. Although these laws were significant forerunners of national legislation, they covered less than one-quarter of the country's urban population and no rural sanitary authority had a local act in place.[5] This situation was swiftly transformed when the permissive 1889 act (though compulsory in London) was widely taken up. By the time the mandatory 1899 law came into effect, notification reached almost all corners of the country.[6] This chapter concentrates on the period before notification became so commonplace (the mid-1870s to late 1880s), and when adoption depended very much on local circumstances, the precise details of which have largely escaped close attention.[7]

One crucial factor in any locality's decision to approve notification was the existence of hospital accommodations. It was widely recognized that notification was of limited use if the infected could not be sequestered in a specially designated facility. This feature of infectious disease surveillance will be discussed in more detail in chapter 3. Put briefly, in London from 1867 the Metropolitan Asylums Board built and maintained a network of infectious disease hospitals.[8] In the provinces, the 1866 Sanitary Act and the 1875 Public Health Act gave local authorities similar powers and allowed them to borrow money for the purpose. The 1875 Act also enabled the LGB to compel the combination of smaller urban and rural districts to provide hospital accommodations.[9] However, by the end of the 1870s, less than one-quarter of all local authorities had any form of provision for the reception of smallpox or fever patients.[10]

Although the lack of hospital beds, or the political willingness to supply them, provided local authorities with a ready excuse not to enact notification, there was in fact much more at stake. Political weight had to be balanced over arguments about liberty and compulsion; the freedom of individuals to take care of themselves vis-à-vis the biological safety of the community; the right to enjoy property and conduct business without constraint; and the privilege afforded to doctors to practice medicine privately. Indeed, much hostility to notification came from GPs, who, being in possession of the requisite diagnostic knowledge and access to patients, were seen by MOHs as the only true custodians of disease reporting to the local authority. However, according to many doctors, notification disrupted the sanctity of private practice, and their support was limited to notification by the householder and not by the physician himself.

This distinction between doctor and householder had wider political ramifications. To begin with, it chafed against the arguments of radical liberals, who protested the burden of compulsory notification on *all* members of the community (not just doctors) and its inevitable association with the mandatory removal of poor and working-class patients to hospital. Experience with compulsory vaccination and the medical examination of suspected prostitutes under the Contagious Diseases (CD) Acts meant that radical liberals took a dim view of the medical profession in general and of public health doctors in particular: the machinery of state medicine robbed individuals of their basic freedom, their independence of action, and personal responsibility for their own health and welfare.

It is important here to stress the diversity of liberal opinion.[11] Though radical liberals were most vocal in their disdain of state medicine, the separation of patient and family during an episode of illness was an issue on which many liberals could unite. Family-patient separation violated the sanctity of private domestic space, and it threatened the moral collateral of "character."[12] In short, it compromised the capacity of the poor to exercise full citizenship. Conventional liberal opinion more readily accepted the trade-off between community health and individual freedoms. Before the permissive notification law of 1889, some liberals complained that municipal administrations overreached by adopting notification through local acts. According to this critique, a local council's role was to implement and manage laws agreed upon by central government. Councils should act as a buffer against the interfering tendencies of central government and not create new laws of their own that impinged so heavily on people's livelihoods. It was in this context that Charles Bell Taylor, a well-known ophthalmic surgeon, antivaccinationist, antivivisectionist, and Contagious Diseases Act repeal campaigner, wrote about the pending notification laws in Nottingham in 1883: "It is under the guise of gas, water, highway and street bills that our liberties are stolen away, by men no doubt well-meaning enough, but who represent nobody and are responsible for nothing, who simply bring forth these bastard laws, and affiliate them onto the Corporation."[13] Later, I will make more of Bell Taylor's allegation that Victorian municipal councilors were unrepresentative and "responsible for nothing." But it is important to recognize that similarly vehement critiques of notification were fairly commonplace and raised wider questions about the acceptable limits of local urban government to interfere with the lives of individuals in the name of public health. So, while notification perhaps did not attract the popular furor of other compulsory health laws such as the vaccination of babies and the Contagious Diseases Acts, it crystallized fundamental questions about Victorian citizenship.

Notions were diverse about precisely what practices should constitute a "liberal" public health. Rhetorical extremes caricatured opposition and support for notification as allegiance to one of two competing freedoms: freedom from state interference (central or local) on the one hand, or freedom from disease on the other. Of course, like liberalism itself, the reality was much more complex than this dichotomy allows.[14] Public health administrators could be as unsure as any other citizen about the intrusive reach of infectious disease surveillance; meanwhile, some working-class people trumpeted public health interventions as loudly as the most vocal councilor. Understanding the spectrum of views requires an examination of the rationales, practices, and technologies of power that were negotiated and played out on the ground.[15] Doing so reengages with the question of agency, because, as Simon Gunn argues, recent historical studies of governmentality, in which the focus is on the exercise of rule through freedom, tend to leave "unanswered the question of how historical change occurs and who or what contributes to it." This is particularly important "in areas such as political rights or public health where the intervention of institutions, groups or even individuals clearly had a significant part in changing the relevant discourse."[16]

In one sense, Gunn's separation of politics and public health is needless. Infectious disease surveillance in Victorian Britain demonstrates that public health *was* political rights. In 2004 Philip Harling tracked the historiographical renaissance of the local in Victorian society when he wrote that "it was the locality and not the central state that became the chief site where the moral intrusiveness that we rightly associate with 'collectivism' and 'national efficiency' exerted itself and was contested."[17] This and subsequent chapters therefore draw inspiration from venerable traditions in urban and public health history to focus on the specificities of place and burrow beneath the "top-down" analytic that, despite claims to the contrary, is so common to historical studies of governmentality. Examples are taken from a variety of places. In Liverpool and Birmingham, compulsory notification was delayed until the national act was passed in 1889. In Nottingham, it was adopted in 1883, while Leicester was one of the earliest cities to legislate for notification in 1878 as a plank of its antivaccinationist policy to "stamp out" smallpox. Limitations of space make it impossible to provide a fully detailed political history of public health in each of these cities. Contextual background is necessarily brief. Yet these accounts need not be read as exclusive case studies. Taken together, they demonstrate the multiple and complex pathways taken to infectious disease notification across the country; how national and local networks of knowledge and expertise mutually constituted one another and permeated discourse; and how the manifold arguments concerning "freedom"—freedom from infection, freedom of individuals from the state, and freedom of the local state from central government—shaped debates about infectious disease surveillance.

## Infection, Inspection, and Compulsion

Historians who have sought to explicate the numerous ways that people were governed "though freedom" in Victorian Britain have steered clear of infectious disease. The main exceptions have been studies of common lodging house inmates, prostitutes who were suspected of having venereal disease, and smallpox vaccination. Otherwise, the history of public health has intersected with the history of governmentality mainly through mapping, the collection of statistics, and what Chris Otter has termed "inspectability." Otter uses "inspectability" in *The Victorian Eye* to capture the strategies, networks, and materials that rendered some aspects of the urban milieu—water mains, sewers, the supply of food for mass markets, for example—amenable to inspection. Otter is at pains to stress the limits to the inspectorial state, its geographic unevenness, and the necessary preservation of individual privacy.[18] Particularly in the domestic realm, water closets and bedrooms were spaces where "private and intimate habits were entirely invisible to outsiders"; privacy was a fundamental aspect of liberal subjectivity.[19] Indeed, maintaining such blind spots was intrinsic to the practice of liberal government. Nevertheless, by the end of the nineteenth century, Otter identifies a brace of "inspected entities": human subjects and technological systems. The smooth operation of the latter—which basically involved regular and routine inspection and transparency of the built environment—secured the conditions in which private individuals functioned.

The inspection of human subjects occurred "only once in a lifetime, at critical organic passage points or 'milestones' (birth, vaccination, death), or else are carried out on sections of the population requiring particularly intense institutional inspection." As a result, writes Otter, "Victorian government, at multiple levels, was turning its rather blinking, squinting, myopic eyes away from it subjects and onto the mammoth technological systems that sustained them."[20] It is therefore significant that infectious diseases were one aspect of public health's inspectorial responsibilities that Otter chooses not to consider. Infectious disease surveillance was a telling assemblage of public health practices precisely because it shifted the government's eye onto humans.[21] However, infectious disease notification did *not* institute the inspection of humans at "critical organic passage points." Rather, it was calibrated to identify and scrutinize the passage of organic crisis points—that is, to individualize the bouts of infection that were part and parcel of urban life. Notification piloted the gaze toward how the vast majority of individuals—and not just socially deviant, marginalized groups such as prostitutes and common lodgers, nor just paupers—behaved in public and private space in ways that encouraged the transmission of infection. Indeed, it was the power of notification to reconfigure such subjectivity that made critics so distrustful of it.

This distrust originated in part with the experience of legislation that already regulated the socially deviant. The Victorian state, says Philip Harling, "was armed with significant powers to discipline the 'residuum' into a mode of personal comportment that befitted the regnant social virtues of the age: self-reliance, orderliness, sexual decency, and sobriety."[22] One strain of the residuum was common lodging house inmates, who, as Tom Crook notes, "were regarded as displaced, residual figures, whether as exiles or human rubbish." By and large temporarily housing "casual labourers, prostitutes and petty criminals," common lodging houses were in turn characterized by contemporary observers as "'sinks,' 'receptacles' and 'human sewers.' Common lodgers were thus the 'lowest of the low.'"[23] The powerful combination of sexual licentiousness and dangerous bodies in repugnant spaces attracted several iterations of regulation.[24] The Common Lodging Houses Act of 1851 required all the keepers of lodging houses to give notice of any lodger ill with fever or a contagious disease to the local authority or Poor Law medical officer. The keeper was liable to a fine of 40s. in the case of negligence. The act of 1853, meanwhile, made it possible for such lodgers to be removed to hospital with the consent of the authorities. Confirmation by the medical officer of health that the disease was indeed infectious or contagious placed a further burden on lodge-keepers to ensure that the clothes and bedding of patients were properly disinfected, although they received financial compensation from local authorities for this. Both the 1851 and the 1853 acts were compulsory rather than adoptive and eventually were incorporated into the 1875 Public Health Act, but local authorities could also create their own bylaws to further regulate common lodgers through clause 33 of the 1866 Sanitary Act.

The Contagious Diseases Acts of 1864, 1866, and 1869 attempted to limit the spread of venereal disease among men in the military who were stationed in garrison towns and ports in England and Ireland.[25] The CD Acts focused on the regulation of "common prostitutes" (identified as such by plainclothes policemen and magistrates) who were subjected to a medical inspection on a fortnightly basis. The inspection was "voluntary," but could be compelled by the order of two magistrates. If inspection revealed evidence of syphilis or gonorrhea, a woman could be incarcerated in a lock hospital for a period of not more than nine months. By 1869 the acts extended to eighteen "protected districts" with a ten-mile radius of supervision around each. In her groundbreaking study of prostitution in Victorian society, Judith Walkowitz suggested that the acts "reflected a new enthusiasm for state intervention into the lives of the poor on medical and sanitary grounds."[26] Opposition centered predominantly on the "double standard" of regulation—that is, the medical surveillance and control of female prostitutes on the one hand, combined with the official sanction of male promiscuity on the other. The acts were suspended in 1883 and struck off the statute books in 1886.[27] Instrumental in the successful repeal campaign was opposition from the National Anti-contagious Diseases Acts Association and the breakaway Ladies National Association. As Frank Mort notes of the repealers, "a common culture . . . bound many of them together." That culture was predominantly urban, radical liberal, and nonconformist.[28] As we shall see, these binding traits were also refracted through networks of opposition to notification.

A further area of contention over compulsion in public health was infant smallpox vaccination, which was provided free of charge through the Poor Law from 1840. The 1853 Vaccination Act made vaccination compulsory for infants within three months of birth, but historians agree that this legislation was ineffective and failed to increase vaccination uptake.[29] Identification and prosecution of noncompliant parents was given backbone by further acts in 1867 and

1871, and it was the exercise of these powers of compulsion that fueled the antivaccination movement. Antivaccinationists were a variegated bunch, but concerns about violations of the body, individual liberty, and state intrusion over parental care of children were fundamental grounds for opposition.[30] Despite the popularity of antivaccinationism—working-class towns in the industrial northwest were a notable stronghold—many were suspicious of antivaccinationists as single-issue campaigners. Yet this suspicion in and of itself is insufficient reason to explain why many in the liberal movement, including John Stuart Mill, were silent on the question of vaccination.[31] As Mill himself wrote, "Objection to the interference with personal liberty begins when the age of education properly ceases," thus carving out a space for public health interventions directed at the young.[32] It was also well within the limits of liberalism to believe that interference with individual liberty was legitimate in the case of collective self-protection: if the medical argument that infant vaccination was necessary to restrict an individual's ability to spread infection was accepted, then vaccination could be, and was, interpreted as a liberal measure for community prevention.

Another significant piece of legislation was the 1866 Sanitary Act (itself an amendment to the Nuisance Removal Acts of 1846 and 1855), which outlawed the public exposure of infected persons or clothing and empowered an MOH to remove infected people to hospital.[33] The 1866 Sanitary Act signified a shift in attitude toward local compulsion. Under the act, whenever health was imperiled by the failure of a local authority to maintain its sewers, to provide a supply of fresh water when one could be had at reasonable cost, to fulfill its duties under the Nuisance Removal Acts, or to enforce the Local Government Act of 1858, a complaint could be made to the secretary of state, who might then institute an inquiry. In five years, fifteen such inquiries were made.[34] According to John Prest, it was because of the 1866 Sanitary Act that "adoptive legislation began to be reinterpreted as a compromise forced upon the legislature by the strength and obduracy of local interest" and its passage helped lay the ground for the Royal Sanitary Commission in 1869 (as discussed in the previous chapter).[35]

All the legislation mentioned above gave local public health authorities the means by which to manage and prevent individual cases of infectious disease through compulsion. A powerful public discourse was provoked by these laws, revealing multiple interpretations about Victorian sexuality, gender, and the human body. In practice, however, historians have shown that their impact was variable, their enforcement at times tentative, and their geography decidedly patchy. First, they were hardly panoptic in an omniscient sense, and their limitations as liberal tools of epidemiological control were all too apparent.[36] To reiterate, the focus of the Common Lodging Houses Acts and CD Acts was primarily on relatively small segments of the public: lodgers and prostitutes. Second, in the other more widely applicable laws such as the 1866 Sanitary Act, the discovery and removal of a diseased person depended on either the action of concerned individual citizens or the vigilance of local government officials, such as nuisance or sanitary inspectors and MOHs.[37] The possibility for the concealment of disease by the community was high. Third, the wording of some clauses was ambiguous and open to interpretation. In particular, the 1866 Sanitary Act stated that an infected person could only be removed to hospital if he or she were "without proper lodging or accommodation." Of course, a patient's lodging may have been sufficient for *accommodation*, but insufficient for domestic *isolation*. In the opinion of many public health professionals, the proper medical management of the case was therefore impeded.[38] The act also stipulated that sufficient hospital accommodations had to be available if removal of the patient were to be enforced. While the act itself gave local government the power to build a hospital if it so desired, when the act became law many places did not run a hospital specifically for the reception of infectious cases.[39]

## Infectious Disease Notification: Was National Legislation Inevitable?

The Huddersfield Water Works and Improvement Act of 1876 was the first local legislation to contain a clause enforcing infectious disease notification, but, as with the 1866 Sanitary Act, it stipulated that notification was only required in cases where there were "inadequate" domestic accommodations for isolation of the patient.[40] This specification came to have deep significance when the class stratification of notification was contested: for the most part, poorer people were unable to isolate a family member in their homes. As it turned out, Bolton was the first town to introduce compulsory infectious disease notification proper. The town's Improvement Act of 1877 made notification of smallpox, cholera, or any other contagious or infectious fever incumbent upon both the household head and the medical attendant. This came to be known as the "dual system" of notification, because it divided responsibility between families and doctors. Doctors were not compelled to notify in person. Dual notification was clumsy: the medical attendant passed a certificate of disease to the householder for transmission to the sanitary authorities. Doctors in Bolton were paid 2s. 6d. for each certificate issued by them, and any householder not complying with the act was liable for a £10 fine.[41]

As the number of towns using notification grew, pressure increased on Parliament to put forward legislation for the country as a whole. In January 1877, between the passing of the Huddersfield and Bolton laws, and only a few months after his speech to the Society of Medical Officers of Health on "Citizenship in Sanitary Work," George Buchanan led a deputation from the society to the LGB demanding a national law for infectious disease notification.[42] A year later, in February 1878, Birmingham MP Joseph Chamberlain introduced to the LGB a deputation from the Association of Municipal Corporations that urged the compulsory notification of infectious disease by medical practitioners. Probably referring to the Royal Sanitary Commission's deliberations on sickness registration, LGB president George Sclater-Booth countered that the "question had been discussed when the Public Health Act was under discussion; and at that time there was no disposition to deal with the subject," but he hoped that it would be introduced in time. The medical profession was "naturally touchy," he acknowledged, and measures would need the consent of the "heads of the profession."[43]

The pressure in Parliament was intense, if relatively short lived. Three private bills were put forward in the early 1880s, all sponsored by MP George Woodyatt Hastings, with the support of fellow Liberals from the medical profession, Sir Trevor Lawrence and Dr. Robert Farquharson.[44] Meanwhile, in February 1880, representatives of the BMA participated in deputations to the president of the LGB advocating a national system of disease registration at which Arthur Ransome urged dual notification. On this occasion, Sclater-Booth acknowledged that interest was growing and the government was monitoring local developments with interest.[45] The pleas of yet another deputation in 1881 were rejected by Sclater-Booth's Liberal replacement, John Dodson, on the grounds that adequate hospital capacity did not exist. In 1882 John Livy, a Bolton medical practitioner sympathetic to the need for compulsory notification, told his BMA colleagues that there had "been numerous petitions in favour of Bills presented to Parliament, but very few against them."[46] Nevertheless, those "few" protests against notification proved effective. Significant opposition was lodged by some northern MPs who were well-known antivaccinationists, supporters of women's suffrage, and affiliated to the radical antistatist Vigilance Association for the Defence of Personal Rights (VADPR).[47] The VADPR presented a memorial to the LGB in March 1883 describing compulsory notification as "a violation of personal freedom and domestic privacy." Notification and isolation, it said:

> tends to sap personal responsibility and that sense of personal freedom and independence that are the essential factors of social and national progress. . . . That with the continuous growth of human knowledge, its ever increasing spread among the people, and their growing capacity to exercise self-control, it would be unwise and mischievous to put . . . the physical conduct of life in subjection to the bias of and dictation of a professional class.[48]

The LGB resisted the pronotification lobby with a variety of counterarguments: the requisite hospital space to accommodate large numbers of infected people did not exist; the public itself was not clamoring for notification; and "local authorities could not be trusted to carry it out with any zeal, or to consent to have it imposed on them."[49]

Parliament's stubbornness on this issue was perplexing. After all, it continued to allow local authorities the power to bring forward their own legislation in other matters. One anonymous writer demanded to know that if "the thing is presumably right because a Town Council asks for it, why should they have to come to Parliament at all?"[50] Charles Bell Taylor made the point to readers of the *Nottingham Journal* that town councils should exist to superintend the business arrangements of the town and carry out existing law, not make laws of their own that differ in each town, or contravene or exceed the statute law of the land: "Time was," he wrote, "when local government guaranteed the rights of the individual and meant freedom, justice and equality before the law." In the same letter where he railed against local notification acts as "bastard laws," Bell Taylor decried the loss of freedom that they invited:

> It is to local letting that the English owe their liberties. . . . Local government has become a curse, a new terror for the poor, and a constant menace to the rights of the people. . . . By the modern system of private bills . . . the meddlesome philanthropist and compulsory fanatic have been enabled secretly to undermine the constitution, and set at naught the just rights and legal liberties of the people. . . . There is no evil so great as loss of liberty; nothing can ever compensate us for.[51]

The only way that a local council truly could have represented the opinion of a town's inhabitants was for it to be constituted entirely by the simultaneous election of all of its members. However, municipal electoral procedures merely allowed for the turnover of part of the council in any one year (usually one-third). It was on these grounds that libertarians believed a council was not morally entitled to enact legislation of its own accord, but should simply implement existing laws.[52] Despite extension of the local franchise in 1869, the rate-paying electorate's hands were somewhat tied if it wanted to administer swift and fatal retribution to a disliked council. Thus, the evils of localism were just as pernicious as the evils of centralization, which libertarians also criticized as the precursor of medical despotism and the loss of autonomy.[53]

By July 1884, thirty-four towns across England and Wales had some form of disease notification in operation, although the schedules of disease and reporting systems differed from place to place.[54] In 1882 the parliamentary Select Committee on Police and Sanitary Regulations (SCPSR) believed that the desire to introduce notification had become so commonplace that it formulated model clauses for insertion into local acts. Chaired by George Hastings himself, the SCPSR had been set up to consider all private bills promoted by municipal authorities that proposed powers "which deviate from, or are in extension of, or repugnant to, the general law."[55] These bills dealt with a whole range of local government matters from gas and water works to drains, street improvements, and the regulation of dairies. The aim of the select committee was to impose some measure of uniformity on public health regulation in particular.[56]

Dual notification now took its place alongside these other urban concerns.[57] Neither the Liberty and Property Defence League nor the BMA's Parliamentary Bills Committee was impressed with this way of doing things. The latter unsuccessfully urged the SCPSR to consider notification as a separate issue or through a Royal Commission.[58] The former, which was set up in 1882 to protect individuals from state interference, mocked local improvement bills as "ill-digested medlies [*sic*] . . . bent upon stamping out infectious diseases."[59] To the horror of both libertarians and doctors, the SCPSR procedure made it easy for councils to sideline potential disagreement over notification.[60] Homeowners could protest to the select committee if "they could show that their rates or charges would increase, or that they would become liable to fresh sanitary regulations or other new burdens."[61] However, because of the strict parliamentary rules on *locus standi*, non-homeowning ratepayers and electors were assumed to be represented by their local council. The SCPSR found it easy to marginalize opposition voices using this stipulation. Furthermore, parliamentary agents, who were responsible for promoting and defending private legislation, preferred to settle the terms of such legislation among themselves with as little outside interference as possible.[62] In 1882, for example, the select committee completely ignored an antinotification petition from Newcastle that contained one thousand names.[63]

In fact, a municipal council could avoid having to defend itself in front of the SCPSR altogether and instead apply to the LGB for permission to repeal or amend a local improvement act. If it agreed to the change, the board issued a provisional order for an amendment. Provincial orders were then passed into statutory law through a "confirming" act. Mostly this procedure was used to manage finances or property, such as increasing borrowing powers to construct gas or water works, manage stocks, or confirm the lease of parkland for public use.[64] However, the LGB allowed Manchester Corporation to use a provincial order when it inserted dual notification clauses in its Waterworks and Improvement Act of 1881.[65] Overall, as Christine Bellamy concludes, despite the oversight of the SCPSR, local councils knew where their legislative bread was buttered when they took the private bill route, because "the balance of initiative and control over local powers lay more positively with the local authority than if the authorities had gone to the central administration."[66]

The LGB finally decided to sponsor notification legislation when its then president, Charles Ritchie, visited Sheffield during a smallpox epidemic in 1888.[67] The Sheffield Town Council itself petitioned Ritchie to support notification as a way of circumventing local opposition in Sheffield and to improve the city's system of voluntary notification, which was dismissed by the city's mayor as "neither one thing nor the other."[68] Just as it had a decade earlier, in March 1888 the Association of Municipal Corporations urged the government to pass a national law. In May, Salford's MOH John Tatham arranged for thirty-eight MOHs in towns with notification to memorialize the LGB, attesting to notification's benefits. By this stage, the variability of notification uptake was regarded as a biological liability. Protected towns were left vulnerable to importations of infection from their unprotected rural hinterlands or from other towns that did not have notification.[69]

Another Hastings-sponsored private bill languished in the summer of 1888 due to the crowded docket of public business, but the board finally gave Hastings and the SCPSR the green light to prepare the Infectious Diseases (Notification) Act. Speaking at the annual meeting of the Ladies National Association in July 1889, MP Walter McLaren described the resulting bill as a "suspicious measure."[70] Nevertheless, it became law on October 1, 1889.[71] The act preserved local autonomy and was optional outside London, where it was compulsory. The LGB argued that legislation would be ineffective in the capital if it was not adopted by all the sanitary authorities there, but the situation was different in provincial towns where a single authority controlled the whole of the urban area.[72] Both the *Sanitary Record* and the *Saturday Review* suggested this concession to localism made it an imperfect step in sanitary regulation.[73] In fact, Hastings himself said that he tried to make notification applicable across the country, but he dropped the idea when he found out that Irish MPs had resolved to defeat a mandatory law.[74] Compulsory notification remained optional until further legislation was passed a decade later.[75]

These, then, are the broad contours of how notification became a national law. In some ways it is a familiar story in nineteenth-century British public health. It was piecemeal and hesitant. Standardization was gradually imposed from the center. Legislation was resisted on practical and philosophical grounds. But in other ways, it is a quite distinctive account. To begin with, notification dragged medical practitioners into an uneasy relationship with the state in a manner that other public health legislation did not, and for which GPs were largely unprepared. Furthermore, despite the commonly held and generally appropriate impression that public health in Britain was an intensely "local" practice, very few public health policies could in fact claim notification's trajectory, whereby it was transformed from a patchy local activity to a mandatory national law.[76] Most public health policy was the product of what Bell Taylor described as "local letting"; that is, permissive laws were passed by central government that allowed local authorities to do a job if they so wanted. However, the national law for compulsory notification was very much the outcome of what might be termed "local wanting." At one point, in the early 1880s, it seemed that this transformation from local to national would happen almost overnight. In the end, it took almost a quarter century, from Huddersfield's foray in 1876 to the mandatory national act in 1899.

## Medicine and Liberalism in the Provinces

Why did it take so long? The only way to answer that question is to chart the uneven geography of local obstruction to notification. Even with a fairly limited number of urban case studies, it is clear that no single blueprint for stalling and preventing notification existed. One common element, however, was the opposition of medical practitioners who protested being compelled to notify under the threat of financial penalty. The most prominent and celebrated case was Liverpool in October 1881, when the council planned to introduce compulsory notification and to close infected schools and dairies. The local bill proposed a payment of 2s. 6d. to the practitioner for each notification certificate issued. Medical professionals successfully prevented this. Pivotal to this episode was the organizational capacity of the Liverpool Medical Institution (LMI), which had been in existence since the late 1830s.[77]

Two Liverpool doctors, Robert Hamilton and Alexander Bligh, sat on the city's health committee and alerted the LMI, which in turn persuaded the town clerk to postpone a health committee meeting about notification until November 10.[78] Meanwhile, the LMI drew up a statement opposing the compulsory notification clauses. A supportive letter from Manchester's Dr. Arthur

Ransome, chair of the BMA's Registration of Disease Committee, confirmed its policy that notification should be the householder's responsibility and not the physician's.[79] An LMI deputation eventually addressed a meeting of the health committee on November 24. One member of this deputation was Josephine Butler's personal physician, William Carter. In 1875 Carter had helped establish the Working Men's National League for the repeal of the Contagious Diseases Acts, and he became a vocal critic of notification on the national stage.[80] Back in the health committee, Hamilton and Bligh managed to secure yet another adjournment of the debate. In the meantime, a conference of twenty-three medical men from north Liverpool rejected the compulsory notification clauses.[81] On December 1, 1881, the health committee voted to drop them, on the grounds that space could not be found in the council's sessional timetable. The motion was seconded by Hamilton and carried by eight votes to four.[82]

The Liverpool Medical Institution's delaying tactics had worked well and were pressed into action again soon enough. During a typhus outbreak in August 1882, the MOH complained to the health committee that doctors were refusing to grant certificates of infection for the hospitalization of patients. Arthur Forwood, chair of the health committee, recommended the introduction of the model compulsory notification clauses as drawn up by the SCPSR.[83] A rider from the medical members of the health committee that "such notification shall not be compulsory upon the medical profession" was blocked. The LMI again rejected compulsory notification by medical practitioners, and a petition declaring physicians' opposition to Liverpool's private bill brought into the House of Commons secured more than 250 signatures.[84]

Meanwhile, Forwood wrote to all local authorities that had obtained any form of notification through a local act and asked for their opinion as to its operation.[85] Deputations were sent to some of these towns to gather evidence.[86] Forwood's ploy was vindicated at the end of September when the health committee voted to send the clauses imposing compulsion on the medical profession to a full meeting of the council.[87] However, the council debate was adjourned until after the local elections and the formation of a new council in November 1882. Thus the opportunity to introduce notification in that session was lost and did not resurface again until the national legislation of 1889, when local doctors eventually endorsed notification.[88] This story emphasizes the crucial role played by the LMI and its members in averting the perceived threat of compulsory notification; the fact that some of its members sat on the health committee helped stall council procedures and provided a platform for the organization and articulation of medical opinion.[89]

During the debate about the notification clauses in Nottingham's 1878 local improvement bill, the city's MOH Edward Seaton paid a visit to Bolton in March to inquire about the workings of notification. Seaton himself favored notification, but like many other MOHs at the time, he was also struggling to establish a private practice in Nottingham. When the contractual terms of his appointment were discussed in late 1877 and early 1878, he had told the health committee that his two responsibilities dovetailed rather well: "If I were to become restricted to what is usually termed sanitary work I should lose the opportunities I at present possess for the cultivation of medical knowledge which bears directly on matters relating to preventive medicine. Exclusion from private practice from this point of view is to the disadvantage of the public."[90] Seaton persuaded Nottingham's health committee to abandon a plan to appoint him under the LGB's terms and conditions, whereby the board's payment of 50 percent of an MOH salary would have prevented him from private practice. Overnight this would have doubled Seaton's income to £800. But by the end of February 1878, Seaton had convinced his health committee that independence from the LGB was something to be valued, as was his right to practice medicine privately. The health committee raised Seaton's salary to £600 plus £50 expenses, paid in full by the council.

So, the timing of Seaton's visit to Bolton in mid-March was extremely significant. His commitment to private practice freshly renewed, he was in no position to coerce his fellow practitioners to notify.[91] He returned from Bolton, where dual notification operated, and recommended a system that relieved doctors altogether from the responsibility of notifying and placed it solely in the hands of householders.[92] As an indication of the failure of this approach, in March 1881 the local authority demanded that Seaton write a letter to all GPs, the Nottingham Medico-Chirurgical Society, and the Midland Branch of the BMA pleading with them to take on the burden of notification.[93] That month, Seaton also attended a meeting of the medical profession on the topic of notification, but told his health committee employers that the meeting had been "of a private character and he could not therefore enter into the nature of the discussion which took place."[94] Eventually, Seaton relayed the medical profession's reactions at a health committee meeting on July 15, 1881:

> Whilst admitting their duty as citizens to aid the state in whatever it may deem necessary for the public welfare and whilst satisfied of the importance of the notification of infectious diseases [the medical practitioners] deem it to be undesirable that the duty of notifying infectious diseases should be laid upon them until the difficulties associated with such notification have received full consideration in Parliament and such duty is sanctioned by being the law of the land.[95]

A smallpox epidemic in February 1882 presented the health committee with an opportunity to have the disease compulsorily notified for a limited period of twelve months. In fact, the full council decided to extend notification to include scarlet fever as well as smallpox, despite concerns over the lack of hospital accommodations.[96] Later that year when the corporation put forward clauses making notification of all cases of infectious diseases compulsory on physicians, thirty-eight members of the local medical profession petitioned the town council in protest.[97] The list of signees included Charles Bell Taylor, who, as we have already seen, referred to local notification legislation as "bastard laws."[98] Seaton found this memorial so hostile that he was left with little choice other than to rebut his colleagues publicly, a task that he found both difficult and unpleasant.[99] Approval for a one-year trial finally was given at the town council meeting in July.[100]

When the trial period neared its end in April 1883, the city's medical profession voted against its continuation, but the majority was reduced to just one doctor.[101] Council debate centered on whether compulsory notification equated to compulsory removal. The chamber echoed the sound of liberal chimes about the enlightened power of persuasion:

> The [health] committee did not approve of compulsory isolation, and did not want it at all. It was very easy to isolate in a rich man's house, but most difficult in a poor man's. A poor man with a large family had no chance of doing it. What they required therefore was that their officials should go and discharge their duties in a kindly manner. They did not want them to play fantastic tricks because they were in brief authority, but they ought to go as ministering angels sent by a Liberal Corporation (cheers and laughter). They wanted their officials to advise the poor what was best to be done. He meant as their counsellors and advisors, and not to compel. What they wished to use was moral force and moral suasion.[102]

Rather than lead to compulsory isolation, notification enabled the MOH to give educational lectures "in the factories and in the localities" where infection broke out. Liberal alderman (and former sheriff of Nottingham) Henry S. Cropper said that an employee from one of his factories had voluntarily stayed at home after contracting an infectious disease and "danger to perhaps 2,000 men was averted. This was the spirit in which the resolution should be carried out . . . but the instant it went beyond that he promised the health committee all the opposition in his power."[103] One surgeon who had not signed the memorial in 1882 publicly supported Seaton and claimed that compulsory removal was nothing but a "bugbear to create prejudice against notification." He argued that it was exceedingly difficult to remove a patient under the 1875 Public Health Act but that coercion was hardly ever used. The public have "an undoubted right to every protective which legislation can afford," he said.[104] Proponents of notification won the day, and the adoption of compulsory notification for smallpox, typhus, typhoid fever, and scarlet fever was carried in council by thirty-five votes to seven.[105]

One medical opponent accused Seaton of "secretly" influencing the health committee while at the same time taking a ringside seat at medical practitioners' meetings.[106] Not long after this, and perhaps tiring of the "good deal of friction" caused by the introduction of the act, Seaton wrote to Nottingham's town clerk—Mr. S. G. Johnson, who interestingly was himself a member of the VADPR and an admitted opponent of notification[107]—requesting a raise in salary to £800 under the LGB's terms.[108] One month after this arrangement was approved in January 1884, Seaton's wife died, and he subsequently accepted the vacant MOH post in Chelsea in June 1884.

In contrast to Seaton, Birmingham's MOH Alfred Hill possessed a salary and tenure that probably was greater and more secure than any of his provincial colleagues. Peter Hennock long ago pointed out that Birmingham resisted employing an MOH until its hand was forced by the 1872 Public Health Act, and even then it made the appointment in bad faith.[109] Indeed, Hill's was only a part-time appointment, but nonetheless it was at the staggering rate of £650 per year. By the end of 1873, Joseph Chamberlain was mayor, and the council sought to make a full-time appointment. The health committee negotiated a salary of £1,000 with Hill (£150 as analyst and £850 as MOH), on the condition that he relinquished his private practice. The city of Birmingham accepted the LGB's 50 percent contribution to Hill's salary.[110] The salaries of Hill's inspector and assistant inspector of nuisances were similarly settled, representing an overall saving to the council of up to £600 per annum. As with so much else that characterized Birmingham's corporatist brand of gas-and-water socialism, this was a smart financial move and at the same time promoted the "efficient discharge" of the MOH's duties.[111]

Barring Hill from private practice meant that potential friction about him poaching patients was neutralized by the time notification arose as an issue in the city. A system of voluntary notification of scarlet fever and smallpox operated from mid-1875.[112] Hill was disappointed in 1877 that only 17 of the 200 medical practitioners in the town reported cases, though he praised these few for their "high sense of professional duty" and "truly unselfish and philanthropic action."[113] Although the voluntary system fell short of what was anticipated and hoped for, the health committee judged that there had been considerable success in isolating infected members of the community.[114]

The very progressiveness of Birmingham's public health administration after the Liberal electoral landslide in 1873 was problematic for local GPs. Although not fearing a loss of patients directly to Hill, they did worry about their shrinking incomes once patients were removed to hospital and domestic visits dried up.[115] By 1875 the council had tripled the number of sanitary inspectors to thirty-eight and had controversially secured ward accommodations on the workhouse grounds for the reception of infectious patients, which came to be known as the Borough Hospital.[116] In February 1878, the health committee asked doctors if they wanted to continue attending their patients after they were admitted to the Borough Hospital. A joint meeting of the Birmingham and Midland Counties branch of the BMA and the Midland Medical Society agreed to this proposition, so long as it came with the assent of the patient or his or her friends. In order to offset the GPs' economic loss, the health committee introduced an innovative fee structure. It offered a standard rate of 2s. 6d. per notification, which doubled whenever the GP undertook "to use his influence to obtain the removal of the patient to the Borough Hospital."[117]

Instantly the number of scarlet fever admissions to the Borough Hospital shot up, from 43 in 1877 to 424 in 1878.[118] Hill, a persistent advocate of the benefits of compulsory infectious disease notification, wavered between praising and admonishing the medical profession on the question of voluntary notification. In 1882 he noted:

> Such information [on cases of infectious diseases] as is furnished is purely voluntary, and is due to the good feeling of a considerable number of the medical profession, about eighty in number, and constituting roughly about one-third of the medical practitioners of the town. This is certainly a considerable proportion, and quite sufficient to show that the difficulties in the way of a general system of notification of infectious diseases are by no means so great as represented. It is only just to say that the medical men in Birmingham have displayed as great liberality of view in this matter as those of any town in England, if not greater. Without compulsion of any kind, they have to a large extent shown themselves willing to assist the sanitary authority in coming to a knowledge of the existence of preventable disease, and it is reasonable to believe that they would willingly fall in with a proposal for universal notification were they only protected from the consequences by the aegis of a parliamentary enactment.[119]

Proposals for compulsory notification in Birmingham's November 1882 Corporation Bill garnered vocal backing from the nationally famous gynecological surgeon Lawson Tait. As a radical liberal councilor and former chair of the health committee, he lent an important voice of support, perhaps even more so given that radicals such as Tait tended to align themselves with antivivisectionists, antivaccinationism, and repeal of the CD Acts (think of Bell Taylor in Nottingham and Carter in Liverpool).

Notification also caused an interesting split within Birmingham's liberal elite. Members of the city's influential Martineau political dynasty were on opposite sides in the council debate. The notification clauses that Tait supported were put forward by Thomas Martineau, but opposition was led by his younger brother, Robert Francis (Frank) Martineau, who argued that evidence from other cities about the effectiveness of notification was inconclusive and that notification resulted in the concealment of disease from physicians.[120] He also articulated a common feeling among radicals that the role of a local council should be to lead people rather than to drive them.[121] Fearing that the popular resistance to vaccination would be replicated by a fight against notification, Alderman Richard Chamberlain—whose brother Joseph, as one of the city's MPs, had introduced a deputation to the LGB in favor of notification in 1878—also thought that by seeking coercive powers the health committee would destroy the relationship it had with the public.[122] In what George Hastings later described as "an evil hour" in Birmingham, the council struck out the notification clauses by a 27–20 vote.[123]

The limits on voluntary notification meant that Hill inevitably would try to take immediate advantage of the permissive national law in 1889. When he did so, a petition was presented to the health committee from Birmingham's "Anti-variole League" expressing its distrust of notification and asking the council to wait and see how the act worked out in other towns before adopting it.[124] Again Frank Martineau voiced his opposition. He conceded that although the health committee and Hill could be trusted to protect local people and treat them all equally in the eyes of the law, a more doctrinaire administration might replace them at some point in the future. Like the prominent advocate of self-help that he was, Martineau went on to say that "if by this new act the committee estranged the people from themselves, they would remove the very cause which had contributed to so much success in their operations." Echoing the comments of such ultraradicals as women's rights campaigner Elizabeth Wolstenholme Elmy, Martineau's allies continued to portray notification as a system of medical espionage that paved the way for medical despotism.[125] Another councilor "objected to handing over to the doctors the bodies of his fellow-citizens, just as he would object to handing over their souls to the priests."[126]

Obviously, widespread resistance to notification in the Birmingham council had shrunk since the last debate in 1882. The chair of the health committee reckoned that its relations with the local medical profession now were cordial enough to withstand any residual resentment to notification on the physicians' part. The council approved notification—despite the dissenting voices noted above, the vote was unanimous—and after years of successful obstruction, radicals, physicians, and antivariolists alike were forced to acknowledge its place in Birmingham's health contract: people who now posed a contagious threat to others and yet refused to notify were, according to one councilor, "deficient in their conception of the moral duties of a citizen."[127]

Unpacking the vexed question of citizenship is further complicated by events in the East Midlands city of Leicester. By the mid-1870s, Leicester was a prominent center of antivaccination resistance, and the council there turned to the strict isolation of smallpox patients as the only preventive means available. The notification and isolation of smallpox cases and the disinfection of homes came to be known as the "Leicester Method."[128] Even Leicester's provaccination public health authorities were prepared to play down the importance of vaccination. In order to stamp out smallpox, "isolation is the only reliable means at all," said Assistant MOH and Superintendent of the Fever Hospital William Johnston. "There is no other line of action that will prevent the spread of disease."[129] When the Leicester Method was inaugurated in 1877, it became clear that for the isolation of smallpox to succeed in the absence of vaccination, the prompt notification of all cases was paramount. According to the chair of Leicester's health committee, Thomas Windley, various calls on Leicester practitioners to voluntarily notify had fallen on deaf ears.[130] Late in 1878, the town council proposed to insert notification clauses into its local improvement bill the following year, and included a stringent £5 fine for failure to notify. The council did not consult the medical profession beforehand, and a New Year's resolution against the clauses was made by thirty local doctors on January 1, 1879.[131] According to a later report in the *Leicester Advertiser,* these thirty signatures amounted to nearly all the town's medical professionals.[132] The health committee agreed to meet immediately with the petitioners, who protested that proposals were detrimental to the independence and best interests of Leicester's inhabitants. They suggested a requirement for notification only if the GP deemed domestic isolation impossible, thus not risking the loss of income from wealthier patients.[133]

It was brought to the attention of the health committee that one of the memorial's signatories was none other than their own MOH, Alfred W. Crane![134]

Crane's name still was attached to the memorial when it was read before the town council on January 16.[135] The clauses remained in the bill, and a further petition signed by 111 Leicester ratepayers requested a public meeting. It is not clear who the signatories of this petition were, but almost certainly it contained those members of the Leicester Medical Society who had signed the memorial of January 1 (though perhaps with the exception this time of the MOH Crane).[136] Although the statutory public meeting was held on January 16 and the requisite advertisement of that meeting had been given in four local newspapers, the mayor offered to meet a deputation of the disgruntled physicians.[137] This meeting never took place. A formal petition was lodged against the local bill in Parliament objecting to the provisions "as imposing . . . new and onerous and unnecessary obligations . . . both uncalled for and likely to lead to endless mischief and complication."[138] The Leicester memorialists failed to prevent the legislation passing through the House of Lords, and the local bill became law. Pursuing the case this far had cost the Leicester Medical Society dear, and it was forced to appeal to readers of the *British Medical Journal* for financial contributions when it struggled to meet the £160 in legal costs that had stacked up in the course of its attack on the clauses.[139]

Why did medical practitioners in Leicester fail to block notification, whereas in Liverpool, Birmingham, Nottingham, and elsewhere they managed to delay it, if not prevent it altogether? In *Radicalism, Cooperation and Socialism*, Bill Lancaster observes that antivaccinationism in Leicester "tended to affirm rather than question the existing status quo" of radical liberalism in the city, the backbone of which was an alliance between workers in the hosiery and footwear industries and middle-class politicians.[140] The strength of antivaccinationism in Leicester clearly was an important factor in the acceptance of notification, but it is not a sufficient reason on its own. Certainly one key difference between, say, Liverpool and Leicester was that when notification was debated, there were no doctors on Leicester's local health committee, which, according to one Leicester newspaper, left the sanitary committee open to manipulation by Assistant MOH Johnston, who was seen as the real force behind the push for notification.[141] Thomas Windley, the chair of the health committee, needed very little persuading. He was well-known among local doctors as being hostile to the medical profession.[142] In Liverpool, however, the LMI could mobilize opposition on the health committee, even when the chair of that committee was the formidable Tory democrat Arthur Forwood.

Timing was also crucial. The BMA favored the *principle* of compulsory notification, arguing that it was almost useless to attempt to check the course of an epidemic without it.[143] But between the Leicester debate in 1878 and the Liverpool episode in 1881–82, the BMA Parliamentary Bills Committee began to challenge attempts to burden GPs with notification. The committee's chair, Ernest Hart, maintained a close correspondence with GPs in all towns where notification was threatened.[144] The strategy of agitation could be extremely effective. In February 1885, for example, Hart reported that the compulsory notification clauses had been dropped in six of the eight towns where he had recently given assistance. Radical liberals claimed similar credit, noting that when the VADPR was "on the track," some towns dropped their bills' notification clauses, worried that their improvement bills would fail in toto.[145]

In fact, for a fleeting and deeply improbable moment in the early 1880s, medical practitioners and libertarians found common cause against notification across a number of fronts. They agreed, for instance, that notification violated the sacrosanct relationship between doctor and patient. The act of notifying sanitary authorities publicized the patient's illness.[146] The principle of medical confidentiality enshrined in the Hippocratic Oath obliged doctors not to use acquired information for any purpose other than the patient's care. By becoming "two-and-sixpenny detectives," doctors might lose their respected status within the community.[147] As one practitioner said, "The physician ought to be the friend of the family, and he ought, by his conduct, to show that he deserved the confidence of his patient. Would he have this confidence if he acted as the tool of the government?"[148] Although the government granted protection over doctors' right to practice, gave them the right to recover financial remuneration for their services, and endowed titles upon them, the state's claim on doctors to render service for payment in the promotion of public health was dismissed as an abstract concern, overridden by the real need for complete confidentiality.[149]

As they railed against the incremental loss of patient autonomy, radicals co-opted and perpetuated the traditional notion that GPs should perform a gentlemanly role. When it came to deciding on a therapeutic course of action, physician and patient were supposedly on equal footing during the domestic clinical encounter.[150] Patients should have the full confidence of their doctors, but by mandating the intrusion of the "Established State School of Medicine," notification gave MOHs a role in the medical management of the infectious sick, which destroyed "the free-will and independent judgment of the patient as to the treatment he will undergo."[151] This version of medico-libertarian individuality was widespread and had immense rhetorical power. The relationship between a GP and his patient was individualistic. GPs identified themselves as distinct from the social body, not in common with it.[152] John Sykes, MOH for St. Pancras in London, reminded his fellow public health professionals that "the medical attendant's first duty is to his patient, his next to the patient's family, but the public comes last, and that the duties of a MOH are in the reverse order."[153] Compulsory notification threatened the priority that GPs gave to individual patients.[154]

The sanctity of individuality in the clinical encounter was entwined with its spatiality. Doctors were content for MOHs to direct their investigative attention toward the materiality of domestic property, such as sewers, drains, and other culprits of sanitary transgression. This implicitly acknowledged the environmental causes of disease. But doctors saw absolutely no need for the MOH—or, even worse, one of his subordinate sanitary inspectors—to enter the sickroom itself.[155] By this time, it was common for sanitary and nuisance inspectors to be accused of interfering with an individual's right to enjoy private property.[156] But because the Sanitary Act of 1866 and Public Health Act of 1875 reconfigured the infected person as a "nuisance" to be abated just like any other, notification kicked the sickroom door wide open. And, as the Liberty and Property Defence League argued, it did so in order that the patient could be removed from the domestic space to an institutional one.[157] Not all domestic spaces were equal, however. Johnston, Leicester's assistant MOH, admitted that the sanitary authorities there "do not go into the houses of well to do people to look after sanitary conditions. We know that sanitary defects prevail to the highest degree unfortunately among the tenements of the poor. We do not go to men's houses who are in receipt of £150 or £250 a year.[158] For doctors with a reputation for notifying, the prospect of a visit from a sanitary inspector meant that "your good patients don't send for you."[159]

Not surprisingly, medical and radical critics alike branded the MOH as the common enemy. Notification invested far too much power in a single municipal official, power that would be abused. The MOH was variously labeled a "modern dictator," a "medical despot," a member of "our new medical spy-police," a "wire-puller" for tyrannical local authorities, and a priest "of the new religion of compulsion."[160] Notification questioned the credentials of GPs because it implied that the "ordinary medical man" could not direct patients toward the control of infectious disease and that the only medical person competent to do so was an MOH appointed by the sanitary authority.[161]

For doctors, particularly those in places where the MOH also maintained a private practice, the MOH was a professional rival and a financial threat. In 1882 the MOH continued in private practice in at least eight of the twenty-three towns surveyed by Liverpool's health committee.[162] Alfred Carpenter outlined the problems this raised:

> Until all medical officers of health consist of either consulting practitioners or men who are not in practice at all, there certainly will be some [medical officers of health] who will be able to hide for a time the malicious character of their action, and try to injure another man's reputation for the purpose of establishing their own, not seeing that if their own is not capable of being established without the other man is damaged, they are proving their own littleness, and their own incapacity to excel their neighbour in the estimation of the people by simply professional work. I am very much opposed to placing any such power in the hands of professional rivals.[163]

The mid-Victorian GP was economically vulnerable in an extremely competitive market. Undercutting rivals and poaching patients was common, normal even. In 1879, having served two years as a part-time assistant MOH in Leicester and retaining his private practice while also administering the city's new system of notification, William Johnston admitted that "a medical man of course going fresh into a town must always more or less take away some of the patients, otherwise he would stand still—you are bound to do some poaching. There is no question of that."[164] Many provincial local authorities outside the big cities could only afford to employ part-time a newly qualified or even debarred doctor.[165] The registration for qualifications in public health was introduced by the

Medical Act of 1886. This may have gone some way toward silencing the allegations of professional incompetence and assuaging the fears of family doctors.[166]

Of course, doctors wanted to exclude other sorts of practitioners from having access to the infected. If registered physicians were compelled to notify and publicize disease, householders might prefer to call in unqualified healers such as druggists or herbalists.[167] The BMA defended the "semi-closed shop" that the medical register had delivered to general practitioners under the 1858 Medical Act.[168] The BMA's preferred method of dual notification preserved the *registered* practitioner's power over diagnosis. The diagnosis alone represented the full extent of the GP's obligation to the wider community, since under dual notification it was the householder's responsibility to inform the sanitary authority.[169]

During the summer of 1882, doctors in Liverpool sought to solidify their cause by setting up an association in opposition to compulsory notification by medical men: William Carter was appointed president; physician and city councilor Robert Hamilton was treasurer; and Ewing Whittle, a member of the National Anti-contagious Diseases Acts Association and the BMA Parliamentary Bills Committee, was also involved.[170] This prompted the organization of similar associations elsewhere in the country. By August these associations had an estimated six hundred members and in spring 1883, the so-called Anti-compulsion Society claimed a membership of more than one thousand medical men.[171] Though subsequently it seems to have disappeared without a trace, the records show that this hitherto unnoticed society was represented alongside the VADPR in the antinotification deputation that met with LGB president Sir Charles Dilke in March 1883.

Libertarians were encouraged by the existence of the Anti-compulsion Society, and they hoped that doctors' resistance to notification might even lead them to reconsider their broad support of compulsory vaccination. In August 1882, the profession was cautioned "not to fall into the blunder . . . of approving compulsion for everybody else, whilst resisting it for themselves."[172] This proved to be a forlorn hope. Within a month, and in the presence of George Hastings, the annual meeting of the BMA at Worcester approved a resolution that reaffirmed its stance that compulsion should be placed on the householder "as his duty as a citizen." In 1883 the *BMJ* explained that while doctors had a legitimate grievance, the general public could not be excused of its duty:

> We cannot see that there is any undue violation of personal liberty in the sanitary authority acting for the whole community, requiring to be informed of the existence of diseases dangerous to others. If a man's house is on fire, and he refuses to have it put out as quickly as possible on personal liberty principles, we should entirely excuse the municipal or fire brigade authorities acting as energetically as possible without his consent. A man's liberty is not to involve risk to others. This is already abundantly admitted in law and in common sense. A man with smallpox has the natural liberty to travel in a cab or an omnibus; but society has a right that overrides his natural liberty, and says he shall not. He may equally convey disease to others through his house or his business; and society will certainly not rest till it has reduced this personal

> liberty to a minimum in the case of grave diseases. It should do so with greatest consideration for the individual, but with more for the community in which he is only a unit.[173]

This tendency of doctors to draw a distinction between themselves and the general public was heavily criticized. Were medical professionals not citizens? The VADPR complained that "pains and penalties shall be imposed upon everyone except the members of the sacrosanct profession, who must be protected, at any cost to the public, from the slightest worry, inconvenience, or odium themselves." The view that GPs were citizens just like everyone else was shared by MOHs. Medical professionals had business interests; as such, they had wider social obligations and duties that they were no less able to escape than other businesses. The mayor of Blackpool asked, "Where is the right to immunity of doctors over mill owners, manufacturers, shopkeepers, and others to contribute their quota to the public good?"[174] One MOH observed that doctors made "no objection . . . to the proposal to put compulsion on the householder or guardian, though I fail to see that compulsion as such be considered more objectionable by a professional than by a non-professional."[175] At the time of the Liverpool dispute, the *Sanitary Record* called on the medical profession: "to remember that all citizens are liable to compulsory service of one kind or another, and would beg them to remember that from several of these they are themselves exempt. Is the sentimental grievance involved in compulsion worthy of being opposed, for an instant, to so simple and beneficent measure as the notification of infectious disease?"[176] The delivery of health care as a commodity reduced each medical encounter to just one of the many financial transactions secured in a buyer's market. The "contractual" nature of private practice (that is, payment for a service) meant that doctors were obliged to differentiate between classes of society upon their capacity to honor this contract (that is, the ability to pay). Fees might be weighed according to occupation or housing tenure.[177] Not only did this expose the claims made in the name of Hippocratic ethics—which one might expect to be applied regardless of the patient's class—it inevitably led to a judgmental differentiation between the moral character of these classes. Carter of Liverpool—as we have seen, a noted opponent of compulsory notification by the family doctor—told the Literary and Philosophical Society of the city that if it *did* have to exist, then notification legislation should apply only to the "sanitarily dangerous and reckless classes . . . while the respectable artisan and small shopkeeper, as well as the classes above them, would be protected from the annoyance of an inquisitorial surveillance and domiciliary visitation."[178] For Carter, distinction between the classes could be made because the wealthy were more capable of preventing disease in the home and possessed the means to do so. Liverpool's *Liberal Review* accurately interpreted the consequences of drawing such distinctions:

> We are told in the first place that people suffering from infectious disease may be divided into two classes—those who are anxious to avoid the spread of the infection, and those who care nothing at all how it spreads; and we are also told that doctors are anxious to give all the assistance in their power to the

> *first* of these classes, leaving it to be inferred that dealing with the second, or careless class, is anybody's business who chooses to attend to it, but certainly not the doctor's . . . who is to be left to devote his exclusive attention, as an amateur medical officer of health, to such persons or families as may be in a position to retain his exclusive services.[179]

In places where there was ample institutional provision, the consequences of removal to hospital could spell either grave financial difficulties or social stigma and embarrassment for a working-class family.

The conflict over notification was played out in multiple political, civil, and medical arenas and at various scales. The integration of medical elites into municipal politics, the influence of an overbearing health committee chair, and the persuasiveness of libertarian arguments in council chambers intersected in complex ways with the authority and status of the medical officer, the political clout of local newspapers, and variable access to knowledge. Effective networks were crucial for the circulation of knowledge about notification because they linked national political entities to local ones; they connected one set of local interests to others; and they brought together like-minded individuals. For example, the LGB acted as a central repository for knowledge about infectious disease notification, liaising with municipal authorities and local MOHs on the one hand, and Parliament's SCPSR on the other. These sorts of networks made up what theorists of urban mobility now term "the informational metabolism" of the city.

Nongovernmental organizations, notably the BMA and the VADPR, were also important conduits of information. The former's Registration of Disease Committee promoted a consistent message to GPs that notification should be the householder's responsibility and not the physician's. It was a one-stop shop for doctors seeking ways and means to obstruct local legislation. The VADPR used disease surveillance to articulate the libertarian belief that state medicine emasculated individuality. This was important because it put ideological opposition to notification alongside opposition to other health laws such as the CD Acts and infant smallpox vaccination, each of which contained an element of coercion. And just like the BMA Registration of Disease Committee, the VADPR tried to exploit its influence in local debates about disease surveillance. Though there was some common ground between physicians and libertarian opponents—look at Liverpool's William Carter, for example—by and large they were distrustful of one another and together they lacked a broad coalition of power in the localities to consistently block notification. Despite notable success in large cities such as Liverpool and Birmingham, in the long term they were unable to withstand conventional liberal support of the dominant public health doctrine that championed community health over individual freedom.

Nonetheless, resistance to, and negotiation over, notification at the local level indicates that it was a problematic feature of public health policy throughout the 1880s. Not least, professional identities were at stake. Precariously tenured MOHs knew full well that notification would transform the extent and depth of their interventions. Their professional authority was cemented by notification's legality, but notification certainly did not deliver MOHs a panoptic field of vision over infectious disease. Through the agency of the medical practitioner, notification trained a spotlight with relative ease onto those who were biologically dangerous and those who, by virtue of bodily proximity, might become so. No less significant was the way in which notification recast the identity of GPs by compromising their freedom to practice privately and placing the trust of health care into the hands of the state. It violated the ancient mores of Hippocratic teaching that sanctified the confidential nature of the doctor-patient relationship; under the fear of exposure, notification deterred some patients from calling in the doctor; patients removed to hospital no longer required follow-up visits; and it gave sensitive medical information to either professional inferiors or rivals in the medical marketplace.

These professional concerns found wider resonance in liberal disquiet about the loss of freedom, the trimming of individuality, and the denunciation of self-help.[180] This occasionally propelled notification to the forefront of national and local political debates that questioned the legitimacy of municipal activity. Victorian Britain is no longer regarded as the most laissez faire of European nations when it came to the propensity to interfere with the lives of its citizens. In a salient comparative review of public health and taxation policies, Peter Baldwin finds that Britain was a far stronger and more effective state (in these areas at least) than its major European counterparts, Germany and France.[181] For most people, this "state" was not down in London, but down the street in the town hall. Some activists complained that municipalities overreached by legislating for public health at all. Partly because of the model clauses formulated by the Select Committee on Police and Sanitary Regulations, notification became emblematic of excessive local interventionism. But for others who promoted moral duty and responsibility to the community as norms of civic participation, notification presented an opportunity to formulate citizenship through localism.

Notification also reconfigured the self and a traditional locus of health care, the family. It should be remembered that bouts of infection—smallpox, scarlet fever, diphtheria, enteric or typhoid fever, whooping cough—were fairly routine household occurrences, particularly when large family sizes were the urban Victorian working-class norm.[182] It is almost inconceivable that a child living in Liverpool, Birmingham, Leicester, or any one of the large industrial cities of Victorian Britain in the 1870s and 1880s could reach adolescence without contracting at least one of these diseases. For most families with children, notification meant there was a fair chance that infectious disease would invite a visit from the local health department that, with its focus on the threat posed by the human body, was unlike other inspectorial visits.

As Edward Seaton's remarks that opened this chapter demonstrate, technological deficiencies in a building's sanitary infrastructure remained a possible source of disease that had to be ameliorated. Indeed, "as soon as notification became law . . . ," wrote Leicester's MOH in 1883, "the greatly increased information received . . . enabled the Sanitary Inspectors to visit and report immediately any sanitary defect."[183] But culpability for broken drains, leaky pipes, and malfunctioning water closets lay at the door of the property-owning ratepayer, not the rent-paying tenant and his or her family. In contrast, the transmission of disease was unambiguously identified with the name of the person written on a GPs' certificate of notification. Infectious disease notification exploited the legal, humanized definition of a *removable* "nuisance" to assign risk to the diseased body, the spaces in which that body was located, and the spaces through which it moved. The task of notification was to locate as many diseased bodies as possible so that their freedom of movement could be restricted or denied, and their interaction with family members and others circumscribed. The most effective, yet traumatic way of doing this was to hospitalize them.

*Part Two*

# Spaces of Risk and Opportunity

# Chapter Three

# *Sequestration and Permeability*

## *Isolation Hospitals*

On the cover page of his 1872 report to the influential Manchester and Salford Sanitary Association, entitled "A Paper on the Duty of Municipal Authorities to Provide Hospital Accommodation for Cases of Infectious Diseases," James Hardie, MD, quoted from John Stuart Mill's *On Liberty*: "The sole end for which mankind are warranted, individually or collectively, in interfering with the liberty and action of any of their number, is self-protection."[1] Isolation hospitals for infectious disease were required, argued Hardie, because unlike diseases of the hip or inflammation of the lungs, ailments such as scarlet fever and typhus were unresponsive to medical therapies. In other words, as the only available "cure" for infectious disease, sequestration of the biologically dangerous represented nothing less than the community's "instinct of self-preservation."[2] One can imagine that Hardie would have approved of Mill's opinion, expressed but one year earlier, that "the health of the community is a subject now considered, I think with reason, to be within the province of Government."[3] Hardie rejected a role for philanthropy in the provision of hospital accommodations for the infectious sick and asked the following questions:

> Why should I not be taxed to prevent the spread of fever—to prevent its attacking my family, or spreading from my house to that of my neighbour? I do not wish fever to enter my household, but would sacrifice a great deal to prevent it. As an individual, however, I am powerless. I may meet with the germs of the disease the next time I shake hands with an acquaintance in the street. As a member of the community—of the civilized community of Lord Derby—I expect to be protected from such risk. Why should I not pay a rate to be afforded such protection?[4]

Though Mill himself was prepared under certain conditions to accept interference with individual liberty by the state in the name of health, he consistently denied a legitimate role for compulsion to undergo hospitalization. Compulsion, he reasoned, degraded the moral character of the person subjected to it. As referred to in chapter 2, this was the fundamental concern of libertarians: that notification would lead to coerced hospitalization.

Removal of an infectious person to hospital was compulsory under the terms of the 1866 Sanitary Act if the person was "without proper lodging or accommodation, or lodged in a house occupied by more than one family."[5] This requirement was consolidated by the 1875 Public Health Act. Almost twenty years later, the Isolation Hospitals Act of 1893 enabled county councils to build an isolation hospital and, if necessary, force local authorities under their jurisdiction to do so.[6] Taken together, these laws prompted something of a boom in isolation hospital provision. Ultimately, however, admission policies varied from place to place, depending in part on a local authority's judgment on the capacity of a family to isolate a patient in the home, and in part on the existence of hospital facilities.[7] Historians have been aware for some time that isolation hospital provision was inconsistent and that utilization differed between places.[8] As Sally Sheard has noted, however, "there have been few examinations of the primary data available to substantiate this view."[9] Apart from the odd occasion when central government carried out one of its implausibly ambitious public health data collection exercises, the evidence does not exist to carry out a comprehensive historical evaluation across the whole period. This chapter has the more modest aim of exploring for a limited geographical area some broad variations in rural and urban provision to assess the extent to which rural areas were underserved and cities struggled to keep up with demand. The question of efficacy also is judged at the local level from MOH reports.[10]

Although the public's enthusiasm for removal to hospital was understandably muted, local authorities reported that resistance was gradually ebbing away and that force—in the form of a magistrate's order, for example—was rarely required to induce a member of the community to go into a hospital ward. Historians have tended to accept this point of view.[11] I take issue with this anodyne official version of events. While prosecutions for refusal were seemingly uncommon, local authorities used less obtrusive, but equally threatening, methods of coercion than magistrates' orders, particularly toward the working-class and poorer members of the community. In the same sense that Pamela Cox has suggested there was extensive "hidden" compulsory treatment for VD patients after the repeal of the CD Acts, equally there was much hidden coercion involved in the removal of patients to isolation hospitals.[12]

Though questions of liberty and intimidation were undeniably important, they were not the only reasons members of the public were reluctant to go into an isolation hospital. At least in the early years of the rise of isolation hospitals, at a time when local authorities were leveraging finance, putting up new buildings, and sorting out admissions policies, there continued to be a fear of association with pauperism. People were also afraid of cross-infection in the hospital; that is, once inside the walls of the hospital because they had one disease, patients were frightened that they would contract yet another.

It is, of course, probable that favorable reports of personal experiences in the isolation hospital got around by word of mouth, and the public's antagonism toward these feared institutions consequently waned. It is also undoubtedly likely that greater scientific understanding of disease transmission endowed the rationale for isolation.[13] Yet, such explanations of how isolation hospitals came to be relatively uncontentious places are only partially satisfactory because they tend to downplay the obvious fact that local health authorities implicitly recognized that hospitals were extremely dangerous places, biologically speaking. Though isolation hospitals tended to be physically remote places, health authorities spent a great deal of money, time, and energy making them safer, regulated, and sealed environments. Constantly evolving knowledge from the domains of architecture, bacteriology, and epidemiology were mapped not only onto the almost-closed space of the hospital, but also onto the associated social relations of domestic and family life.

## Compulsion, Coercion, and Class

By the early 1870s, public health administrators firmly believed that sequestration in a hospital environment was the most suitable way to deal with infected patients. Edward Smith's reports for the Poor Law Board gave this conviction added impetus when he showed that there were massive numbers of infected patients being attended to as outdoor paupers in appalling domestic conditions.[14] Nevertheless, the main locus of bed provision for infectious patients were the fever wards in Poor Law institutions. Some general hospitals also had separate accommodations for fever patients, but in most places, this never amounted to more than a handful of beds. A small number of private fever hospitals were founded in Liverpool, London, Manchester, and Newcastle-upon-Tyne between 1800 and 1804.[15]

The 1866 Sanitary Act, the 1875 Public Health Act, and the 1893 Isolation Hospitals Act granted local governments authority to finance the building of their own isolation hospitals. They were also empowered to remove forcibly people to hospitals if they deemed it necessary. It was this legislation and the concurrent development of notification that drew the ire of many liberals, for whom compulsion posed a clear threat to freedom. It damaged the moral character of individuals by denying them choice, and it represented an infringement of personal liberty.[16] Even public health professionals were prepared to accept that this was the case. By the early twentieth century, experience had taught Stockport's MOH Meredith Young that there was a considerable downside to "the indiscriminate and wholesale removal to hospital of scarlet fever cases" in that it "weakens that sense of individual responsibility which is at the root of good citizenship."[17] This was apparent in a variety of ways. First, hospitalization interfered with the parents' right to care for their sick child.[18] Historian of the sickroom Miriam Bailin underscores how central this was to the Victorian sense of identity: "The Evangelical valorization of suffering coincided with the mid-Victorian domestic ideal—the care of the sick being one of the primary duties and supposedly instinctive capacities of the angel in the house. Illness thus became one of the principal objects of sentimental pieties about family life and family nurturance. . . . Nursing the sick was, for both men and women, as sanctified an act as suffering itself."[19] The removal of children to isolation hospitals ran against traditional ways of treating sickness in the domestic sphere and drew families into unavoidable contact with the state. As Lucinda McCray Beier has shown, public health authorities used their statutory powers to intimidate working-class parents in northwest England to hospitalize their children, and parents who preferred to nurse their children at home resisted such tactics.[20] The second argument against sequestration was that, quite simply, it was a form of temporary imprisonment.[21] Third, the hospital deprived the patient access to the freedoms enjoyed by participating in the therapeutic market:

> What shall we say of compulsory *treatment* in these enlightened days? Are those of us who prefer homeopathy to be treated invariably by allopathy? Thinking persons are beginning to know that there are better, safer and simpler modes of healing than those offered by the State school of medicine. They know something of homeopathy, of the water cure, of American modes of "packing" to bring out blood poisoning, and something too of the simple force of the Swedish movement cure to act on the blood through organs of respiration and absorption. . . . And what of our hospitals? Again we must answer: These are sometimes turned into human shambles.[22]

These were all undeniable concerns. The sequestration of children was, nonetheless, broadly characteristic of two countervailing trends in Victorian society: the state's increasing willingness to intervene in family life, and the shaping of separate spheres of existence for adults and children.[23] Furthermore, the bottom line was that in the eyes of people like James Hardie in Manchester, hospitalization did not violate the harm principle; that is, the compulsory regulation of infected individuals' actions was acceptable, since it protected the whole community. As we shall see in the next chapter on infectious disease and schools, some have argued that this sort of stance and the corollary inculcation of moral character "justified a kind of despotism over the child."[24]

When he gave evidence to the Royal Commission on the Contagious Diseases Acts in 1870, Mill argued for the state administration of institutions for the prevention of ill health based on equality in the face of disease:

> Supposing the opinion of Parliament was that contagious diseases generally, all sorts of infectious and contagious diseases, were proper subjects for the Government to take in hand administratively, and to provide means for curing, I should say there was no objection in including this [venereal disease] among the others. . . . As long as hospitals are not peculiarly for that class of diseases, and do not give that class of disease any favour as compared with others, they are not liable to objection, because their operation consists in remedying the effects of past evils; they do not hold out a special facility beforehand to practising illicit indulgence with a security which it would not otherwise enjoy. The interference is not preventive but remedial.[25]

In other words, government provision of hospitals for all infectious diseases was acceptable for two reasons. First, it ironed out the exceptional case of having hospitals only for one infection, venereal disease. Second, from the individual patient's point of view, these hospitals did not seek to condition activities that *produced* the diseased state, which would have been an infringement of liberty. Rather, they acted remedially on the individual patient.[26] This is extremely interesting because it seems to accept implicitly an argument that infectious disease hospitals had the capacity to remediate the course of infection in an individual, even though there was little or no concrete evidence that this was the case for all the types of disease that were admitted to fever hospitals at the time.[27] In fact, the question of hospital efficiency—that is, did they actually do what they were supposed to do?—barely was addressed and did not receive sustained critical attention from public health administrators until the turn of the century. I will return to this question later.

Nonetheless, the timing of Mill's interjection was significant. It was just around this time—the late 1860s and early 1870s—that local authorities across the country were beginning to weigh the implications of legislation that allowed them to build isolation hospitals, funded by tax revenues. Within a decade, 296 local authorities—about one-quarter of all local authorities—made some sort of provision for the reception of patients suffering from an infectious disease.[28] By World War I, there were 755 isolation hospitals and almost 32,000 beds available nationally for infectious diseases (Poor Law infirmaries had nearly three times as many beds).[29] As with notification uptake, the geography of hospitalization was very uneven across the country. Table 3.1 summarizes information from a large government survey on hospital provision undertaken in the early to mid-1890s. It shows that the rural districts of three Midlands counties were comparatively underserved. Just 13 percent of Leicestershire's rural population was served by an isolation hospital. In comparison, 98 percent of Warwickshire's urban population was covered (Warwickshire includes Birmingham).

Table 3.1. Provision of isolation hospitals, ca. 1894, in the rural and urban sanitary districts of three English Midlands counties

| | | | Population covered | |
|---|---|---|---|---|
| | District type and number | 1891 Population (thousands) | Number (thousands) | Percent |
| Leicestershire | RSD (10) | 138 | 17 | 13 |
| | USD (10) | 230 | 197 | 86 |
| Nottinghamshire | RSD (7) | 153 | 35 | 23 |
| | USD (16) | 352 | 268 | 76 |
| Warwickshire | RSD (12) | 158 | 100 | 63 |
| | USD (11) | 687 | 671 | 98 |
| Total (average) | RSD (29) | 449 | 152 | (34) |
| | USD (37) | 1,269 | 1,136 | (90) |

*Source:* House of Commons Parliamentary Papers, C. 28 (1895) LXXXIV.589, *Sanitary Districts (Accommodation for Infectious Diseases).*

New isolation hospitals took on a variety of forms. In rural areas, a cottage might serve the surrounding countryside. Elsewhere, old Poor Law buildings were converted. In larger cities, if an existing building could not be retrofitted, the urban periphery was scoured for suitable grounds. Besides cost, local authorities had to balance a variety of factors when making their choice of a site, including reasonable proximity to the city, accessibility via road, drainage, and the availability of space for recreational activities for both medical staff and patients. More often than not, arriving at the ideal location involved a certain amount of trial and error and could take decades. The experience in Nottingham is instructive. Its health committee began to explore options for an infectious disease hospital in response to the 1875 Public Health Act. The only other nonpauper accommodations for infectious patients was a sixteen-bed ward attached to the general hospital. The most convenient possibility was the rededication of a group of buildings known as the Garden Hospital (so named because they were sited in the gardens of Windsor Street workhouse). The Garden Hospital had been used to accommodate more than four hundred smallpox patients during the 1871–72 epidemic. On the advice of the MOH, Edward Seaton, the health committee had these buildings thoroughly cleaned to expurgate any lingering smallpox infection. Consisting of eight timber buildings on brick foundations and containing eighty beds, the doors opened in the autumn of 1875.[30]

A special subcommittee was set up to deal specifically with issues relating to the hospital. Patients were allowed to have their own medical attendants or dispensary staff, which obviated that particular point of friction. The most pressing questions the hospital administrators faced were financial ones. The health committee encountered persistent problems extracting payments from the Poor Law guardians for paupers sent to the hospital.[31] Sometimes private citizens were pursued for payments. The hospital had a scale of charges for nonpauper patients, which was waived in some circumstances. However, abuses were rooted out assiduously. In 1881, for example, a Charles Smith was chased when he neglected to pay for the time his two servants spent in the hospital.[32]

Within a few short years of the opening of the Garden Hospital, Seaton was complaining that the number of beds was insufficient. There were more than 300 scarlet fever cases during the outbreak of 1879. While the city hospitalized as many as it could (60 in all), Seaton estimated that domestic isolation was adequate for only 34 patients; for another 184 it was deemed grossly insufficient, with sick children lying about in houses or parts of shops.[33] The search for an alternative site began in 1883. The city found a site about two miles from the center and purchased 126 acres of land from the vicar of Basford in 1884 at a cost of £25,475 (at least £2 million today). The health committee then visited other isolation hospitals (including one as far afield as Newcastle) and began to draw up plans. Protracted negotiations between the committee, the borough engineer, and the LGB ensued, delaying construction until 1889.[34] The new Bagthorpe Hospital eventually opened on July 15, 1892.

Even when a modern, up-to-date hospital existed, the negative popular perception of isolation hospitals militated against the sequestration of cases.

Local authorities used hospitalization rates as a rough-and-ready means of assessing community acceptance of, and satisfaction with, its isolation hospital. In 1891 Sheffield's medical officer of health regarded the city's scarlet fever hospitalization rate of 29 percent as a dismal figure.[35] Although hospital accommodations in the city were "exceedingly well adapted to the requirements," and that "every day it is found less difficult to persuade" people to go in, the MOH puzzled at parents' lingering reluctance to utilize the city's hospital.[36] But Sheffield was not an outlier. One survey of ninety-three towns by the county MOH of the West Riding of Yorkshire, James Robert Kaye, showed that more than a quarter of his sample isolated fewer than 20 percent of the reported scarlet fever cases.[37] Another forty-two of the ninety-three towns isolated between 20 and 50 percent, while only 10 percent sequestered more than 80 percent of scarlet fever cases.[38] Birmingham consistently managed to quarantine between 80 and 90 percent of scarlet fever cases by the turn of the twentieth century, even during the 1902 epidemic when more than five thousand cases were notified (fig. 3.1). Once the Bagthorpe Hospital opened, Nottingham was not far behind this number, though it struggled to keep pace during the 1899 epidemic (fig. 3.2).

Regardless of the proportion of diseased patients hospitalized, the overwhelming impression is that isolation hospitals tended to serve the working classes and poorest members of the community. This is undoubtedly true, since legislation that sanctioned removal to hospital stipulated that it need only take place in instances where domestic isolation was not feasible—that is, in the majority of poor and working-class homes. When George Buchanan was dispatched by the LGB to make an investigation into the smallpox epidemic in Birmingham and Aston in 1874, he took the opportunity to estimate the level of need for isolation for the main infectious diseases. With 800 annual deaths from smallpox, scarlet fever, diphtheria, and enteric fever, and with an estimated attack rate of ten cases per death, Buchanan reckoned that there were about eight thousand potential patients in the city in any one year. Clearly this sort of back-of-the-envelope calculation could easily overemphasize the magnitude of the problem, given the temporal cycles of epidemics. But Buchanan's main point was that an as-yet unknowable proportion of these cases lived in the sort of circumstances that encouraged the increased transmission of disease.[39] Sheffield's MOH indicated precisely why isolation hospitals came to be portrayed as the "poor man's spare bedroom":

> It is quite impossible that proper isolation can be carried out in small houses where there are several members of a family, and where the room containing the patient is in close proximity to that used by others, or where the mother, no matter how careful in the use of disinfectants, has both to nurse the patient and superintend domestic arrangements. Efficient isolation consists in completely cutting off the sick room with all it contains, including the nurse, from the rest of the house and family, and, except in special cases, this is quite impossible in private houses.[40]

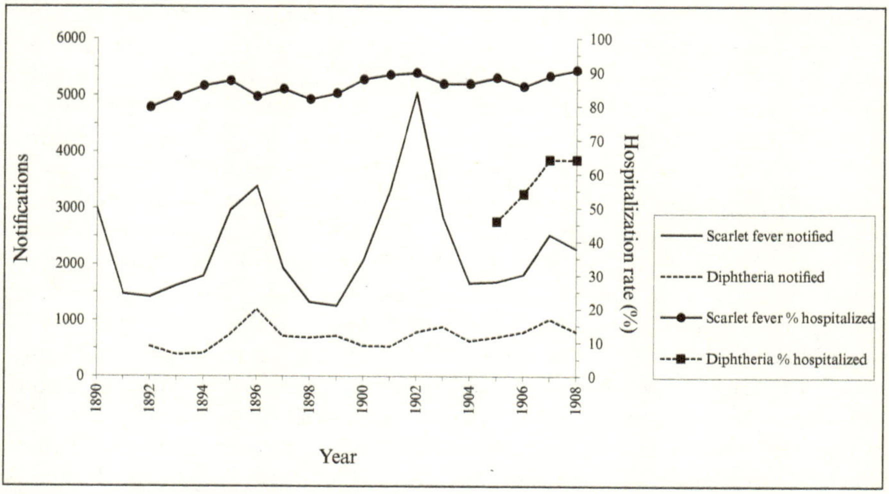


Figure 3.1. Scarlet fever and diphtheria notifications and hospitalization rates, Birmingham, 1890–1908. City of Birmingham, *Annual Health Reports.*

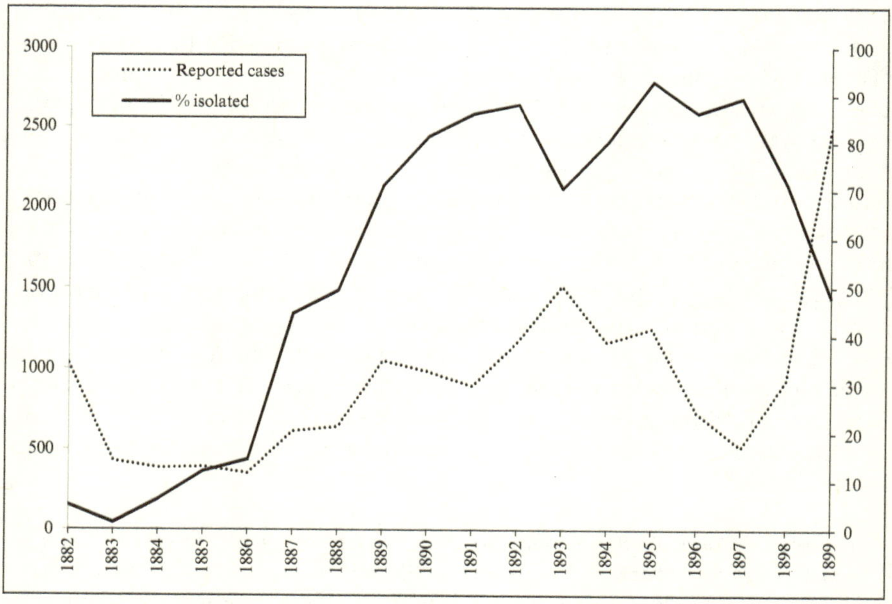


Figure 3.2. Scarlet fever notifications and hospitalization rates, Nottingham, 1882–99. Borough of Nottingham, *Annual Health Reports.*

One critic from the Vigilance Association made no bones about the barefaced class discrimination of this approach. "What sanitary officer," he asked, "would enter the mansion of my Lord Tom Noddy, and order the removal of the eldest daughter, or the youngest son? None. But the sanitary officer would go to the abodes of the humbler classes, and would there do what he dare not in the upper circles."[41] Even though some medical officers argued that middle-class families were also incapable of ensuring complete isolation, the general assumption held that hospital isolation was intended for poor people.

These class fissures were reflected and deepened in other ways. Some local authorities opened their hospitals with the intention of charging patients. It did not take them long to realize that this acted as a deterrent to their use. In Warrington and Huddersfield, removal to hospital was acknowledged to have been more fully complied with by the working classes once the charges for hospital admission had been dropped.[42] Pauperization was a more pressing issue in the capital. Until 1889 in London, where the Metropolitan Asylums Board (MAB) was a constituted authority of the Poor Law, those unable to secure domestic isolation and submitting to hospital admission were immediately pauperized (and thus disenfranchised).[43] In other places, many people considered that associating with paupers was something to avoid.[44] Some local authorities contracted with the local guardians to admit paupers with an infectious disease, especially where separate accommodations did not exist in the workhouse infirmary. In the late 1870s, around 40 percent of Salford and Manchester's isolation hospital patients were paupers.[45] Securing the isolation of patients unwilling to cohabit wards with paupers was a recurring issue in many places, while some authorities refused to admit paupers altogether.[46] A minority of hospitals reported that no troubles were encountered with the admission of outdoor paupers, particularly if their ragged or dirty clothing was replaced with a hospital-issue uniform.[47] Another solution was to provide private rooms that the more well-to-do parents might pay for, saving their children from having to commingle with the lower classes and paupers.[48] Wealthier patients might be induced into the hospital by being allowed, again at their own cost, to call in their GP.[49] The fear of pauperization on the one hand, or the prospect of a substantial payment to the hospital on the other, undoubtedly led to a certain amount of concealment of disease by poorer families.[50] Such apprehensions were conveniently misrepresented as working-class ignorance by all strands of the medical profession.

Ultimately, of course, these concerns could be dismissed as an inconvenience by a local authority; in the face of a recalcitrant patient, officials had recourse to legally enforced compulsion. Take this colorful example from Birmingham in 1875:

> The chairman [of the health committee] reported that a man named Henry Hawkley had escaped from the City Hospital while in the desquamation stage of scarlet fever. He had put the matter into the hands of the police. The man was found at Leicester by an assistant inspector of nuisances who had been despatched in search of him. He was taken to the Medical Officer of Health

> there, who allowed him to be brought to Birmingham after prescribing certain precautions to be observed for preventing the spread of infection. On arriving in Birmingham the man was at once taken to the hospital again.[51]

Casting Hawkley in the role of dangerous fugitive, the chairman's weaving together of crime and infection, and of medical and legal authority, makes for a compelling hide-and-seek escapade.[52] Overall, however, the sparing use of compulsory removal orders was cited as evidence that working-class citizens gradually were submitting to the increasingly clear benefits of isolation hospitals. In his substantial national inquiry into isolation hospital provision in the early 1880s, for example, Local Government Board medical inspector Richard Thorne Thorne stated that he came across no more than three dozen cases of removing patients to hospital by force.[53] Protests against compulsory hospital isolation never registered on the scale of agitation against compulsory infant smallpox vaccination.[54] But this does not mean that resistance was absent altogether. No less than 16,000 signatories to Nottingham's "Rights and Liberties Defence League" petition reacted vocally to the council's resolution to adopt the 1890 Infectious Disease (Prevention) Act:

> We the undersigned inhabitants and ratepayers of the town of Nottingham, pray that your honourable Council will take such steps as may be necessary to rescind the resolution recently passed by the Council, which converts our hospital into a prison and deprives us of our right to nurse our sick and claim our dead. We consider that the powers conferred upon certain officials under this resolution are greatly in excess of any that ought to be granted, that they are absolutely uncalled for, certain to be abused, and calculated to create a spirit of prejudice against an institution which has cost the ratepayers very dear.[55]

Under this act, medical opinion (either that of an MOH or of another registered practitioner) was authorized, if the authority saw fit, only to release the body of a deceased patient from the hospital if it was to be buried immediately. A magistrate could also order the detention of a patient in the hospital if he or she could not be discharged to homes applying "proper precautions" for the prevention of disease. These issues brought a great deal of raw emotion to the surface and reopened old sores for at least one parent. "As a ratepayer of Nottingham I am diametrically opposed to any further compulsory powers being granted to our town officials," wrote C. J. Welton, recounting his own child's death just ten hours after admission to the isolation hospital:

> What would the world be without sentiment? What can be better than kindness and happy endearing surroundings for a person who is suffering from some foul disease? Your cold, callous doctrine of isolation and separation from all friends, even if directed against all adults, is unbearable when applied to children, who are to be dragged away from their parents, perhaps never to see them alive again. . . . I would suffer imprisonment sooner than I would allow another child to be cruelly dragged from its parents to die in a hospital.[56]

Sometimes resistance was expressed more or less covertly, and not without the occasional connivance of the family physician. Leicester's sanitary inspector, Sergeant Francis Braley, reported on one couple who were in the habit of sending their sick children to their grandmother, and had initially refused to allow their child to be taken to hospital after the family practitioner had advised them that it would be treated equally well at home.[57] It was also in Leicester around this time that one letter-to-the-editor writer with the pseudonym "An Englishman" observed: "Who amongst us would think of running to the Sanitary Inspector and saying 'Please, sir, my child has the whooping cough; come and fetch it from its mother, and take it to the fever hospital; it will be quite safe under Dr Johnston [Leicester's medical officer of health], for they say he can cure all diseases.'"[58] It was believed by some that the concealment of disease to avoid hospital admission was as common among the wealthy as it was among the poorer classes.[59]

Returning to Nottingham, we might contrast Mr. Welton's experience with that of local surgeon Thomas Burnie:

> Without any compulsion, I was glad to avail myself of the opportunity of sending to the Bagthorpe Hospital one of my boys who, some three months ago, began with scarlet fever. He has recently come home in good health and excellent condition, and no other member of the family has taken the disease. During his stay in the hospital he was treated with the utmost care and kindness by everyone connected with the institution, and everything that could conduce to his recovery or well-being was provided for him without stint. . . . I am fully conscious of the grave objections there must always be to a parent parting with his or her child, especially when the child is seriously ill, but I am able, from my own experience, to assure my fellow townsmen that if they do send their children when ill to one of these institutions they will be tenderly and gently cared for, and will have provided for them everything necessary to their comfort and welfare.[60]

Because he was a practicing surgeon, we should perhaps treat Burnie's account with more skepticism than if he were, say, one of the city's lace makers. But anecdotal accounts such as these probably did have a positive impact on the regard in which isolation hospitals were held. Thorne believed that admission rates were aided by "the steady diffusion of the reports made by previous patients as to the comforts and excellence of nursing obtained with the several hospitals."[61] In advocating the extension of its isolation hospital, Birmingham's health committee used patient evidence to show the hospital was becoming increasingly popular. The committee told the city council in 1884 that the hospital had received letters from discharged patients, thanking them for their kindness and attention, arguing they had little difficulty inducing the relatives of the sufferers to send patients to the hospital.[62] In Nottingham, the health committee reported in 1891 that it had *never* needed to use its powers of compulsion to remove a patient. Mostly, it seems, medical officers and hospital administrators believed that word of mouth increased the popularity of isolation hospitals, and they were confident that any unwillingness would dissolve once parents realized that by sending their child to the hospital they would be free from keeping their child at home, enabling them to go to work or to keep their businesses running.[63]

Compulsion in the form of a magistrate's order was, however, substituted by a more subtle form of coercion that involved informing employers about the existence of infection in the homes of employees. In the first week of compulsory infectious disease notification in Leicester (September 12–19, 1879), eighty reports of infectious illness were received by the health department from local doctors. As was customary whenever the medical officer was informed of an infectious disease, a sanitary inspector was dispatched to investigate and remove the infected person to hospital if need be. The health committee was concerned to learn from the sanitary inspectors that some of those who had taken ill continued to go to work. The committee's response to this news was to issue the following statement: "In such cases where persons refuse to allow the patient to be taken to the Fever Hospital the Sanitary Inspectors be authorized to inform their employers of the existence of disease in the home." On the face of it, the health committee might have argued that its was a rational attempt to restrict disease transmission in the workplace. Yet, it is worth paying close attention to the wording of this edict, for it displays a blatant willingness to play on the economic fears of working-class people. The refusal to succumb to hospital removal triggers the potential disclosure.[64] It does not say that the employer will be informed should an adult employee decline hospital removal, though that is certainly one possibility; rather, it refers to "persons" who obstruct the hospitalization of the "patient." These "persons" could be parents and the "patient" their child. The crafting of the statement further allows for this possibility when it instructs that the employer be informed of the presence of infection "in the home"; as such, the infection need not belong to the adult employee him- or herself, but to another member of the employee's household altogether. So, it is well within the bounds of the health committee's resolution to imagine a sanitary inspector gently—or perhaps not so gently—reminding an obstructive mother of a four-year-old with scarlet fever that the father's boss might hear about the illness if she did not comply with a removal order.

Leicester was not a typical example in the sense that the imperative for removal and isolation was marked in an environment that was so vehemently against vaccination. The success of the city's policy for smallpox control relied heavily on prompt notification and sequestration of individuals in hospital, and it is easy to imagine that this approach could be transferred seamlessly to other infectious diseases. Yet, other cities doubtless practiced equally coercive methods. Readers of the *Nottingham Daily Express* heard of threats meted out to the "respectable" parents of a girl with scarlet fever that their small shop would have to be closed and the father prevented from going to work if they refused removal.[65]

Increasingly, then, the official creed was that popular opposition to isolation hospitals was on the wane and that parents were gradually acquiescing to the state's requirement that they act out their duty toward community well-being by giving up their children for removal. But with the legally enforceable weapon of compulsion lurking ominously in the background, underlined by the rather unsubtle hint at severe financial loss, working-class parents were faced with relatively little choice but to submit to the local state's interference with traditional modes and spaces of familial caregiving.

## Separation and Observation

Of the several barriers to the acceptance and utilization of isolation hospitals, the fear of cross-infection was perhaps the greatest. The best way to avoid patients infecting each other was to make sure their direct encounters were minimized. Where possible, this question was resolved architecturally. Patients with different diseases were kept apart through the adoption of pavilion-style wards, which eventually became the standard recommended design.

Pavilions operated in conjunction with other aspects of internal hospital design, such as robing rooms, in which medical and nursing staff changed outer garments before entering a different ward. Other planning and architectural devices included intricate yet easily operable window systems such as the Combination Collapsible Ventilator Company's "CC" window that literally streamlined the air coming into the wards so that it was forced upward and did not cause a through draft. The use of wooden floors was phased out because the joints between boards opened up and became a haven for dirt, dust, and other germ-retaining materials that could be unwittingly moved between wards (for more on dust and germs, see chapter 5). Jointless flooring systems such as British Doloment flooring were favored in British and German hospitals because the edge of the floor could be carried up the wall to form a dado rail. Solid doors were simply designed without detailing, again with the purpose of avoiding the accumulation of dust. Various openings were made in the external walls of wards in order to allow the safe removal of soiled linen in disinfecting trolleys. One leading architect of isolation hospitals advocated that the inspection windows between the nurses' duty room and the ward should be built without a sill, making it impossible for the staff to obscure the view with plants or other ephemera.[66]

These strategies worked most effectively when the patients had a clear-cut and confirmed diagnosis and were settled into a ward. But as the number of hospitals grew, GPs were pressured by local authorities to notify cases as soon as possible, and larger numbers of doubtful cases were inevitably sent to isolation hospitals, many of which found their way onto the main wards of the hospital.[67] Arthur Whitelegge, Nottingham's MOH in 1888, wrote about this pressure:

> Much of the value of notification depends upon promptness. A certain amount of delay is inevitable, even when there is no intention of concealment. Time is required for the recognition of the case, and slight cases are often unrecognised until many days have elapsed, or even until suspicion is

> aroused by the occurrence of other cases. When the diagnosis is made, some hours usually elapse before the notifications reaches [*sic*] the health department through the post.[68]

Whitelegge constructed tables that showed the speed with which Nottingham's health department received scarlet fever notifications and the speed with which cases were removed to hospital (table 3.2). The vast majority of cases—almost 80 percent—were notified within the first week of the rash's appearance. Almost 90 percent of those cases that were taken to hospital were institutionalized within a week of the clinical diagnosis. While in general terms this urgency was seen as a positive thing because it made the domestic environment safer, at the same time it heightened the risks of cross-infection in the hospital itself. Sometimes when the patient first arrived at the hospital it was too early to tell if the case really was scarlet fever, diphtheria, or enteric fever. Some patients suffering from scarlet fever or diphtheria developed another infectious disease the symptoms of which had not been obvious at the time of admission. The problem with such cases was that they could possibly transmit the infection to other patients in the ward, causing complications and, sometimes, death. Such instances were a managerial nightmare because all the patients on the ward had to be treated as contacts for the newly introduced disease. This stopped the admission of new cases to the ward until all patients had been declared free of that infection; nor could any of these patients be transferred. A ward of twenty beds could be locked down for weeks.[69]

The somewhat remarkable response to this aspect of cross-infection was to treat *every* case as doubtful and hold all cases under observation until the identity of the patients' infection(s) was confidently established (for the role of diphtheria bacteriology in this process, see chapter 4). Consequently, observation wards—frequently, and confusingly, called isolation wards—came to be seen as an architectural signal of the most modern isolation hospitals.[70] As early as 1890, the MAB hospitals in London were urged to provide observation wards for patients with an uncertain diagnosis, who could be immediately discharged if a bacteriological examination proved negative. Such provision was made in both New York and Paris hospitals as well.[71] The Bagthorpe Hospital in Nottingham, opened in 1891, used observation wards to monitor the progress of doubtful scarlet fever diagnoses. In 1899 twenty-three patients were sent home after being declared free from the disease—a conclusion that was reached after they had been detained in the observation wards for an average of sixteen days (discharged and deceased scarlet fever patients were hospitalized for an average of fifty-nine and ten days, respectively).[72] By the early twentieth century, Birmingham's MOH was advocating an observation period of up to twenty-eight days for doubtful scarlet fever cases.[73]

It soon became accepted good practice to include observation wards in the planning of new infectious disease hospitals, particularly ensuring that they were well isolated from the other wards in the hospital.[74] In 1902 the LGB's model plans for isolation hospitals included recommendations for isolation pavilions.[75]

Table 3.2. Scarlet fever notifications received and patients removed to hospital following the appearance of a rash, Nottingham, 1887–88 and 1889

| | 1887–88 | | | | 1889 | | | |
|---|---|---|---|---|---|---|---|---|
| | Notified | %[a] | Removed | %[a] | Notified | %[a] | Removed | %[a] |
| Same day | 79 | 6.5 | 64 | 10.7 | 124 | 11.4 | 114 | 15.3 |
| 1 day later | 202 | 16.6 | 111 | 18.5 | 223 | 21.6 | 152 | 21.7 |
| 2 days later | 223 | 18.3 | 120 | 20.0 | 223 | 21.2 | 138 | 18.5 |
| 3 days later | 172 | 14.1 | 79 | 13.2 | 147 | 14.0 | 122 | 16.3 |
| 4 days later | 132 | 10.8 | 67 | 11.2 | 75 | 7.1 | 54 | 7.2 |
| 5 days later | 81 | 6.7 | 47 | 7.8 | 45 | 4.2 | 31 | 4.1 |
| 6 days later | 48 | 3.9 | 18 | 3.0 | 31 | 2.9 | 18 | 2.4 |
| 7 days later | 30 | 2.5 | 19 | 3.2 | 19 | 1.8 | 23 | 3.0 |
| First week[b] | 967 | 79.5 | 525 | 87.5 | 891 | 85.2 | 652 | 88.8 |
| Second week | 118 | 9.7 | 46 | 7.7 | 78 | 7.4 | 43 | 5.7 |
| Third week | 53 | 4.4 | 15 | 2.5 | 39 | 3.7 | 22 | 2.9 |
| Fourth week | 32 | 2.6 | 11 | 1.8 | 28 | 2.6 | 11 | 1.4 |
| Later | 21 | 1.7 | 3 | 0.5 | 11 | 1.0 | 7 | 0.9 |
| Interval unknown | 26 | 2.1 | 0 | 0.0 | 0 | 0.0 | 0 | 0.0 |
| Total | 1,217 | | 600 | | 1,047 | | 735 | |

*Sources:* Nottinghamshire Archives, CA/HE/2/1/1, Borough of Nottingham, B. Arthur Whitelegge, *Annual Report of the Medical Officer of Health for 1888*, 38–40; Nottinghamshire Archives, Open Shelves, Borough of Nottingham, Philip Boobbyer, *Annual Health Report for 1889*, 30.

[a] Percentages might not equal 100 due to rounding.

[b] The totals provided for the "First week" in fact relate to notifications on the "Same day" plus those occurring up to "7 days later."

For the most part, these pavilions contained between two and five beds. Two observation pavilion designs were included in Liverpool's new isolation hospital that opened at Fazakerley in 1906. One had two wards with four beds each (see fig. 3.3, Type "A,"), while the other had two distinct sections, each with two wards for two beds (see fig. 3.4, Type "B,").[76] More demanding versions incorporated cubicle wards to separate patients individually. In 1890 the Plymouth town council sought permission from the LGB to build a hospital with compartments subdivided by glass panels (permission was refused).[77] During the mid- and late 1900s, some wards in the MAB hospitals were adapted as cubicles, and new cubicle wards were constructed in hospitals run by councils in Croydon, East Ham, Enfield, Norwich, and Walthamstow.[78] While cubicles were primarily used to monitor uncertain cases of infectious disease, particularly scarlet fever, they were also used if the diagnosis was confirmed but still required isolation, if the patient had been exposed to another disease prior to admission and was

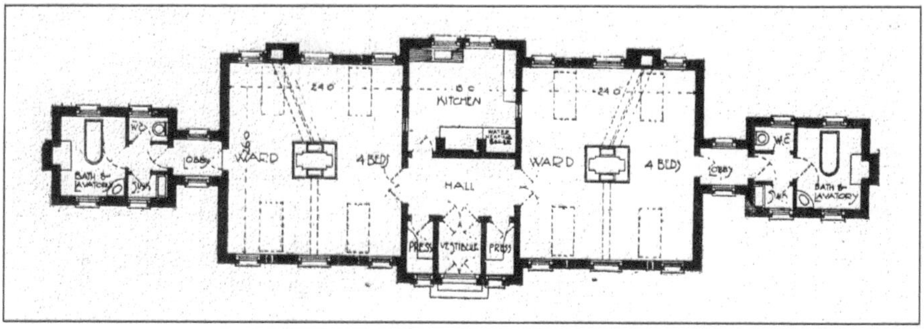


Figure 3.3. Type "A" isolation block, Fazakerley Hospital, Liverpool. Freeman, *The Planning of Fever Hospitals*, 78.

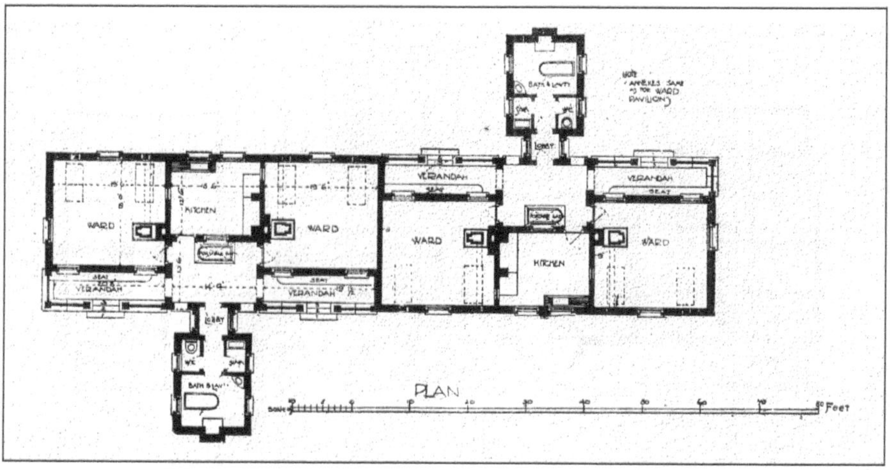


Figure 3.4. Type "B" isolation block, Fazakerley Hospital, Liverpool. Freeman, *The Planning of Fever Hospitals*, 79.

therefore possibly incubating a second disease, if the patient was suffering from more than one infectious disease, or if the disease was not infectious.

Developments in Britain were influenced by the opening of cubicle pavilions in Paris at the hospital of the Pasteur Institute and the Sick Children's Hospital.[79] Theodore Thomson, medical inspector at the LGB, took a tour of the cubicle wards of these two hospitals in 1903, where the cubicles were termed "boxes" and *all* diseases were admitted to the cubicle wards indiscriminately.[80] The cubicle system in Britain developed three slightly different forms: one in which the cubicles were completely separated from each other and entered from an external verandah; a second in which compartments were separated by a glass partition from floor to ceiling but could be accessed via a common corridor; and a third in which the cubicles could also be entered from a common corridor, but the dividing wall did not reach to the ceiling.[81] The MAB in London adopted the third system, and by 1907 the Northeastern MAB hospital had thirty-four cubicle beds and the Southwestern MAB hospital had thirty-two.[82] Each cubicle contained a single bed and was separated from adjoining cubicles by a dividing wall. It is noticeable, and significant, that the dividing wall did not extend to the ceiling. The glass window between the rooms gave "the nurses a better control and the patients a means of making the isolation less irksome."[83] Strict, and admittedly "laborious," procedures were followed by the medical and nursing staff—some of whom were chosen especially for the duties of cubicle attendance.[84]

Sinks in each cubicle provided for the washing of hands after touching the patient or the bedding. A separate overall was provided for wearing inside each cubicle (though in other hospitals the overall hung outside the door).[85] Every instrument, syringe, spatula, and medicine glass was sterilized following each use, as were cutlery and crockery. Brushes, combs, flannels, soap, toys, and books were reserved for individual patients. In the first months of the cubicle ward opening in Walthamstow—where the glass partitions rose to the ceiling—both definite and doubtful cases were housed in the cubicles. Staff were alerted to the difference by a white disc hanging outside the cubicle of a definite case, while a red disc and an overall hung outside the cubicle of a doubtful case.[86]

In his report to the LGB in 1912–13 on isolation hospitals, Parsons noted that the form of the cubicle tended to depend on the dominant beliefs about the mode of disease transmission. The system in use at the MAB, where the wall only went part of the way to the ceiling, was thought to be of limited use in cases where the disease turned out to be smallpox, chicken pox, or measles in its infective stages. These diseases, it was believed, could carry more than a few feet in the air. For other diseases, especially scarlet fever, the limited partitions were considered to be adequate in preventing infection, but only if aseptic practices were adhered to faithfully. Medical superintendents at these hospitals believed that the cubicles and protocols ("loyally carried out," according to Medical Inspector Thomson; and "as careful as human beings can be made to be," in Dr. Foord Caiger's opinion) were highly effective in reducing the risks posed by doubtful cases.[87] Medical superintendents in isolation hospitals that successfully practiced bed isolation (also known as barrier nursing) were less sanguine, suggesting that the partition wall merely offered a false sense of security: "the attention of the nurses becomes fixed on the partition as the safeguard," presumably causing them to neglect other safeguards such as hand washing and sterilization.[88]

## Managing Permeability

The strenuous efforts to implement observation of doubtful cases were an implicit acknowledgment that isolation hospitals were complex and dangerous biological spaces. Individuals were being removed from one risk-laden environment (the home) to another. Another form of regulation was visiting rules, which were part and parcel of creating a highly ordered community that encompassed outsiders as well as patients and staff. Hospital authorities frowned on violations of visiting rules that represented a potential threat to the moral and hygienic order of the hospital environment.[89] Visitors might unwittingly contract a disease in hospital and contaminate either other areas of the hospital or, even worse, the outside world by taking it with them into the local community. Isolation hospitals were spaces laden with infectious risk. Visitors were dangerous not because, like patients, they had contracted a disease with visible signs; nor even because they harbored a disease asymptomatically. Rather, visitors constituted a danger because they carried no imprint of disease and were susceptible to the biological risks present in the isolation environment. Consequently, visitors were expected to submit to rules and regulations that acted as strategies to underline the exclusionary nature of infectious disease isolation both to them and to the patient.

In his report, Thorne could point to no examples where ward visiting by family and friends was freely allowed in isolation hospitals. Visiting took place in most isolation hospitals under tightly controlled conditions. Nowhere, at least in the official rhetoric, was it possible for a parent to turn up, walk onto a smallpox, scarlet fever, or diphtheria ward, and take a seat next to their sick son or daughter. If daily, weekly, or even monthly ward visiting times were ever posted, they never made their way into Thorne's report. In fact, Thorne only came across two provincial locations (Alcester and Bradford) where the visiting rules were committed to paper; the MAB also published visiting regulations. Perhaps this in itself reflects a reluctance to entertain the idea of visitors: there was no need to produce a set of rules for a constituency that was not supposed to exist in the first place.[90]

Typically, mothers were portrayed as problematic. I have already alluded to the ways in which mothers became the hospital authorities' focus of outreach activities. This recognition of the need for tactful handling of parental feelings extended to allowing mothers to accompany children in the ambulance and make sure that they were settled in bed. Thorne's review of his evidence indicated that it was "general policy" to admit a mother along with her child "if isolation could not be secured domestically."[91] Except in cases where the mother was breastfeeding, her length of stay ranged between a few hours and three days. However, the picture is more complicated than Thorne's summary of his own survey would have us believe. To begin with, at least one hospital (Aberdare) forbade mothers from accompanying their children. According to Medical Superintendent William Gayton, the MAB's Homerton Smallpox Hospital adopted this policy in 1881, much to his apparent regret.[92] In Aberdare's case, Thorne was prepared to admit that this practice probably caused resentment among the local population and contributed to the perceived failure of the hospital. At the other extreme, parents in Sunderland were admitted with their children when their objections were sustained and where their occupation was "of such a nature as to facilitate the spread of infection from their homes or shops."[93]

Alternative techniques were adopted in places where parent-child separation on removal was considered draconian. When a financial charge was levied on accompanying parents, they were reclassified as hospital inmates, not visitors. In Blackpool, resident mothers were billed at the same daily rate, 3s. 6d., as paying patients.[94] In Carlisle, it was the custom to admit a parent, relative, or nurse along with the patient and a weekly payment of 10s. 6d.[95] These costs were clearly prohibitive for the average working family, particularly when lengths of confinement for scarlet fever were between six and nine weeks.[96] Not surprisingly in Carlisle, where the 10s. 6d. payment also procured a private room, only the better-off could afford these fees, so the "arrangement is thus not applicable to the lower classes": no money, no mother.[97] In addition to these financial disincentives, hospital officials were confident that the rituals of isolation were ample enough to discourage parents from wanting to stay in hospital for any prolonged length of time. In Oldham, parents were permitted to go in with their children, but "the restrictions to which such parents are necessarily subjected when in the hospital soon induce them to leave their children, and there are but few who have not within a few days returned to their own homes." Being required to take a bath and have their clothes disinfected may have proved deterrent enough for many parents.[98]

While the presence on the ward of parents and close relatives was not necessarily an unusual occurrence, it was a portentous one. In nearly all the instances where visiting rules and practices are known, visitors were only permitted when a patient was deemed to be so "dangerously ill" as to be close to death.[99] For Mancunian patients, the chance even of this final comfort was slight, since "visitors have only in one or two very special cases been admitted even when fatal results were anticipated."[100] According to the oral testimony of one fever nurse who worked at the London Fever Hospital as late as the 1930s, there was no visiting at all except for patients in the private wards.[101] In Alcester, dangerously ill patients were allowed to see only one of their nearest relatives or intimate friends for no more than fifteen minutes, although in very urgent cases two visitors were allowed and the time was extended.[102] One four-and-a-half-year-old patient at a Kent isolation hospital during World War I later recalled that when one girl died "the gardener had to walk to her house to inform her parents."[103] The terms of hospital rules were open to interpretation, and ultimate authority lay at the top of the hospital hierarchy. The medically qualified staff deemed when a patient was dangerously ill or not. Evidence also suggests that it was not lodge-keepers or junior nurses who decided whether visitors met the bloodline or intimacy criteria. At the Queen's Memorial Infectious Diseases Hospital, in Australia, this gatekeeping power extended to the matron.[104] In Edinburgh no visitor entered the City Hospital's wards without a pass issued by the medical superintendent himself, and this was also the case at the MAB's smallpox hospital in Fulham. Also at Fulham, the name of each visitor was recorded, presumably to prevent multiple visits by the same person on the same day.[105]

Once admitted, the behavior of visitors was highly circumscribed. In almost all the hospitals where details of visiting are known, relatives and friends were required to wear some form of special clothing, typically described as a "wrapper," an "overall," a raincoat, or some other "impervious covering."[106] Such rituals existed well into the twentieth century.[107] Visitors *were* allowed to sit at the bedside, but at "some little distance from the patient" in order "to avoid touching the patient, or exposing themselves to the breath or to the emanations from the skin."[108] Contact with bedding was also forbidden.

Unless every visitor was closely monitored by the staff, it defies belief how these strictures on nonbodily contact could be enforced, especially when hospital wards teemed with patients during an epidemic outbreak. One witness to the Royal Commission on Small-Pox and Fever Hospitals cited a flagrant breach of the rules at the MAB's Deptford Hospital, where a wife in borrowed items of clothing spent the afternoon with her infected husband's head on her breast.[109] In the absence of infection-proofing garments, visitors had to remove their clothing for fumigation once the visit was over, and regardless of attire all visitors were requested to wash hands, face, and head with a disinfecting agent, usually carbolic soap.[110] In Huddersfield, this cleansing stage extended to a full bath.[111] The epidemiological rationale behind these procedures was obvious. The most pressing need was to minimize the possibility of visitors acquiring infection.[112] (Alexander Collie, medical superintendent at the MAB's Homerton Hospital, made the otherwise unacknowledged point that it would be highly unlikely that the most common visitors, mothers and wives, would not already have been exposed to the disease in the domestic environment.) This explains the wrappers and the prohibition of contact with the patient. Nonetheless, the possibility of infection remained, and the cleansing of garments and bodies provided an additional barrier to the escape of infection from the hospital. These regulations were also employed as a management tool to deter visiting in the first place. In Huddersfield, the tiresome rituals associated with visiting had served practically to do away with relatives' and friends' demands to enter the wards.[113] The disinfection of clothing and the washing procedures had "the unquestionable advantage of indicating to the public the views which are entertained by the hospital authorities as to the danger likely to result from needless visits."[114]

The pointed use of "needless" here betrays the dismissive official attitude toward visitors; the ordeal of entering the ward only took place, it should be remembered, when the patient was perilously close to death. It is also striking that in the few instances where visiting regulations were formalized, various attempts were made to condition the behavior of the visitors well beyond the boundary of the hospital, both before and after their encounter with isolation. Entry as a patient visitor into the MAB smallpox hospitals required physical evidence of successful vaccination.[115] With the warning that "they run a great risk when entering the hospital" still ringing in their ears, visitors to both metropolitan and provincial isolation facilities were advised not to enter the wards if they were "in a weak state of health, or in an exhausted condition." This stipulation certainly can be understood in relation to a visitor's potential susceptibility to infection when in a compromised physical state, but for reasons that I am unable to fathom, eating food before entering the hospital was also frowned on.[116] A further exhortation not to use a train or any other form of public transport "immediately after leaving the hospital" is, at first glance, wise advice. However, given the state of knowledge regarding incubation periods of infectious disease, allied to the relative inaccessibility of many isolation hospitals by any means other than public transport, the dispensation of such advice was practically pointless. Once again, the laying down of these rules served more than just an epidemiological purpose. Since the hospital was doing all in its power to reduce the possibility of infection being exported, and since families were openly warned of the risks of entering such a contaminated environment, responsibility for an epidemic outbreak subsequent to a visit could be legitimately directed at the visitors themselves.

As such, a variety of alternative management strategies evolved that allowed relatives and friends to *see* patients but further underlined the exclusionary nature of isolation. One concession was the operation of what can be termed "window appointments."[117] Relatives and friends were allowed to view the patient through the ward windows for brief periods, at set times, on specified days of the week. Alcester Hospital set aside one hour for this activity on Tuesday and Friday afternoons. One hour once a week was the norm at Broadstairs.[118] It is not clear whether the windows were open or closed during such visits; in Broadstairs, a window appointment was thought to have caused scarlet fever to spread in the district on one occasion, so it might be guessed that the windows were open on that occasion at least. In Aberdeen, however, the stated practice was to keep the windows shut.[119] This system of window appointments endured until after World War II. Quoted in Margaret Currie's book on fever nursing, this is Jean Bell's list of the worst aspects of her job at West Lane Fever Hospital, Middlesbrough, in the late 1950s: "Deaths in young and small children; looking after septic abortions, and VD. Seeing a dead foetus. Doing loads of sluicing and emptying mugs from TB patients. Seeing children upset when relations could just look through the window at them when visiting."[120] During the war itself, visitors could see very little inside one hospital as the windows were protected by sandbags.[121]

Many authorities successfully kept potential visitors at arm's length simply by providing daily updates on the welfare of each patient. In Nottingham, Leicester, and London, parents and relatives were told that information could be had at the hospital lodge. At Fulham's smallpox hospital, a daily list of dangerously ill patients was kept by the gate porter, and appearance on the list qualified patients for visitors.[122] For most working-class parents and relatives in places where isolation hospitals were located on the outskirts of the communities they served, such information was quite literally beyond their reach.[123] As James Gray has described, a system of daily newspaper bulletins was developed in Edinburgh. This involved ascribing to each patient a number on admission. The number was known to the family of the patient but otherwise preserved anonymity. Each patient's number was then classified into one of four categories, according to his or her condition, as follows:

1. Dangerously ill, friends requested to come out
2. Seriously ill, no immediate danger
3. Ill, making satisfactory progress
4. Not quite so well, no cause for anxiety

The list then was published in the local daily newspapers. As well as providing an indication of the well-being of all patients, the list acted as a signal to relatives of dangerously ill patients to come and visit.[124]

Accessibility to patient information was a long-recognized problem. Sheffield's health committee lamented the lack of communication at its hospital and would have envied the situation in Manchester, where ward visiting to the Monsall Hospital was practically unheard of.[125] The Mancunian isolation hospital's telephone connection with the more centrally located Royal Infirmary acted as a line of communication to the outside world and saved some inquirers a journey of several miles. Thorne witnessed this system in operation and was highly impressed:

> Whilst at the hospital I could not fail to note that the answers sent to inquirers, instead of being merely formal or limited to monosyllables, afforded some detailed information as to the progress of the patients in question, and to this is probably due the fact that the arrangement has to a very great extent done away with the difficulties which might otherwise have attended the rule which prohibits visiting.[126]

Thorne's official rubber stamp of approval can be read alongside John Burdon Sanderson's recommendation to the Royal Commission that telephones should link each ward to the outside world to render visiting superfluous.[127] All these channels of information provision were designed to prevent visiting and conferred privilege on those in possession of the means of transport and communication.

Did it work? Did sequestration reduce the number of cases, case fatality rates, and death rates? For historians, the answer is that we will never really know. The irony is that, despite the flourishing of isolation hospitals from the 1870s onward, contemporaries could not work out the answer either. Apart from the vexed question of return cases of scarlet fever, there were relatively few attempts to properly assess the effectiveness of hospitalization in reducing the incidence, mortality, and case fatality rates of infectious disease.[128] The most voracious and tenacious critic of the notification-isolation system was Daniel Biddle. A practicing doctor in Kingston-upon-Thames, Biddle initially was against the dual system of notification that effectively put the onus of reporting disease on the family physician, even though in theory the householder was also responsible.[129] Between 1888 and 1894, Biddle wrote about ten times each to the *British Medical Journal*, the *Lancet*, and the *Times* in an attempt to highlight the fact that notification had not resulted in a reduction in mortality from the diseases that were reportable in most towns and cities.[130] Biddle was a credible critic. He was elected to the Royal Statistical Society in 1891—sponsored by Noel Humphries, an important background figure in the General Register Office[131]—but there is no evidence to suggest that he was regarded as anything but a minor irritation to the proponents of notification and sequestration. After one protracted exchange, the *BMJ* simply refused to continue printing his letters.[132] Newsholme called the statistical efforts to discredit notification and isolation "puerile."[133]

Such exercises to prove the value of notification using statistics were futile, because until 1899 at least there was far too much variation in the coverage and methods of notification and the availability of hospital accommodations to make the comparison between different places meaningful.[134]

Killick Millard was probably the most influential critic. He was medical superintendent of Birmingham's isolation hospital and went on to become the nationally known MOH for Leicester. His detailed analysis of Birmingham's hospital data concluded that the isolation of scarlet fever had not substantially reduced the attack rate or case mortality of the disease.[135] Other local MOHs conducted their own analyses and came to conclusions that helped satisfy their political masters. When Nottingham's MOH and hospital superintendent pleaded for more investment for the Bagthorpe Hospital at the beginning of the twentieth century, the town council demanded to know what difference the hospital made to mortality rates. MOH Philip Boobbyer's response was to make a retrospective calculation for the percentage of deaths to cases for hospital and home patients. The disease was just beginning to undergo a secular decline, with the difference between hospital and home mortality of cases starting to narrow, but the rates did show that a hospital patient had a much better chance of recovery than a home-based one (fig. 3.5).

This sort of data interpretation was crucial for the continuance of isolation practices for scarlet fever. Millard's counterevidence was taken seriously, but the isolation of scarlet fever continued unabated, pointing us toward some of the less obvious motivations for sequestration. The removal of biologically dangerous individuals from their community surroundings and into confinement was as a strategy of government power. In common with penal incarceration and confinement of the mentally ill, isolation of the infected demonstrates a central contradiction of liberal governance that has been studied under the rubric of "freedom":[136] freedom was a means to govern because practices such as isolation created, in the words of Nikolas Rose, "the conditions in which subjects themselves would enact the responsibilities that composed their liberties."[137]

Taking their cue from critical studies of governance, historians Carolyn Strange and Alison Bashford have noted that "isolation was not an aberration from liberal governance but central to its internal logic."[138] Put simply, ensuring the liberty of the many necessarily meant restricting the freedom of the few. They go on to observe that "the 'dangerous' became those who did not deserve, or those who could not be trusted with, the freedoms that responsible and healthy citizens enjoyed. In both liberal and totalitarian regimes, experts and government bureaucrats stretched the definition of 'dangerousness' to capture individuals who had not yet committed offences."[139] Noting the amount of human traffic coming out of and going into these institutions, Logie Barrow has lamented "how prematurely historians label these institutions as 'isolation' hospitals."[140] Certainly we need to be conscious of not taking at face value the reports of medical officers and interested officials who pointed to rising rates of hospitalization as a measure of the isolation hospital's acceptance. Some of the concerns expressed by inhabitants of towns where it was felt the local public

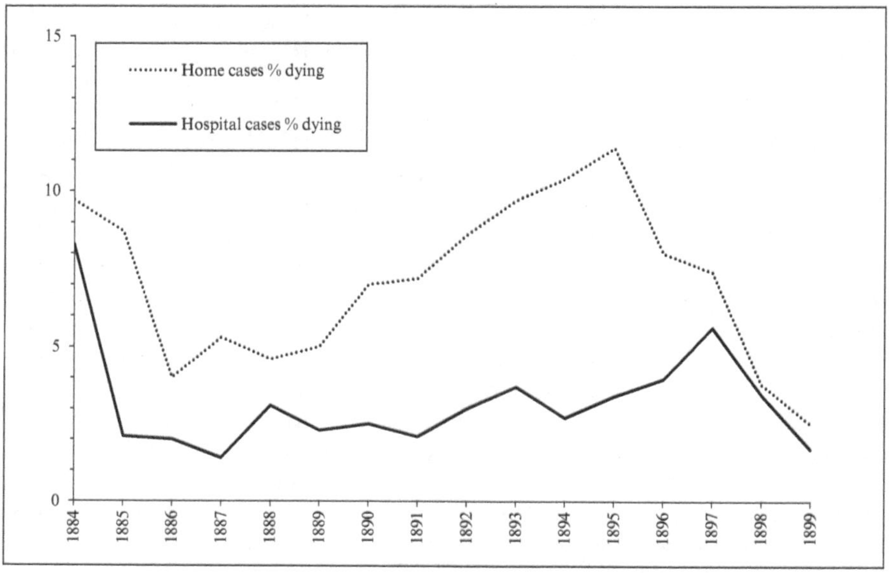


Figure 3.5. Scarlet fever hospital and home deaths, Nottingham, 1882–99. Borough of Nottingham, *Annual Health Reports.*

health authorities were adopting coercive methods of removal are indicative of some unrest, if not outright protest.

The general public was prepared to voice resistance to stringent public health measures—in this case hospitalization—even if the legal threat of coercion usually proved to be persuasive enough for most parents to allow the state to hospitalize their children. The restriction of visiting to all but the most dangerously ill served to underline to the public the dangers of infection and the authorities' desire that these hospitals be put out of reach of all but the most desperately worried parents.

For the most part, hospital authorities tried to keep parents at arm's length. Once inside the hospital, authorities impressed on parents, other relatives, and close friends their responsibility toward the rest of the community not to engage in behaviors that might facilitate the spread of disease. Restrictions were not simply directed to how parents should act inside the hospital, but also what they may or may not do before and after crossing the hospital boundary. As such, the disciplining of visits need not be interpreted as a "means of producing terrorised slaves without privacy." It is worth remembering that some public health authorities recognized the injuries caused to autonomy, responsibility, and independence by removing people to hospital. The regulation and education of visitors was a way to counteract these damaging impacts and presented public health authorities with an opportunity to mold "self-managing citizens capable of conducting themselves in freedom . . . according to norms of civility."[141] The regulation of visiting was about encouraging responsible behavior in the healthy in order to secure for everybody in the community the freedoms that good health bestowed.

Chapter Four

# "Combustible Material"

## Classrooms, Contact Tracing, and Following-Up

It has long been argued that the introduction of elementary schooling in 1870 shaped the identity of the English working classes by reinforcing their station in the social hierarchy.[1] Strict discipline, obedience, and the maintenance of order were the foundations of moral reformation and spiritual salvation that drove the mid-nineteenth-century creed of social obligation.[2] The curriculum in elementary schools came to be heavily influenced by ideas about national identity and imperialism, particularly against the background of national decline in the 1890s and 1900s.[3] The economic threat posed by Germany and the worrisome physical condition of Anglo-Boer War recruits prompted a reshaping of the Board of Education and the elementary school system in the early twentieth century under the rubric of "national efficiency."[4]

Family and domestic space were accorded privileged status in elementary school reading books in the early twentieth century. According to historian Stephen Heathorn, the campaign of "national efficiency" urgently promulgated a sense of Englishness. The English idea of home, Heathorn says, "implied both a sense of natural order and a genealogical and historical rootedness."[5] A stable and structured ordering of home and familial relations was scaled up to represent the nation as an extended family and a web of obligations. Domestic femininity, Heathorn argues, was posited as the natural foil to civic masculinity: "The professional middle-class construction and projection of an idealized femininity and its association with 'traditional' domesticity and motherhood should be considered as a correlative to the fabrication of the active, worldly, and virile imperial-nationalist masculinity evident in the understanding of 'good citizenship'."[6] Competent and effective child rearing became a national duty, not just a moral one.

As we have seen, earlier in the nineteenth century the middle-class ideal of domesticity was a foundation for social morality, electoral reform, political participation, and public health intervention. The dominant model of the nuclear family was based on the notion that the moral and spiritual values of women held sway, though financial security and decision making ultimately lay in the hands of the male head of household.[7] By the end of the century, however, the complexion of this domestic symbiosis was changing. The male "flight from domesticity" was accompanied by female challenges to patriarchal power. The woman's role as wife and mother alone came to define the domestic sphere, whereas the man became predominantly a public creature.[8] This shift was strongly influenced by medical discourses that reconstructed the identities of women based on reproductive functions and biological cycles.[9]

A particular set of gendered assumptions were reflected in classroom materials, where girls were taught to be homemakers, wives, and mothers while boys were encouraged to lead a productive public life in support and defense of family and home.[10] Though implementation and adherence was patchy across the country, the elementary school curriculum was segregated from the beginning, and the separation of girls and boys only intensified over time.[11] Girls were obliged to take needlework (beginning in 1870) and theoretical domestic economy (1878), while cookery (1882), laundry (1889), and general housewifery (by 1900) were optional grant-earning subjects.[12] Domestic economy became more important early in the twentieth century because the home was perceived to be the cradle of the empire. In 1903 Alice Ravenhill, an experienced and influential proponent of the household science movement and an inspector of hygiene and domestic economy for West Riding of Yorkshire County Council, wrote that

> the home constitutes the centre of interest in any study of present social and economic progress, for it is no exaggeration to say that on the happy, healthy maintenance of family life hinges the political, commercial, and industrial welfare of the Empire. . . . Good homes are the basis of the highest and most fruitful civilization; to secure them for the British Empire depends on her women, her schools, and her educational zeal.[13]

The reification of "home" and a woman's place in it was central to the education of the working classes. But not all of this education in domestic economy was "useful"; nor did it always bear any relation to children's sense of national identity, as Heathorn readily concedes. In other words, books themselves did not, and could not, convey all that schoolchildren needed to know about the significance of home to the national enterprise.

According to some influential activists and child-welfare professionals, there was an experiential way of knowing about home that was accessible through hygiene and a deeper understanding of the self. In 1903 the London School Board medical officer, James Kerr, outlined how learning-through-doing had the potential to transform a child's psyche and conduct. In a section of his report, tellingly titled "Right Living as a School Subject," Kerr claimed that

> the rules of healthy living which each should know for the good of all, requires also to be taught by example as well as precept. . . . As the young children learn not only from the spoken word, but much more from the thing seen and done, and automatically stored away in their subconscious memory as a part of the warp which gives bias to their character and action for ever, it is essential that the whole conduct of the school should be influenced by healthy ideals.[14]

Yes, the basic rules of health *could* be taught from books, and Kerr supported the progressive and graduated classroom teaching of hygiene throughout a pupil's elementary school career. But for Kerr, this sort of formal instruction was subordinate to the broader needs of child development and physiology.

Kerr's previous position (1893–1902) had been as school medical inspector in Bradford, where he initiated an innovative program of pupil examinations. One member of the Bradford School Board at that time was Margaret McMillan, the influential socialist educational theorist who later sat on the national executive of the Independent Labour Party. According to McMillan's biographer, Carolyn Steedman, Kerr's ideas about the determinants of children's ill-health and the neurological basis of a child's unconscious development had an "important effect on her development of an educational theory," a theory that later shaped the Labour Party's policy on childhood.[15] McMillan's thinking was very much derived from the educational and physiological theories of Édouard Seguin and European writers on psychology that comprehended the mind and intelligence through their relation to the material body; for McMillan and Kerr, this individuality was very much nested in the social relations of domestic space.[16] Alice Ravenhill, whose time at the West Riding County Council overlapped Kerr's and McMillan's in Bradford by a couple of years, similarly pointed out that bookish instruction alone was wasted on the very young:

> An important part of the process [of a liberal education] is to acquaint children with some conditions of their environment, present and to come, and to give them sound principles for their guidance in the right conduct of life, which, when apprehended, conduce to render compliance with restrictions more willing and self-control more consistent. . . . Acquaintance with its [hygiene's] elementary principles should be made along lines which would from the first actively influence conduct, and subsequently stimulate to individual observation of the moral, intellectual, and physical results associated with wholesome or unwholesome habits and homes.[17]

To achieve this state of "right conduct," "compliance with restrictions," and "self-control," Ravenhill claimed that young pupils (up to the age of seven years at least) should be asked to make observations on the activities and needs of their bodies and how their senses worked. They should seek to comprehend when and why meals were eaten; when, how, and why humans sleep; what dirt was and how it was made; about the home and how its constituent parts were used; and how the home and the people in it were kept clean. In sum, young children should develop "the conception of health as a treasure to be carefully guarded and spent" through activities that went on predominantly in the home.[18] It is probably too much of a stretch to say that the writing and works of Ravenhill, McMillan, and Kerr together represented a "Bradford School" of thinking that determined the shape of public health intervention in domestic life through the classroom; but, as we shall see, in the realm of infectious disease at least, Kerr's philosophy thoroughly permeated central government policies.

This chapter seeks to demonstrate how public health reached into the home via the school. At one level, epidemiological tools were used to analyze the role played by elementary schools in the propagation of infectious diseases, aligning them with poor ventilation, inadequate buildings and defective plumbing.[19] It was almost inevitable that the attention of public health authorities would be drawn to the congregation of young children in confined, overcrowded, and underventilated spaces. In 1851 the General Board of Health had attempted to give MOHs the power to enter a school whenever a pupil was found to be suffering from smallpox or another infection. Edwin Chadwick wanted MOHs to inspect the school itself and the pupils for any signs of illness.[20] However, the tracing of individual pupils was relatively neglected, and the midcentury focus was more on the sanitary condition of the buildings and the surrounding environment as a breeding ground for disease.[21]

When the foundations of free and compulsory elementary schooling were laid in a decade punctuated by the Education Acts of 1870, 1876, and 1880, there was precious little, if any, agreement on how schools acted as a factor in disease transmission, though it was generally believed that they *did* pose a risk. Social class played a role in these debates. It was common for MOHs to argue that diseases were more likely to be spread through public elementary schools attended by working-class children, since the parents of middle- and upper-class pupils were aware of the dangers of sending an infectious child to school.[22] The Local Government Board codified this bias in its policy on school closure and pupil exclusion, which in the early 1890s stated that it was "rarely possible to provide effectual separation of the sick from the healthy within the homes of children of the class attending public elementary schools."[23]

Opinions about the most appropriate means of action when a case of infection came to light were diffuse: should individual pupils be excluded; should particular classes be suspended; or should the whole school be shut down?[24] The LGB's approach toward the end of the century tended to favor class or school closure, a policy that was based on precious little evidence but was a common practice in Europe and North America.[25] In the early twentieth century, epidemiological methods were used to arrive at a more "scientific" solution that excluded individual pupils according to their immunological status rather than suspend classes or shut down schools altogether. National policy in this area was heavily influenced by research on cases of diphtheria, scarlet fever, and measles in children attending schools of the London School Board and its successor, the Education Authority of the London County Council (table 4.1). Expert knowledge—still imperfect at this stage—about incubation periods, immunity, and bacteriological causation was integrated into the routine of school management.[26] This integration was by no means seamless. Interventions such as school or class closure and the exclusion of individual pupils were explored, tested, and argued about on a disease-by-disease basis, not least because such interventions had funding implications for individual schools.[27]

Table 4.1. Notified cases of scarlet fever, diphtheria, and measles in London, 1906–14

| | All ages | Elementary schoolchildren | % |
|---|---|---|---|
| Scarlet fever | | | |
| 1906 | 20,333 | 8,371 | 41 |
| 1907 | 25,923 | 12,307 | 47 |
| 1908 | 21,648 | 10,291 | 48 |
| 1909 | 17,389 | 7,716 | 44 |
| 1910 | 10,513 | 4,700 | 45 |
| 1911 | 10,484 | 4,640 | 44 |
| 1912 | 11,316 | 5,060 | 45 |
| 1913 | 17,552 | 7,969 | 45 |
| 1914 | 25,048 | 11,337 | 45 |
| Diphtheria | | | |
| 1906 | 7,934 | 2,549 | 32 |
| 1907 | 8,597 | 3,170 | 37 |
| 1908 | 7,671 | 2,809 | 37 |
| 1909 | 6,617 | 2,212 | 33 |
| 1910 | 5,391 | 1,861 | 35 |
| 1911 | 7,268 | 2,572 | 35 |
| 1912 | 7,009 | 2,571 | 37 |
| 1913 | 7,564 | 2,663 | 35 |
| 1914 | 9,056 | 3,391 | 37 |
| Measles | | | |
| 1906 | | 18,899 | 100 |
| 1907 | | 26,179 | 100 |
| 1908 | | 19,385 | 100 |
| 1909 | | 20,145 | 100 |
| 1910 | | 25,677 | 100 |
| 1911 | | 31,905 | 100 |
| 1912 | | 19,809 | 100 |
| 1913 | | 15,142 | 100 |
| 1914 | | 18,585 | 100 |

*Source: Annual Reports of the London County Council Medical Officer (Education)*

Of the three diseases mentioned above, this chapter is mostly concerned with measles. Research on measles in London's elementary schools transformed policies on school closure and pupil exclusion across the country. Measles generated the most interest in part because, unlike diphtheria, there was no diagnostic test to confirm its presence or absence, and in part because it was most fatal to the youngest children in the infant classes. This epidemiological characteristic meant that measles had deep resonance in the contentious national debate about the most appropriate age at which school attendance should begin; or to put it another way, whether it was proper for children as young as three and a half years to be spending such long periods of time outside the home. At another level, then, the techniques employed in school-based surveillance underlined how the discovery and monitoring of infection in schools was not just about managing the discrete space of the classroom; it was central to discussions that were taking place about female participation in the workforce and the supposed deterioration of the nuclear family that had been the fulcrum of liberal ideas about domesticity for the better part of a century.

Nor was school-based surveillance simply about identifying individual sufferers and regulating their movements. Rather, contact tracing was concerned with the mediation of disease through the social relations of domestic space, which were themselves being destabilized by mass compulsory education. Local MOHs encouraged teachers and educational authorities to report absent pupils and suspected cases, providing an additional line of defense against the risk posed by parents who had either failed to notice the symptoms of an infectious disease or had not called in a physician. This evidence was the starting point for what, at times, was the painstaking and remarkably intricate tracing of children's contacts. Schools, then, became a sort of interstitial space in which the biological threats posed by the public environment and the private home were observed on the bodies of young human beings in a multiplicity of ways. But public health authorities expressed relatively little concern about the role of the public environment in these bodily inscriptions (though "the street" was a notable exception). Rather, the school came to be an essential space for public health because it opened the gateway to a child's home.

The technique of contact tracing became deeply embedded in the operations of the School Medical Service (SMS), an aspect of the service that has been underappreciated by historians, though Richard Meckel has recently pointed to the fundamental role of school nurses in the development of home visiting in the United States.[28] The final section of the chapter outlines how the SMS procedure of "following-up"—that is, the close monitoring and documentation of inspection, treatment, and outcome for each child—incorporated many components of infectious disease prevention strategies that already existed in schools. Card indexes of medical histories, registers of absence and presence, the co-opting of parental involvement, and an unremitting intrusion into domestic space rapidly became central features of the School Medical Service.

## Administration, Finance, and Attendance

Local administration of rate-funded schools was in the hands of school boards, which were created by the Education Act of 1870. School boards served either a borough or a civil parish. With the exception of London, which had a board imposed on it, a board could be created either by a vote of council, or of the majority of ratepayers, or by imposition from the Board of Education.[29] The size of the board varied between five and fifteen members, who were elected. While the franchise excluded married women, both married and unmarried women were allowed to stand for election.[30]

School boards were commonly formed in places where voluntary education provision was unable to provide a full complement of places. Boards drew upon the rates for all current and some capital expenses; loans for major expenditures, such as the building of a new school, could be secured against revenues from the rates.[31] Attendance committees were appointed in districts without school boards, and they sought to compel attendance. Meanwhile, voluntary elementary schools—predominantly owned by the Church of England and the Roman Catholic Church—were managed by a committee. By the mid-1890s, more than 1.89 million children were educated in schools managed by local school boards, compared to almost 2.45 million in the voluntary system.[32] More than 40 percent of all three- and four-year-olds attended elementary school by the beginning of the twentieth century.[33]

The Board of Education's Code of Regulations allocated school budgets according to examination results, average attendance, teachers' qualifications, and the condition of the schools.[34] The first two of these criteria attracted criticism for health-related reasons. The emphasis on examination results led campaigners to complain about "over-pressure" on children, resulting in mental and physical stress.[35] As far as attendance was concerned, schools were financially penalized whenever pupils were absent, including for reasons of illness. This was especially problematic for a school whenever an epidemic passed through. The code was modified in 1874, when attendances could be recalculated by taking into account closures for infectious disease, thus protecting a school's source of income.[36]

The regulations gradually ceded authority to local health departments. In 1882 school managers were instructed to comply with the MOH's directions to either close the school or exclude individual pupils due to infectious disease.[37] School board managers had recourse to immediate appeal, but this loophole was tightened in 1889 when they were directed to act "at once" on the sanitary authority's decision and could only appeal after the event.[38] From 1893 decisions about closure and exclusion could be taken on the signature of two members of the school board acting on the MOH's advice.[39] Finally, the 1902 Education Act abolished school boards, incorporated voluntary schools into the ratepayer system, and brought education under the auspices of county councils and borough councils through the creation of local education authorities. In theory at least, these councils had simultaneous control over health and education.

David Hirst argues that the incremental nature of these administrative changes indicates that infectious diseases created continual problems between public health departments and school boards.[40] The evidence suggests that while there were instances of cooperation, Hirst's view is broadly correct. The adoption of infectious disease notification in London and many provincial towns in 1889 was a double-edged sword in this respect. On the one hand, it meant that MOHs were less reliant on the educational authorities for information about disease. On the other hand, notification gave the MOH a capability to identify infected children and interfere with their education.

Difficulties between health and educational authorities crystallized over the roles of parents, teachers, attendance officers, and general practitioners. Many local authorities countenanced prosecuting parents for sending infected children to school.[41] By and large, however, they placed faith in educating and persuading parents. In 1880, for example, 40,000 circulars were printed in Sheffield warning parents that they risked a fine of £5 if their children were sent to school while in an infectious state, though the school board refused to distribute them for fear that this threat would cause alarm among parents.[42] In other places, GPs were encouraged to remind parents to keep such children, and their siblings, at home. Also in 1880, Leicester's health committee wrote to four GPs politely suggesting that they had "overlooked the necessity of advising the parents to keep the children from school."[43]

Teachers, of course, were the first line of defense against the spread of epidemics in schools. Under the 1875 Public Health Act, teachers were required to notify the health department of pupils with infectious disease.[44] But the ever-increasing number of schoolchildren not only heightened the risk of transmission; it also made it more likely that individual cases would escape the notice of even the most vigilant teacher.[45] MOHs sometimes incurred the ire of a school board by speaking directly to teachers, providing recommendations about the exclusion of pupils from class, and reminders of the need to inform the local authority, especially for nonnotifiable diseases.[46] One example of cooperation was in London where, from 1878, the LSB's ten district superintendents agreed to forward to MOHs information about cases that came to light.[47] It is clear, however, that many MOHs thought school boards were obstructive and an unnecessary barrier to the speedy receipt of information. They also resented the fact that the school board and not the health department could issue regulations to teachers on health matters.[48]

Although MOHs were keen to be told about cases, they nevertheless complained if teachers made a diagnostic mistake, which wasted time and energy.[49] It was easy to pick holes in the medical judgment of teachers. In 1878 the health committee in Nottingham was delighted that teachers sent notice of absent pupils, but they expressed concern that these notices did not give them "authentic information as to the nature of the disease."[50] A number of problems arose in September 1881. In the same week that one teacher was reprimanded for allowing a student with scarlet fever to attend classes, it was also discovered that nine children had been attending the Sneinton Board School, notwithstanding the fact that a case of scarlet fever was notified at each of their addresses. The upshot of these incidents was that Nottingham's MOH met with the school board chairman and sent him a written statement on the precautions necessary to prevent infectious disease.[51] To avoid ongoing confusion, in 1894 the health committee requested that teachers send home any child suspected to be suffering from infectious disease accompanied by a card notifying the parents of the illness and instructing them to forward the card to the MOH.[52] But even this cautious strategy—which the teachers were not required to obey—was unhelpful for a disease like measles that even experienced doctors had difficulty identifying in its early stages.[53]

Furthermore, these sorts of interventions tended to have a fleeting impact. When Nottingham's MOH visited the houses of 174 notified scarlet fever cases in 1896, he found that thirty-six children from these houses were still attending school—in other words, the teacher had not sent them home.[54] During a measles epidemic in Islington in the same year, the MOH received no information from teachers despite his estimate that there were approximately 3,400 cases and that the London School Board required teachers to inform the MOH.[55]

The most egregious practice was when teachers sent pupils to another child's house to investigate an absence. Arthur Newsholme heard that it was not unknown for the healthy child to be "ushered directly into the living room in which children suffering from scarlet fever or measles, or some such disease, were lying."[56] Such was the pressure on attendance figures in Nottingham that one teacher had even "endeavoured to induce" a pupil to attend even though the child was suffering from scarlet fever.[57] It is not clear from the record what form this particular inducement took, but one-penny bribes were not unknown elsewhere.[58]

School board attendance officers (also known as visitors or visiting officers) were supposed to investigate the nonattendance of pupils.[59] The existence of this post was largely driven by financial concerns. It was in a board's best economic interests to ensure high levels of attendance in order to maintain its funding grant. As with teachers, MOHs called into question a number of aspects of lay AOs' competence. Could they identify a case of infectious disease? (This skepticism was hardly surprising given that some MOHs doubted even the capability of qualified medical practitioners to do the same.) Would they be vigilant in ensuring continued absence during the convalescence period? Did they possess the acuity to separate fact from fiction when encountering parents who were intent on deceiving them about the true cause of their child's nonappearance at school?[60] Though genuine, these sorts of concerns failed to appreciate that faults lay not with AOs themselves but with the system under which they worked. Medical expertise was not routinely put at their disposal, and this lack undermined their authority in the eyes of uncooperative parents. No funds were available to pay for medical assistance or advice. Indeed, such payments to school boards across the country were disallowed.[61]

A further persistent criticism was the length of time that it took for information to reach the MOH.[62] The system in most places operated along the lines described by Jarrow's MOH John Boyd in 1903. There, the attendance officer was provided with the name of a pupil missing consecutive schooldays and then visited the child's home within thirty-six hours. Any health-related information was sent to the headmaster over the next thirty-six hours (in some cases it was presented to the school board). Then the details were passed on to the MOH.[63] As mentioned above, some school boards tried to trim costs by sending pupils to check up on their classmates rather than go to the expense of employing an AO. In July 1883, it was revealed that the Sheffield School Board routinely dispatched healthy children to inquire at the homes of absentees. Even though the board apparently warned the "little messengers" not to enter homes, the MOH was skeptical that they resisted the temptation, stating that one may "as well expect a load-stone not to attract steel, as that the children will not go into the houses whither they are sent. . . . It is hardly credible that children should be thrust into the way of such fatal danger (as proved by the alarming number of deaths among children) in order to save the salary of an official."[64]

There were, of course, variations from place to place and according to disease. Attendance officers in Birmingham only reported infectious diseases on a weekly basis, but from mid-1897 an agreement was struck with the school board that they should notify the MOH each evening of the names and addresses of measles cases.[65] During a 1906 measles outbreak, however, the AOs reverted to reporting on a weekly basis, and the MOH declared that it was only through information from the teachers themselves that "a certain amount of supervision was exercised over such households" by the health department.[66] Leicester's MOH, Killick Millard, thought that being sent daily lists of suspected chicken pox cases by the schools was a far more efficient way for him to gather information than making chicken pox compulsorily notifiable by GPs. It is clear from the available evidence that some MOHs received such daily lists of infectious cases from their local schools but that others did not; the extent of the practice is difficult to gauge.[67]

MOHs were relentless in their quest for access to schools and information about pupils.[68] In 1899 the BMA council was urged to put pressure on the Board of Education to facilitate the entry by MOHs into schools to inspect premises and examine students during epidemics.[69] Some MOHs pressed for the creation of a cadre of school board medical officers to inspect all children who had been reported absent on account of infectious disease.[70] Others suggested that the AOs should be ex officio sanitary inspectors, trained in a variety of tasks: to recognize illnesses when visiting "suspects" at home; to procure details about the family doctor; and to distribute health department leaflets on disease prevention.[71] Whatever their shortcomings, it was widely understood in public health circles that attendance officers played an essential role in enabling the MOH to exercise a certain amount of supervision over households containing a diseased child.[72]

Both MOHs and school authorities depended heavily on the goodwill of general practitioners.[73] When a pupil was struck by infection, some boards required a certificate of ill-health from the GP in order to excuse the child from class; another certificate was needed when the child had recovered from the illness. Other boards were reluctant to require certificates on the grounds that poor families could not pay for them. Practice was uneven across the country. For example, in 1880 Sheffield's MOH provided printed certificates free of charge.[74] However, the certificate system was open to abuse. Leicester's former MOH Alfred Crane was caught red-handed issuing false certificates to the school board management committee in 1884.[75] Five of Crane's sixty-one certificates were signed by him without having any additional information filled out. A further twenty-three were signed by him but had been completed in another person's handwriting. For all but three children, the period of authorized absence exceeded thirty days, and in one case it extended to ninety-three days. It is not clear how the board uncovered Crane's misdemeanor, nor is Crane's response recorded. All we know is that the committee no longer accepted Crane's certificates as evidence that children were unfit to attend school on health grounds.[76] While this incident might reflect the isolated actions of a maverick practitioner, widespread concern about the accuracy of certificates of absence prompted the London School Board to appoint a medically qualified officer to examine cases in which the certificate was considered suspicious by the divisional superintendent.[77]

Crane's shenanigans aside, GPs were in an unenviable position. While it is unclear to what extent public health and school authorities were fully cognizant that the duration of exclusion needed to be different for each disease—the first edition of Arthur Newsholme's groundbreaking manual *School Hygiene* did list incubation and infective periods for the main childhood diseases[78]—the circumstances of each individual had to be considered when deciding whether to readmit the child. Such circumstances included facilities for domestic isolation, the presence of siblings, and the opportunity for disinfecting the house. House disinfection was widely considered to be an acceptable point at which a pupil might go back to school (at least until the introduction of bacteriological analysis for diphtheria). Some school boards required a certificate of freedom from infection that was issued by the council's health department when the house was disinfected.[79]

The concerns articulated by MOHs over teachers, AOs, and GPs were very much part of a battle about prompt access to accurate knowledge. As a small minority of school boards became increasingly interested in their health-related responsibilities, this tussle became less one-sided. London's was the first board to appoint a medical officer, Professor W. R. Smith, in 1890.[80] Before the end of his first year of tenure, he held a meeting with the London MOHs to ensure the exclusion of *any* child coming from a family suffering from an infectious disease.[81] Smith secured agreement on the following: that a copy of the notification certificate of scarlet fever, smallpox, diphtheria, membranous croup, typhoid, enteric fever, and typhus fever cases would be forwarded by the MOH to the headmaster of every school attended by the children of an infected household; that the MOH would send to the headmaster another certificate to acknowledge when disinfection of the infected premises had been carried out; and that the MOH would consult with Smith prior to any school closure.[82]

In return, the LSB sought to limit the spread of disease by regulating the activities of contacts as well as cases. In line with LGB recommendations, it specified that any child "showing symptoms of an infectious disease, or any child coming from a house where an infectious disease exists, must be sent home at once, and the superintendent of visitors must be immediately informed of the case in order that inquiries made with a view to proper steps being taken to prevent the children living in the same house or tenement from attending school."[83] Similar cooperative efforts were made in Edinburgh, Glasgow, Aberdeen, Manchester, Liverpool, Birmingham, Salford, and Bristol. The exchange of information undoubtedly proved useful;[84] however, it is difficult to judge the efficiency of these regulations, especially in London, since regular annual reports from the LSB medical officer were not issued until after Smith resigned in 1901.[85]

## Measles Notification and School Attendance

Measles attracted a great deal of attention in the mid-1890s. Mortality had been increasing since the 1870s, at a time when death rates from other childhood diseases, diphtheria excepted, were heading in the other direction. By the end of the nineteenth century, measles was causing more deaths every year than smallpox, scarlet fever, diphtheria, and other "fevers," and it rivaled whooping cough as the most fatal infectious disease of childhood. Significantly for the youngest elementary schoolchildren, measles was most deadly among two- to four-year-olds.

One fundamental problem for sanitary authorities was, again, a lack of information about cases. Measles was not covered by the Notification Acts, despite the fact that it was popularly understood as a contagious disease with a high case-fatality rate and that its inclusion as a notifiable disease was frequently debated in the 1890s.[86] The LGB's Theodore Thomson investigated the control of measles in thirty-three rural and urban sanitary districts in the early 1890s and found that most local authorities did not make measles compulsorily notifiable because it was highly infective even before the characteristic rash appeared and epidemics tended to be short lived.[87] Parents rarely called in a doctor, since measles was not regarded as a particularly life-threatening disease; indeed, early symptoms were indistinguishable from those of a common cold. It was extremely difficult to isolate young patients at home, especially if there were multiple cases in a household. From the ratepayers' perspective, notification of a disease with high incidence rates would lead to extensive hospitalization and disinfection, which would be far too expensive and place tremendous pressure on hospital accommodations in urban areas.[88]

Nonetheless, it was contended that the high levels of child mortality from the disease made notification imperative. It was acknowledged that measles was indeed highly infective in the early stages when it was difficult to diagnose, but it was also believed to be infectious *after* the appearance of the rash. Notification would at least enable isolation and removal at that point, thereby constraining an outbreak, if not stamping it out altogether. The interventions set in train by notification, including isolation and disinfection, would underline the gravity of the condition and encourage parents to think of the disease as something other than "only measles."[89] Leicester's MOH mentioned that despite all its difficulties, the notification of measles "would certainly bring about a closer relationship between the Health Officials and the mothers who might in this way be educated to look upon these diseases as serious and requiring careful treatment and isolation."[90]

Thomson declared himself in favor of measles notification (in the long term, few local authorities heeded his advice).[91] He cautioned that any knowledge gained from it was just the starting point for deeper probing about the chain of transmission. Whenever a case did come to light through notification, MOHs were encouraged to investigate its origin and conduct an intensive search for additional cases. Thomson devoted most of his attention to the role played by schools, both as a source of information about incidence and patient contacts and as an agent in the transmission of the disease. MOHs were instructed to provide schools with a list of pupils known to have measles in the hope that this would encourage schools to return the favor and let the MOH know when a pupil was absent with the disease.[92] Thomson found that this sort of exchange rarely happened, but cooperation was not entirely unheard of.[93] For example, following fifty-three deaths from measles toward the end of 1884, Leicester's health committee drew up 15,000 circulars describing symptoms of the disease and the precautions parents should take to prevent it from spreading. The school board assisted in distributing the circular to every house in the town containing school-age children.[94] In Birmingham in 1890, 63,000 handbills on the prevention of measles were distributed to students, taking directly into homes a message that also appeared on 1,000 placards across the city.[95]

The question of school closure was fiendishly problematic. To those who accepted that measles was communicable, it made intuitive sense that schools drove up prevalence by mixing infected children with those who had never had the disease. In line with LGB policy, Thomson encouraged MOHs to put pressure on schools to exclude *all* children from households containing a case of measles. Indeed, he went even further and recommended that exclusion should extend to "children inhabiting houses not yet invaded but in close relation with houses already invaded, and to children in homes which there may be reason to regard as likely to become invaded, by reason of personal communication with houses in which measles is known to have broken out."[96]

Having said this, Thomson concluded that the balance of evidence pointed toward the utility of school closure, even though definitive proof was elusive; even Thomson's own subsequent reports on measles outbreaks in Burton-on-Trent and Lancaster came to divergent conclusions.[97] Local MOHs were similarly perplexed. During an epidemic in Nottingham in 1896, pamphlets were circulated, the attendance registers were opened to the MOH, and schools were closed either singly or in groups. Yet, the final observations of Philip Boobbyer, Nottingham's MOH, were typically equivocal:

> I have endeavoured to ascertain whether the closure of the schools could be shewn (statistically) to have checked the extension of the disease, but, owing to the irregularity of the epidemic wave, both in time and place, and the consequent irregularity in the school closure, I have not succeeded as well as I could have wished. The general effect, however, of this preventive measure, in checking the spread of the disease in particular localities, as indicated by the reduction in the number of deaths during the month following the closure, as compared with those in the corresponding period preceding it, has been unmistakable on many occasions.[98]

Even when the number of new cases dropped following a closure, as happened in Nottingham, this could be explained by other factors, such as the seasonal downturn of the disease or, as Thomson put it, the "exhaustion of susceptible human material in the locality."[99] And when the number of cases failed to come down after the closure of a school, this, too, pointed to various possibilities: that closing a single school in a district might be insufficient while other schools remained open; that children from closed schools still met and played together on the street; or that the disease was passed around between siblings at home.

By the early twentieth century, school or classroom closure for measles was widely practiced. In 1901 more than fifty schools or classes in London were shut down in response to measles outbreaks.[100] A survey of more than one hundred urban MOHs across the country confirmed that closure was very common. Francis May, the MOH who distributed the questionnaire, claimed with an air of certainty that closure checked the spread of disease, limited the area of the outbreak, and delayed attacks in children until they reached an age at which the disease proved less fatal.[101] Yet, as we have seen, school closures took place in the absence of any solid evidence that the measure reduced the disease. Indeed, it was contrary to the opinions of many other commentators, and a *BMJ* editorial tagged it a "clumsy and unscientific" procedure.[102]

Matters were complicated by developments in education regulations. In 1903 the Board of Education removed Article 101* from its Code of Regulations.[103] Ever since 1892, Article 101* had ensured that a day school would not forgo any part of its annual grant incurred by a reduction in pupil attendance due to a school ordered closed by the sanitary authority. It also required that a medical attendant certify absences.[104] The announcement of the removal of this article "came upon everyone interested in epidemic disease as a perfectly incomprehensible decision," since it removed any "inducement to officials or teachers to increase attendance at the risk of health."[105] However, the 1902 Education Act brought the local control of education under the auspices of a town council education committee. No longer would an MOH face resistance or personal criticism from a school board when deciding to close a school or department on health grounds. In theory at least, health and education were placed on an equal political footing. Article 57 of the 1905 Education Code simply required the signature of two council members to secure a school closure. Even though this meant that one committee of a town council (health) interfered with the interests of another (education), in practice it guaranteed the more rapid closure of a school whenever it was thought to be required.[106] In other words, school closure was bureaucratically less contentious, but financially more injurious.

## "Combustible Material"

The dominant thinking about classroom and school closure was transformed in a few short years by research on measles in London. The immediate context was that school medical authorities had begun to exert some control over diphtheria, over and above the utility of the diphtheria antitoxin that had been used in London from the mid-1890s.[107] Many provincial councils and districts in London had their own bacteriological services (or contracted them out), which were most heavily used to culture throat swabs for diphtheria (along with sputum tests for tuberculosis).[108] In his *First Annual Report* as the London School Board's medical officer (indeed, this was *the* first annual report of an LSB medical officer), James Kerr expressed the hope that the provision of laboratory tests would mean that children were safer from infection in school than on the streets.[109] Between July 1903 and December 1908, a total of 5,983 cultures were taken from children showing *any* sign of diphtheria, including aural or nasal discharge, enlarged glands, or nothing more than an undue pallor.[110]

It soon became known that "mild" cases of diphtheria, either too slight to be infective or perhaps not recognized by parents, teachers, and even doctors, represented the most danger to schoolchildren. The repeated testing of school-age children became the norm. In the first year of the board's laboratory's operation in 1903, two children were excluded from Lewisham Bridge School after having been bacteriologically tested. One, a boy, was examined three times between September 29 and December 8, and diphtheria bacilli were present on each occasion. The MOH had wanted to close the whole school at the commencement of the outbreak, but Kerr demurred: "It was felt a more scientific procedure would discover the carrier cases, and exclude them only. . . . The closing of schools for diphtheria should be looked upon as a confession of impotence and defeat."[111]

Testing for diphtheria is one of the clearest examples of the rapid and successful translation of bacteriological knowledge into public health practice.[112] There was, of course, no comparable laboratory test for measles, yet the school closure/pupil exclusion debate was no less pressing for a disease that exacted such a heavy toll on youngsters and caused havoc with schools' attendance records. So the London School Board pursued alternative ways of investigating the measles question. In autumn 1902, Dr. Sydney Davies, the MOH for Woolwich (in southeast London), began to work closely with the school board's Dr. C. J. Thomas to monitor all cases of measles in the district for one year. Teachers in the infants' departments kept a list of children who had already had measles upon admission, those who contracted measles while at the school, and those who left school and were not known to have had measles. The measles history of each child was recorded on a card. Whenever a child caught measles, particulars of the attack were noted on the card, which was taken home by the child. The school then informed the MOH, who arranged a domiciliary visit to investigate the spread of the disease among the child's family and in the immediate vicinity.[113]

Early analyses revealed that 54 percent of three-year-olds in Woolwich's infants' departments had already had measles. The figure rose to 83 percent at seven years of age, which indicated a steady transition to immunity through early childhood.[114] This observation led Kerr to believe that the "combustible material in each classroom"—that is, the proportion of children vulnerable to measles—was the most important factor in the spread of the disease through schools.

The time period of the study was extended so that the efficacy of class and school closure could be explored. This was achieved by turning the elementary schools of Woolwich into a sort of epidemiological laboratory whereby the district was split in half: rigorous class closure was practiced in east Woolwich; in the west, reliance was placed on the exclusion of pupils and contacts coming from infected families. Within three years of the beginning of the experiment, Kerr confidently claimed that "the usual sanitary idea of results in measles prevention by school or class closure is mere imagination."[115] Due to the high infectivity of measles, closure was only effective if applied at the occurrence of the first case, and because measles was so difficult to diagnose, this was practically impossible. In east Woolwich, closure proved little more effective than pupil exclusion in the west. During 1904–5, for example, 38 percent of unprotected children were attacked by measles in the eastern "closing" schools. The corresponding figure was 46 percent in the western "nonclosing" schools. More important, the difference between the two districts in the amount of "combustible material" remaining after the ravages of measles was minimal: 7.7 percent of the children in the east were left unprotected versus 9.0 percent in the west.[116] "Scientific" results such as these meant that by mid-1908, decisions about closure or exclusion could be taken with quantifiable accuracy and at substantial financial savings. On June 2, 1908, four cases of measles were reported in three classrooms in Atley Road School, but the knowledge that 82 percent of the children had already suffered measles indicated that no spread would take place, so no action was taken.[117]

The Woolwich inquiry revealed that measles was most likely to spread through a class when between 30 and 40 percent of the pupils were immunologically unprotected. Diffusion continued until between 80 and 85 percent of the class had had the disease. One striking diagrammatic representation illustrated how varying amounts of "combustible material" precipitated the progression of measles in a classroom (fig. 4.1). In the youngest age group (Class VI, three-and-a-half- to four-and-a-half-year-olds), 38 percent of the children (each represented by a square) were unprotected (white squares; those who already had the disease were shown as crosshatched). After the outbreak in 1904, thirty-three of the fifty-two susceptible children caught measles (black squares). More children

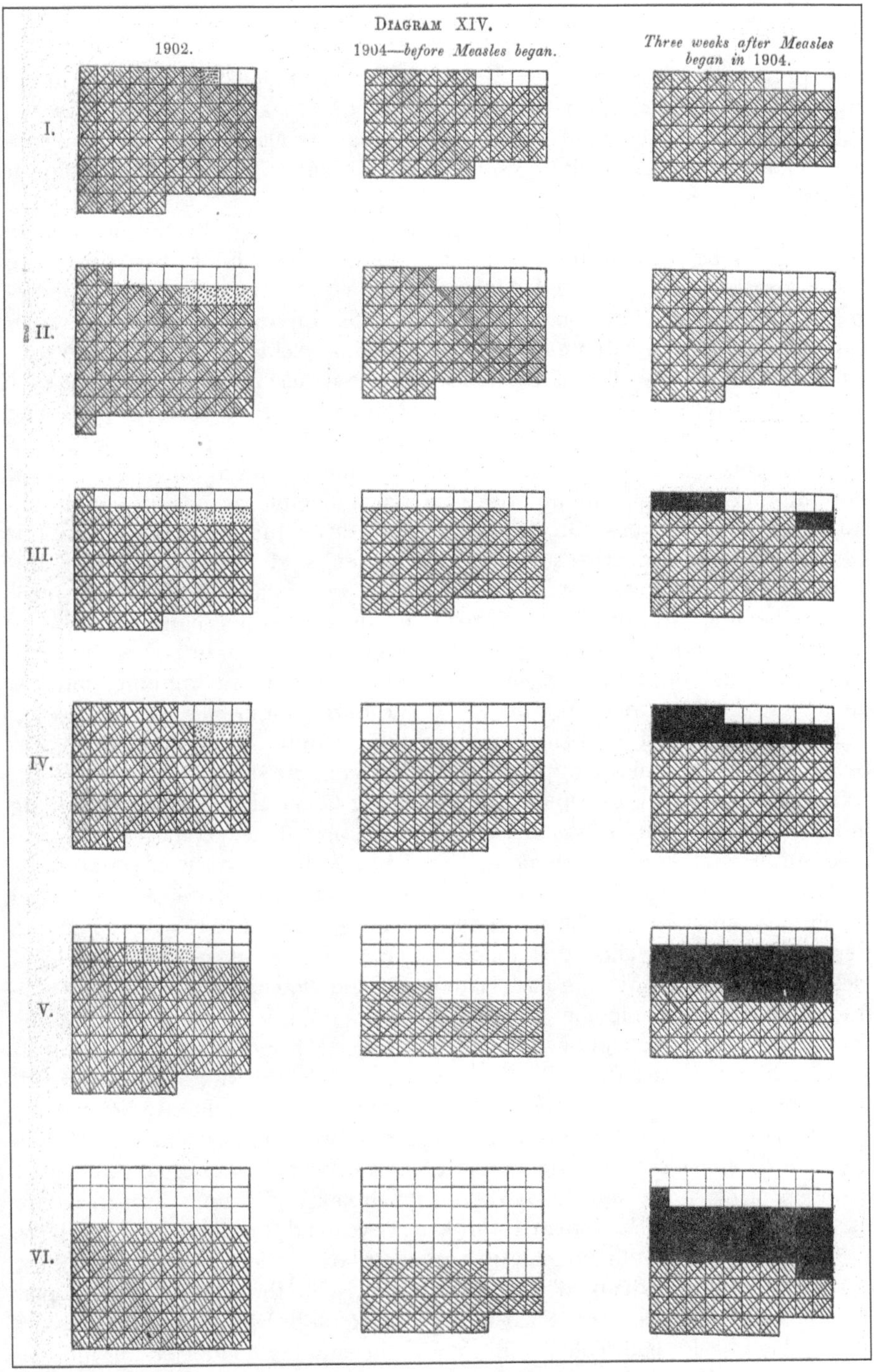


Figure 4.1. Measles "combustible material" in an elementary school's classrooms. Kerr, *Report of the LCC* (1905), 48.

were protected as they got older, and there was less chance of an outbreak in the classrooms of older children. In this particular outbreak, there were no cases in Classes I (eight years of age) and II (seven years) because so many of these children had acquired immunity, even though the immune status of some children was unknown (dotted squares).

A number of important points need to be made here. Bacteriology made no direct contribution to the evolution of the London School Board's thinking about measles policies, though it might be argued that the example of diphtheria had a strong influence on the belief that exclusion was more efficacious than closure. The same, incidentally, can also be said of excluding children with scarlet fever. The novelty of what the LSB was trying to accomplish meant that Kerr and Thomas were scratching around for an appropriate vocabulary to describe the characteristics of their models. On the one hand, the language was, shall we say, inflammatory. The metaphor of combustibility conveyed the seriousness of nonimmunity and the rapidity with which an epidemic of measles could consume vulnerable victims. On the other hand, this vulnerability was borne out by the more familiar terms such as "unprotected" and "susceptible." Kerr and Thomas's empirical findings in the classroom were establishing the terrain of "herd immunity" in human populations, but the language for that field of epidemiology did not yet exist.[118] Most significant in my opinion is that this polychotomous model of diseased/unprotected/protected cast immune status as an attribute of *populations* (in this case, classrooms), not of *individuals*. Students were either excluded from class or allowed to continue attending because they belonged to a particular group, categorized by immune status.

Besides causing less disruption and increasing financial savings, another thing in favor of pupil exclusion was that it facilitated more efficient contact tracing and follow-up in the home environment. Revealing the disease status of contacts was crucial for untangling the knots of when, where, and how the disease was passed around among children. The infectious disease sections of Kerr's *Annual Reports* were replete with detailed descriptions of tracked cases. Take the example of Nellie I., aged five, of Maryon Park School near the Woolwich dockyard, who contracted measles on September 16, 1905. Intensive inquiries concluded with some confidence that Nellie had been directly or indirectly responsible for no less than eleven additional cases (fig. 4.2). Kerr's account of Nellie's witless generosity with her germs is riddled with sarcastic asides about the parenting abilities of her mother, and wry amusement at the unrestrained nature of working-class children's friendships. First Nellie played with her cousin Charles B., who then infected three other members of his family and "his next-door neighbour and chum" Chris C. Before she was isolated, Nellie also played with her five-year-old "bosom friend" Gertie W. and, after a week of confinement, with her "other bosom friend," Lily S. Once these other two became "exhausted" with the disease, Nellie then "descended" to play with a toddler of three years, Ellen R., who also took to bed. Exactly three weeks after Nellie's health had "failed" with measles, her mother conducted "an interesting experiment" by allowing Nellie to see her two-week-old brother, Henry George. Needless to say, little Henry contracted measles and then "happily recovered."[119]

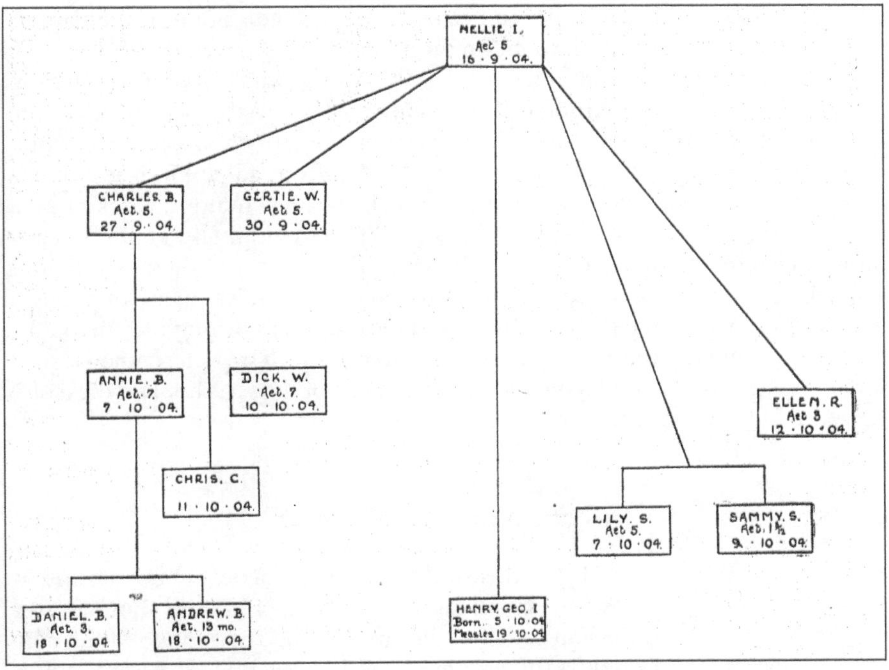


Figure 4.2. Diagram showing the measles cases traced to Nellie I., aged five years. Kerr, *Report of the LCC* (1905), 52.

Kerr's pejorative tone and language characterized mothers' innocuous actions as reckless. The perils of intimacy are communicated through the choice of tender terms such as "bosom friend" and "chum" rather than simply "friend." This passage implicitly conveys exasperation at the daunting task the medical department faced. It also underscored the importance of keeping the children within reach. Nellie's was one case out of 115 that occurred in the Maryon Park student body. The forensic approach to contact tracing revealed that almost one-third of these cases was "definitely" contracted at home; closing schools and sending children home en masse risked missing these cases, which put the brakes on any sort of control the MOH may otherwise have had over the outbreak.[120] Furthermore, it was difficult to know whether children returning to previously closed schools were still infectious or incubating the disease.

The relative ineffectiveness of school closure highlighted the importance of identifying a case of measles as soon as possible. In this respect, it was easy to scapegoat mothers for not detecting the early signs of measles. From 1905, whenever the first case of measles was noticed in a classroom of Woolwich infants, circulars were sent to all the pupils' mothers, "begging" them to keep surveillance on their little ones, and to keep a child at home for a day on the slightest suspicion of coldlike symptoms.[121] In January 1908, this approach was adopted across London in order to ensure “a gradual education of the parents to a sense of their responsibility and to the seriousness of the disease.”[122]

The Woolwich study continued until 1908, during which time it revolutionized ideas about the prevention of measles in schools.[123] As a direct result of the Woolwich inquiry, all children suffering from measles in schools across London were compulsorily excluded for one month. Moreover, all children in infants' departments coming from *any* house in which measles, mumps, chicken pox, or whooping cough existed were excluded. This restriction also applied to any unprotected older children in other classes.[124] The efficacy of these regulations was helped in subsequent years by the more rapid communication of knowledge. In 1912 AOs began to telephone suspected measles cases through to the public health department, and these homes were favored with a preferential visit. In some instances this shaved ten days off the amount of time a school medical officer waited for the notification.[125]

## Infection and Mothercraft

Kerr triumphantly declared that this study of measles made “school closure as a sanitary measure as obsolete as quarantine. . . . School closure should never be necessary; it is a confession of failure, a throwing up the sponge in the contest with disease.”[126] Certainly the lessons of the Woolwich inquiry were rapidly absorbed and reproduced as central policy. In 1909 the Board of Education and the LGB issued a joint memorandum on school closure and pupil exclusion detailing the circumstances under which schools should be closed and detailing the procedures to be deployed for individual diseases. The Board of Education's chief medical officer, George Newman, reported that the actions that had been routine in London for some years were also now common practice in other urban areas.[127] That is, on some occasions classrooms might need to be shut, but it was far more effective and economical to exclude individual pupils or groups of pupils based on their immune status. This was also the conclusion of a consultative committee of the Board of Education set up to explore the desirability of sending children under the age of five to elementary school. Having listened to the evidence of school medical officers (including Kerr), local MOHs (including Newsholme from Brighton and Niven from Manchester), local education authorities, school inspectors, teachers, and even some “representative” working-class parents, the committee “agreed that one of the most efficacious methods of preventing the spread of infectious disease in school is the prompt exclusion of individual children . . . [which] also causes the least amount of interference with the education of the majority of the children in a school.”[128]

The consultative committee favored the provision of some form of education for children under five years of age. The medical contingent that gave evidence to the committee was not in full agreement with this conclusion; neither were other quarters of public health opinion. John Sykes, MOH for St. Pancras in London, who wrote extensively on the infectious diseases of childhood, argued that the defenselessness of the under-fives against measles provided a prima facie case for their permanent exclusion from school. Sykes made a much deeper philosophical point about how the compulsory public education of such young children drew them away from the nurturing ambit of the home:

> Under modern conditions the father goes to his workplace and club, the children over school age leave home, the elder children go to school, the children under school age are left at the day nursery, and the mother goes out to work. To such, and they are not a few, there only remains a sleeping-place; there is no family life, there is no true HOME. . . . Efforts directed towards the prevention of physical deterioration and sickness and to the amelioration of the health, habits, and character of the individual must commence at the very earliest age.[129]

Sykes was an enthusiastic proponent of the "mothercraft" movement.[130] For him, the exclusion of children under five from the classroom had to be substituted by the provision of facilities and services to advise and guide mothers in hygiene and "maternal and domestic arts, and by assistance in the training of their children, both in special institutions and at home." Sykes hoped to live to see schools of mothercraft everywhere, making a valuable contribution to the prevention of illness.[131] The consultative committee's preference was for the attachment of nurseries to the elementary schools—an idea that Sykes and his ilk deplored because it continued to facilitate the participation of women in the workforce and failed to address the root cause of mothers' failings. It was acknowledged, however, that at least some benefits would accrue to infectious disease control. That is, while there was some risk that the incidence of measles and whooping cough might increase among the under-five population, this was offset by the hope that incipient cases would be recognized by well-trained teachers and that prompt isolation and exclusion could then be enforced. Of equal significance to the committee was the greater amount of attention that would devolve on "uninformed parents," who could be given "advice which they sorely need."[132] Domestic space was central to the guiding ethos of the committee, which asserted that the home was the most appropriate environment for child rearing, provided that there were sufficient opportunities to provide maternal care and training. Unfortunately, according to the committee, these circumstances did not exist for the vast majority of young children in the elementary school system:

> It is not only that there are parents who are not sufficiently alive to the well-being of their children; it is rather that many mothers, however anxious to discharge their whole duty towards their children, are nevertheless unable to train them properly at home owing to various circumstances. They may lack the necessary means or accommodation, or they may be compelled to leave home during the day and go to work. . . . Many homes now exist in which the mental and physical development of young children cannot be properly secured. . . . The ideal scheme for young children is to leave them in a good home. . . . At present this ideal is in many cases not attainable.[133]

Just as the consultative committee issued its report, the brand-new School Medical Service was rolling out a technique to deal with the supposed inadequacies of working-class child rearing. This method was known as "following-up."

## Following-Up

The introduction of the School Medical Service in 1908 was an important milestone in social welfare in Britain. The creation of the SMS was influenced by a variety of factors. Some of these I have already mentioned, such as public health's broader interest in the school environment and the "over-pressure" controversy of the 1880s. The Education Acts of 1893, 1899, and 1902 had encouraged authorities to cater to the needs of deaf, blind, and epileptic children and those with physical and mental disabilities. Some form of medical inspection had been taking place in some schools from the late nineteenth century, though the British also looked to examples from abroad as well as closer to home.[134] In the introduction to this chapter, I also alluded to the question of "national efficiency," and it has been argued that the most pressing impetus for the School Medical Service lay with the Interdepartmental Committee on Physical Deterioration, which made four broad recommendations: first, the establishment of an advisory council to appraise the government of appropriate public health interventions; second, the need for improved measurement of health and sickness; third, changes in the field of environmental standards; and finally, a tranche of recommendations for improving the health of schoolchildren.[135] The committee's report came to be associated with a slew of public health legislation in subsequent years, but it is most closely connected to the provision of school meals and school medical inspection.[136]

Historians' attention has been focused mainly on the content and form of inspections and treatments, as these were some of the most innovative and challenging aspects of the service. John Welshman has pointed out that the SMS was part and parcel of the general trend toward "health education," while Bernard Harris argues the agency was more oriented toward personal health needs compared to nineteenth-century public health measures.[137] Harris suggests investigations into the spread of infectious diseases in schools emphasized that medical officers "would have to devote much more attention to the children themselves."[138] It seems to me that while this individualized aspect of the SMS rightly has been emphasized, it is important not to forget that it was deeply embedded in the rhetoric of familial social relations and domestic space. So, although inspection and treatment in school formed the core activities of the SMS, it was intentionally structured to maximize access to working-class homes.

The medical inspection of elementary schoolchildren involved taking a medical history and clinical examination to reveal existing health problems, including aural, speech, vision, and dental defects; physical and mental disabilities; and ailments including ringworm, adenoids, skin conditions, rickets, various forms of lung infection, tuberculosis, and heart disease. Children were also inspected for signs of malnutrition and uncleanliness, which included infestations of the hair, body, and clothing. By treating many of these conditions, the SMS blurred the boundaries between preventive and curative medicine. Initially it proved extremely difficult to configure patient treatment between private medical practitioners and hospitals, which many families could not afford and had not commonly availed themselves of in the past. This problem was partially solved by the creation of clinics in the schools, but on the eve of World War I, the provision of clinics and the extent of services varied a great deal across the country.[139]

Some aspects of infectious disease surveillance were recognizable in the works of the SMS. This was partly because it became conjoined with the existing local public health administration; more often than not, the local MOH was appointed as the school medical officer. Combining the roles of MOH and SMO met serious opposition in some quarters, not least from James Kerr, who wanted the positions kept separate.[140] The Board of Education pushed all objections to one side, noting that in some places separate appointments might end up being a source of friction (which did in fact transpire).[141] George Newman's first report as the CMO of the Board of Education outlined some of the reasons why uniting the two posts made sense from a broader perspective:

> School hygiene cannot be divorced either from home hygiene on the one hand, or from the health conditions of the community generally on the other. The duties of the School Medical Officer, and the results arising from the effective discharge of those duties, involve of necessity the wider questions of the public health. For instance, there is the whole subject of the certification and prevention of the spread of notifiable and non-notifiable infectious disease, in which the duties of the Medical Officer of Health and the School Medical Officer necessarily overlap. Associated with that are the kindred questions of disinfection and the closure of schools, or the exclusion of children from them, in which the Medical Officer of Health of an area has specific responsibilities. Then there is the external sanitation of the school, the sanitation and hygiene of the home from which the child comes to school, and the whole business of securing cleanliness. Those matters fall by statute within the province of the Medical Officer of Health, but they arise immediately in the work of the school doctor.[142]

The prevention of infectious disease though systems of notification, the role of disinfection, and the regulation of conditions in the pupil's home environment all figure prominently in Newman's justification for integrating the SMS with the wider structures of public health administration. The SMS threw open the doors of domestic space. One of the Board of Education's first acknowledgments of this came in August 1908, when it issued a circular on medical inspection that claimed "it is in the home, in fact, that both the seed and the fruit of public health are to be found." The board also predicted that the SMS would ultimately increase the burden of responsibility on parents, not lessen it.[143]

Emphasis on the home was framed through a system called "following-up."[144] Initially, following-up was used to describe the work of the school nurses, who gave guidance to parents in the home and checked that they were heeding the school medical officer's advice. Nurses routinely helped out with inspections and operation of the school clinic, but more and more they were deployed in the domestic setting, visiting cases of absence due to illness, pursuing the contacts of pupils who had infectious diseases, and acting as the general line of communication between the school and parents whenever a student was excluded on health grounds. In 1910 Merthyr Tydfil's school nurses paid 1,976 visits to 562 homes. Often, this sort of work was complemented by visiting nurses who were already employed by local authorities in other capacities. Over one thousand pupils' homes were visited in Finchley, where the school nurse already acted as a health visitor under the Notification of Births Act. In Croydon, more than 8,000 home visits were made possible by the borough's existing five health visitors.[145]

As "following-up" came to be used more formally—the Board of Education CMO's 1909 report was the first to devote a section to "The Proceeding Known as Following-Up"—teachers, school attendance officers, and parents were brought under its umbrella.[146] Echoing the ethos of Alice Ravenhill, Dr. Barwise, school medical officer for the County of Derbyshire, wrote about how teachers were encouraged to nurture a "health conscience" among children through the performance of regular surveys of bodily cleanliness, tidiness, posture, and breathing. The idea was that the teacher would make the school the model for the home through example, training, and habit. It was the teacher's responsibility to impress the wishes of the school doctor on both children and parents.[147]

As for the AOs, the local health authorities continued to rely on them for information about pupils with nonnotifiable infectious diseases such as measles, and for regular reports of children absent from school through illness. The local health department reciprocated by informing the AOs whenever schoolchildren were admitted to the isolation hospital and furnishing them with lists of all children excluded from school on medical grounds.[148]

In some parts of the country, voluntary care committees were set up to monitor the results of these activities and manage other aspects of the children's social welfare that arose out of medical inspections, such as the administration of recreational play centers.[149] The London County Council (LCC) created a centralized children's care subcommittee to regulate these agencies, and salaried council employees organized their activities across the capital. Representatives of each school's care committee were permitted to attend the medical inspections from 1912. The results of the examination were kept on a special card, which also catalogued subsequent treatments. The care committee used this card to track the progress of each case until the patient was discharged by the attending doctor.[150] Care committees tended to be connected to existing voluntary agencies, such as the local Guild of Help or the Charity Organisation Society. As such, they naturally aligned with the Board of Education's declaration that one of their main duties was "to endeavour to bring about in special cases permanent improvement in the condition of the home by regular visits of a friendly character."[151] It is worth describing in full what the LCC expected of the care committee volunteers:

> The energies of the voluntary worker . . . are devoted to persuading the parent of the importance of obtaining treatment, discussing with her the ways and means of obtaining treatment, deciding which cases are suitable under the Council's scheme, determining the time most suitable to the particular parent, applying for vouchers, assessing the amount to be paid, explaining the necessary preliminaries and impressing the parent with the necessity of observing the times mentioned, doing all that is possible to ensure that all appointments are kept, receiving notices from the centre as to further visits necessary, ensuring, as far as possible, that these visits are made, using further persuasion in cases where there has been failure to keep the first or subsequent appointments, receiving reports from the organisers as to necessary adjustments in the home and environment of the child, ensuring, so far as possible, that these are being carried out, considering the ways and means to be adopted for supplying spectacles to each particular case (in cases of defective vision), advising and helping the parents in every way necessary, and seeing that the school doctor, at the re-inspection, is apprised of what has been done.[152]

This extensive litany of responsibilities conveys a number of important things about what the care committee was supposed to do and the attitudes its existence embodied. Volunteers could potentially spend a lot of time cajoling parents into keeping routine appointments for their children; they had to assist parents in their negotiation of the new administrative layer of red tape that the School Medical Service's inspection, surveillance, and treatment entailed; "parents" in fact meant "mothers" (e.g., "discussing with her . . ."); and what went on inside the home itself, and not just the child's ailments, was a target for "treatment." In other words, a school's care committee was the agency through which the Board of Education tried to make good its promise that more responsibility would devolve to parents.

Parental involvement was seen as the key to the success of "following-up," even though, as Harry Hendrick has indicated, the school medical officer remained very much in the senior role.[153] The Board of Education asked local authorities to encourage parents' attendance at the inspections of their own children, even though their presence was sometimes seen by the doctor as an inconvenience. It was nevertheless perceived as a not-to-be-missed opportunity to educate the parents and the most effective way of ensuring their continued compliance with the doctor's directives. There was, of course, much unevenness in terms of participation rates, and it was accepted that such disappointing outcomes could be due to social circumstances and employment. For every town or city with a parental attendance rate above 80 percent, there was another where it was below 40 percent.[154]

The forced cleansing of children and prosecutions to compel delousing represented the extremes of intervention under the following-up rubric (and were far less draconian than the use of summonses to the defaulting parents of truants).[155] Although, as David Hirst has observed, documentation on parents' reactions is scarce, it is likely that the threat of legal action was far less important to the effectiveness of following-up than was the creation of a bureaucratic repository that married a child's comprehensive medical history to a wealth of information about their domestic circumstances.[156] The records kept by the care committees were one example of this. Another was the school's disease register, which became a valuable part of infection prevention at the local level. Fortified by the results of the Woolwich measles inquiry in London, school medical officers across the country were encouraged to keep not only a measles register but also a register of pupils excluded for all health reasons. Information was kept on each case, and this was often stratified into infectious diseases and long-term illnesses.[157] In Worcestershire in 1909, 7.8 percent of 14,113 medical inspections resulted in exclusion for conditions ranging from "general weakness" to anemia, from ringworm to "scaldhead," and from bronchitis to pulmonary tuberculosis.[158] In Leicester a chronic disease register was made of all children who had been kept out of school for more than six months; at the end of 1911, it contained details of 547 children. Some of the most common ailments appearing on Leicester's register were heart and chest diseases, nervous diseases (such as imbecility, chorea, epilepsy, and paralysis), diseases of the eye, and the vague condition described as "debility."[159] Meanwhile, from 1913 in London a card index was kept of all children absent from school for more than three months. Analysis of 3,560 such cases showed that chorea and tuberculosis of the lungs were the most common explanations for long-term absence, accounting for 10 percent and 11 percent of cases, respectively.[160]

Tuberculosis of the lung was the most frequent reason why children were excluded from school for extended periods. It is no surprise, then, that school medical departments were encouraged to keep separate registers for tuberculosis that were much more detailed than they were for other diseases. The Board of Education's chief medical officer suggested that these registers should enumerate the hygienic condition of the home, overcrowding, family history of the disease, existence of the disease in other family members, opportunities for transmission within the home, and the extent of contact with infected people.[161] By 1910 Liverpool and Bolton maintained a register of all school-age children with tuberculosis so that they could be kept under observation and reexamined periodically.[162] In reviewing activity across the country, the CMO revealed that

> whenever investigations were undertaken the home surroundings, and particularly the sleeping arrangements, have almost always been unsatisfactory, and the need for inspection and supervision of the homes, together with the giving of advice and practical assistance, becomes increasingly evident. Such duties may be undertaken by the School Nurse (if she has time), by Health Visitors working under the Medical Officer of Health, or by a special tuberculosis inspector, as in Sheffield. Or they may be undertaken, with perhaps more success, by the officers of a Tuberculosis Dispensary, working in conjunction with the School and Public Health Medical Services.

The school medical authorities of the LCC closely associated tuberculosis with malnutrition, though the former was seen as a determining factor in the latter, rather than vice versa. Either way, in 1913 almost 20 percent of children identified as malnourished at inspection were found to have tuberculosis as a comorbid condition.[163] Care committees in the capital were issued special forms to document in great detail the home conditions of malnourished and tubercular children, and local authorities used these findings to remove tubercular children from their home environment and place them in open-air schools or sanatoria.[164]

The introduction of compulsory notification of respiratory tuberculosis in 1912 and all forms of the disease in 1913 gave public health departments further access to the homes of tuberculosis sufferers. This topic is dealt with in chapter 6, but it is worth noting briefly here that around this time a Tuberculosis Service was created, the provision of institutional treatment was boosted by the Finance Act of 1911, and the National Insurance Act included a sanatorium benefit.[165] Nevertheless, the vast majority of patients were not institutionalized, and most sufferers were cared for at home, often managed through a dispensary. The notification of tuberculosis was significant for contact tracing because many health departments shared their lists of tuberculous adults with dispensaries, school doctors, and care committees, so that children living in homes with a tubercular parent could be comprehensively monitored.[166] In Sheffield, where special tuberculosis inspectors were employed, the children of sufferers were called "delicate contacts."[167] By the outbreak of World War I, the repeated examination of child contacts—that is, the inspection of any children who had regular interaction with a tuberculosis sufferer—was normal procedure in many urban schools.[168]

To some extent, following-up was a rhetorical device that created an impression of professional unity and a seamless package of treatment at a time when the configuration of the new School Medical Service was still being worked out. Some aspects of following-up did cause professional tensions. It was acknowledged, for example, that teachers frequently resented the disruption to the classroom routine that medical inspections caused. There was also a degree of unease about the potential overlap between the domiciliary visits of nurses and attendance officers, even to the point that the Board of Education became worried about the excessive number of officials with legitimate reasons for visiting pupils' homes. Also, the closeness of the association of the school attendance and school medical departments varied across the country.[169] As the documentary memory of all this activity, registers and card indexes were central to following-up. They were the glue that supposedly held together the many interested parties.

One of the problems with the way the history of public health in the late nineteenth and early twentieth centuries has been written is the beguiling simplicity of its narrative arc. Just as the Victorian age gave way to the Edwardian, public health's preoccupation with the environment ceded ground to notions about the individual basis of disease, a transformation that was driven by advances in bacteriological knowledge. For historians of public health, this signaled a more intense government interest in individuals and their behaviors than before. This trope has often been repeated in the history of child health, but I think it misses most of what that atomization signified. Dorothy Porter pointed out more than twenty years ago—rightly, I think—that "public health officers embracing the bacteriological revolution no longer viewed the individual simply as an isolated health unit; he or she was seen rather as the bearer of the social relations of health and illness."[170] In other words, the *I* of individuation cannot be imagined without the *we* of society or domestic social relations.

This chapter has presented a case that bears out Porter's claim emphatically. James Kerr once recounted the story of a mother he visited who could not recall the ages of her three children, or even the month when her last child was born. She could only tell him that she was expecting another baby next March. For Kerr, who believed that a large section of the population was neglectful of its children, just like this anonymous mother, an enlarged role for the state in child rearing was inevitable: "People subject to disease and dirt, who neglect their children, are an ever present danger to the people, and the state or the authority should step in and do something, both for the sake of the children and for other people. For the sake of the children, because every child born has the right during its helpless time to be protected and looked after by somebody."[171] The biological risk posed by the individual child, no better exemplified than by a case of measles, was to be countered by state intervention in familial practices.

Bernard Harris has argued that if we view the School Medical Service through a political lens rather than a medical one, then it is possible to see how important were questions of rights, responsibilities, and citizenship in its gestation. The appetite for the humanitarian aspects of the SMS—the child's "right during its helpless time," in Kerr's phrase—was whetted by the political climate of the early twentieth century. Harris says that "it would be difficult to argue that the more 'humanitarian' arguments for the introduction of school meals and school medical inspection would still have prevailed, if they had not been reinforced by arguments about national efficiency."[172]

Public health policies toward infectious schoolchildren translated "national efficiency" into "social efficiency" through an appeal to the science of epidemiology. In the case of measles, the policies of pupil exclusion and contact tracing were governed by ideas about incubation and immunity that were more "scientific" than the clumsy approach to school closure that had no secure evidential basis. The forensic identification of "combustible material" did the same work for measles policy that bacteriological examination did for diphtheria.

It is somewhat ironic, then, that measles maintained its high position in the annual records of childhood mortality in London well into the twentieth century, which is probably as good evidence as any that schools played a relatively small part in the incidence and prevalence of the disease. Measles, we now know, is a disease mainly associated with overcrowded living conditions and malnutrition.[173] Its high infectivity during the early stages, difficulties with identification in these stages, and the fact that it was most prevalent at ages before compulsory schooling mean we can say with some confidence that the overall epidemiological course of the disease was probably only influenced to a minor degree by the actions of the educational authorities.

## Chapter Five

# *Disinfection, Domestic Space, and the Laboratory*

A peculiarly Victorian disquiet centered on the materiality of domestic life.[1] The disease-harboring threat of furnishings and decorations had been long acknowledged by medical authorities on the sickroom.[2] Writing in the 1840s, elite physician Anthony Todd Thomson argued not only that infection settled in clothes and bedding made from wool, cotton, and fur, but that it also clung to floors, furniture, and ornaments, especially if these objects had rough and unpolished surfaces.[3] Advice from physicians like Thomson remained a feature of home nursing manuals throughout the Victorian period.[4] Removing superfluous furniture and ornamentation formed part of the ritual that signified the sickroom as a space of separation and seclusion within the home.[5] Domestic patient management both during and after the episode of illness featured the regular cleansing of floors, walls, fixtures, and fittings with soap and water, washing with a solution of chloride of lime or other chemical agents, and fumigation.[6] However, the potential risk posed by furnishings extended beyond the sickroom and included the entire domestic space. According to Eileen Cleere:

> The Victorian home was under increased pressure in the second half of the nineteenth century to appear hygienically inviolable, impermeable, and unassailable. Yet after the development and general acceptance of germ theories in the 1870s, the impenetrable Victorian home became an anxious fantasy rather than a predictable ideological construct. . . . Mid-Victorian sanitary geographies of the city turned inward, eventually producing analogous geographies of the overdecorated, architecturally busy middle-class interior.[7]

One might quibble with Cleere's chronology, the ubiquity of germ theory's acceptance, and its impact on public health policy, but the general point remains. The proliferation of nooks and crannies in the Victorian home gave safe haven to the detritus of life and harbored the threat of death. This preoccupation with spotlessly clean domestic interiors was something of a new twist in the politics of the sanitary home. To understand why, it is necessary to appreciate the complex interplay of multiple "liberalisms": liberal notions about the relationship between the individual and the state; liberal political economy; and liberal governmentality.[8]

The early stages of Victorian sanitary reform and government-sponsored public health initiatives were replete with tacit assumptions about domestic space, issues, and relations.[9] Domestic space and the physical environment existed symbiotically rather than separately; connections between the intimate space of the home and the public space of the environment were several and layered.[10] Edwin Chadwick's famous 1842 sanitary report concentrated on private domestic space as much as the wider physical environment. Sanitarians argued that the degradation of urban places fostered immoral habits and vice.[11] While this seemingly "confirmed the vision of the poor as incapable of exercising citizenship," Pamela Gilbert writes that "it also implied a remedy that might bring such creatures within the pale of those who could develop into citizens over time."[12] The "remedy" was an environmentally based public health that offered the chance to create the conditions under which individuals might achieve *domestic* propriety.

As such, sanitary reform had the potential to reconfigure the relationship between the individual and the state. This potential was harnessed through liberal political economy. Private property was the political link between domestic space and sanitary reform. Public health legislation was based on the rights, responsibilities, and representation of private property.[13] Chadwick hit upon the idea of selling sanitation through the language of political economy, demonstrating that it was a legitimate *public* enterprise given the private market's failure to protect against disease. Local ratepayers—and before the 1867 Reform Act, that meant owners of private property—underwrote this public effort, though not uniformly across the country and not without objection.[14]

Between the 1830s and 1860s, debate about the franchise focused increasingly on the "fitness" of the working class to contribute to the social well-being of the nation as a whole. "Fitness" did not simply mean the ability to pay taxes based on the ownership of property; rather, it signified the capacity of working-class people to procure and maintain a home and demonstrate a degree of prudent household economy that resonated with middle-class norms.[15] Consequently, the definition of the "respectable and independent" workingman dominated the run-up to the 1867 Reform Act. Was such a man capable of exercising the privileges that the vote bestowed?[16] For some, know-how about careful financial management and Friendly Society membership proved the trustworthiness of the working-class and their propensity for character-building self-help.[17] Electoral reform shifted qualification for the vote from property ownership to property rental.[18] The 1867 Reform Act enshrined "respectability" though rate qualifications and residential stability.[19] Reformers hoped that extension of the franchise to the "respectable" working-class man would slowly dissolve the problem of class conflict.[20] Exclusion of the itinerant, dependent "residuum" from the electorate solidified the ideal of the domestic man with "a house, a wife, children, furniture and the habit of obeying the law."[21]

The idealized, respectable home was a haven of domesticity. When he sought to cast light on the homes hidden in the *London Shadows*, sometime editor of *The Builder* George Godwin wrote with pain and desolation at midcentury about the necessity of "obtaining for the suffering thousands of dwelling-places worthy of the name HOME, where the virtues and kindly feelings might be cultivated, and the household gods worthily set up."[22] In this, we see how homes and domesticity are linked. The former denotes a discrete space of attachments and obligations, distinct from the workplace; the latter was associated with a kind of mentality, encapsulating comfort and privacy for members of the nuclear family into a "single commanding concept (in English, home)."[23] Victorians acknowledged the long genealogy of domesticity, but an obsession with it crystallized in the mid-nineteenth century, when liberal visions characterized the English home as a place of retreat and refuge, the locus of strength and renewal.[24] Through the agency of the family, home was a place where self-disciplining parents would nurture their children into upstanding moral characters who might act as rational, responsible citizens of democratic society.[25] The *Manchester Times* summed it up in March 1876 asserting, "Home is not only the home of ratepaying and respectable citizenship, not only a place for enjoying necessary repose, but the home of the sacred and conjugal parental relationships, the neucleus [*sic*] whence spring, or should spring, the influence which intelligent beings exercise on others."[26]

The inclination toward refuge was buttressed by developments in the architectural design of working-class domestic space. Shared facilities (stairways, water pumps, and privies) in English courtyards were inimical to privacy and retreat. Insularity and disconnection meant that slum dwellers were not offered the opportunity to observe and absorb the lessons and habits that their more respectable middle-class peers had to offer. Domestic architecture moved away from this problematic model of communal space. The pattern and form varied across the urban landscape, but after midcentury it was more common to see adjacent housing units constructed along opposite sides of the street, each having enclosed sanitary facilities and separate rooms—the "home within"—that enabled inhabitants to withdraw and perform specific functions (sleep, cook, read, and defecate) in specific spaces.[27] Through the twin instruments of bylaws and slum clearance, shared facilities and spatial disconnection gradually ceded to privatized facilities and spatial connectivity.[28]

It was a typical contradiction of liberal modernity that the intense privacy of domesticity, and the struggle to secure and maintain it, provided some sort of structural stability for public life. "The congregation of families in their sacred separate spaces," note Karen Chase and Michael Levenson, "was identified as the paradoxical foundation of sociality. The delight in being happily apart offered itself as the basis for community."[29] This idealization concealed the layered and unstable complexity of private lives enacted within the home. Furthermore, for members of polite society, the home was not only a space of retreat. It also was an exhibition space for character, virtue, and prudence.[30]

Home was reconfigured as a potential space for the exercise of a third public health "liberalism": governmentality. Privacy itself was central to safeguarding cleanliness, health, and decency. The subterranean sanitary structures that were put in place in British cities from the 1840s neutralized the external threat posed by the filthy domestic spaces of the poor. It was possible to engineer these and other sorts of material technologies in a liberal way, because they were "designed with certain aspects of human freedom in mind."[31] Yet, as this chapter will demonstrate, the intrusion of disinfection into domestic space represented a tacit admission that these infrastructures could malfunction; that they might fail to circulate heat, air, water, and light adequately; or that they were absent altogether (indeed, the elusiveness of the perfect infrastructure propelled the desire for its attainment).

Disinfection also acknowledged the limits of isolation hospitals, which did not necessarily possess the capacity to accommodate all cases of infectious disease, as shown in chapter 4. In fact, the domestic sequestration of a patient in a working-class house was practically impossible without jeopardizing the health status of the rest of the family. Setting aside a sickroom forced a family to live in an even smaller number of rooms, a state of affairs that, according to Sheffield medical officer of health Dr. Francis Griffiths, "predisposes them to receive the infection."[32] Disinfection implicitly acknowledged how difficult it was to secure a domestic environment safe from the threat of infection.

As such, disinfection violated the very domesticity that it sought to shield. Reconsider the sickroom. Though the sickroom was the key repository of infection within the home and a natural focus for disinfection, it was a deeply significant space for other, nonbiological reasons. Miriam Bailin has argued that unlike all the other private spaces in the home, the sickroom was resistant to the gaze of both the household head and servants. It offered a haven to express emotions and thoughts about oneself that were otherwise censured in polite society. In other words, the sickroom was the ultimate *private* domestic space.[33] The state's increased propensity to disinfect took it not only into the sickroom but into other spaces of the home as well. Furnishings, bed linens, clothing, and a multitude of ancillary items of personal property such as books were subjected to the state's disinfecting powers. Through disinfection, the danger of infection was balanced with the accumulation and tidy arrangement of possessions in domestic space, which in itself was representative of moral uplift.[34]

The rest of this chapter explores how disinfection was shaped and reshaped into a technology that negotiated the ubiquitous threat from what was called "the debris of everyday living."[35] Historian William Coleman has observed that disinfection was the primary tool of Britain's antiquarantine position in the mid-nineteenth century.[36] Peter Baldwin argues that disinfection was a remarkably flexible intervention. It was sold as a classic quarantine measure because it admitted that contagious material could be conveyed in clothes and belongings.[37] For sanitarians, however, it neutralized emanations from putrefying matter. Baldwin's survey of the medical literature and legislation suggests that the 1860s witnessed the introduction of disinfection "in a more systematic manner." He describes disinfection as "one of the main strings in the Kochian bow . . . [whose] fortunes were revived with the recognition that it was supported and enhanced by the new [bacteriological] knowledge."[38] Michael Worboys briefly mentions that important changes in the specifics of disinfection took place with the integration of bacteriology into public health.[39] (Yet, he has also subsequently acknowledged that very few histories of Victorian public health reveal how science of a particular technology gets translated into practice.) Barring the odd throwaway comment, broad surveys by Anthony Wohl, F. B. Smith, and Dorothy Porter are silent on the topic of disinfection.[40] Many studies of local public health practice hardly mention disinfection. Neither Hardy's book on public health in Victorian London, Eyler's assessment of Arthur Newsholme's work as medical officer of health in Brighton, nor Niemi's examination of public health in Birmingham say very much about the theory or practice of disinfection.[41] In *The Great Stink of Paris*, David Barnes explores the adoption of disinfection in urban France. As with Baldwin and Worboys, Barnes suggests that from the 1880s disinfection practices integrated bacteriological findings with traditional methods of chemical application. Although by the century's end disinfection's responsiveness, mobility, and safety had achieved partial success, Barnes argues that obstacles and resistance to its implementation in Paris and elsewhere in France were overcome by a combination of educational campaigns and repeated use that familiarized the general public with it.[42]

To some extent, the British story is similar to the French. Part of what follows is devoted to sketching out the places where disinfection was and was not enacted, the objects and spaces that were disinfected, and the means used to free materials from infection. Reliance is unavoidably placed on statistics collected by the central and local state, which superimposed a grid of exactitude and certainty on the municipal practice of disinfection, which was, at best, patchy and incomplete. Disinfection was not practiced systematically across Britain, but it was carried out very intensively in many towns and cities.

## Materializing Domestic Infection

Disinfection has an extremely long history that Victorian scientific and medical writers loved to invoke. They would tell readers how Homer's Ulysses burned "pest-averting sulphur" to fumigate the rooms in which the bodies of dead suitors lay; how, in his 1552 *Boke or Counseill against the Disease commonly called the Sweate or Sweating Sickness*, Dr. John Caius advised the use of fires to purge infected air; and how, until recently, it had been common in criminal courts to place a bunch of rue to either side of the prisoner to purify the immediate surrounding air and prevent the spread of disease from jail. There were also frequent references to the formal adoption of fumigation in Parisian hospitals and British prisons at the end of the eighteenth century.[43] These historical allusions express an important rhetorical duality. In general terms, they augmented the veneration of disinfection and supported the continuation of long-held practices. However, their anecdotal and unprovable quality was equated with the "unblushing quackery" that bedeviled so much of the literature on disinfection.[44] In other words, while history protected the value of a venerable tradition, it also invited a more scientific approach to disinfection. It was hoped that experimentation would establish the ability of chemicals and physical processes to destroy specific disease threats.

Separating out the disinfection of private domestic space and material goods was important. Each required a different approach to the use of technology in spatial settings. It took some time for the reach of disinfection legislation to locate the internal space of the house. The disinfection of streets, drains, sewers, and yards was a common feature of the response to cholera between the 1830s and 1850s.[45] The most popular chemical applications were quicklime, chloride of lime, carbolic acid, sulfate of iron, perchloride of iron, and chloride of manganese.[46] The original intention was to sanitize the public environment in anticipation of an epidemic, although this form of disinfection was not only used during crises.[47] The normalization of disinfection was further solidified by the permissive Nuisances Removal Act of 1845 and subsequent amendments that allowed authorities to clean dirty premises and remove or remediate annoyances.[48]

Disinfection mostly was used to neutralize the nasty smells associated with the accumulation of filth, a product of overcrowded urban living and the unwanted waste of industrial processes. Interventions were made largely at the instigation of complaints from aggrieved neighbors. These limits—permissive legislation and dependence on a motivated citizenry—rendered disinfection paltry compensation for the lack of properly functioning drains and sewers and the infrequent removal of house refuse. The Common Lodging Houses (CLH) Acts of the 1850s therefore represented a key development, since keepers of lodging houses where an "infectious or contagious" illness had been present were required to call in the inspector of nuisances to assess the premises and carry out chemical disinfection of rooms.

Some local health boards confiscated and destroyed household items and clothes during epidemics, often to the consternation of owners. In other instances, bed linens and clothes were boiled.[49] However, the other innovation of the CLH Acts was to routinize the disinfection of material goods: blankets and bedclothes used by the infected lodger had to be cleansed and fumigated at the expense of the lodge-keeper. Financial compensation was given if the articles had to be destroyed.[50] The CLH Acts focused on a relatively small "residual" population that did not fall within the bounds of respectability; but the laws nevertheless marked a departure in that the disinfection of an individual's personal belongings, however marginalized that individual might be, was no longer an intervention that was associated purely with epidemic times.

A more diffuse population focus for disinfection was signaled in 1861 when John Simon, chief medical officer of the Medical Department of the Privy Council, detailed the measures that local authorities should take when threatened with epidemics. Simon argued that pursuance of interventions like disinfection in noncrisis times made prophylactic sense. He reiterated that lodging houses "always require particular attention," but that "proper precautions are equally proper for all classes of society." Vigilance, information, and advice needed to be especially forceful with poorer populations crowded into courts and alleys. Simon made some general recommendations about overcrowded living and ventilation that were little more than routine exhortations that lacked legislative teeth. He also set out to clarify a set of standard practices for the abatement of rotting organic matter, filthy cesspools and middens, and unclean premises. Such steps were already available to local authorities through the nuisance laws, although these, of course, remained permissive and uptake was far from uniform. Most revealing for the context in which disinfection became a routine municipal practice, Simon set out an agenda for the special precautions of cleanliness and disinfection of patients in a domestic setting:

> Discharges which it is proper to treat as infective, are those which come, in cases of small-pox, from the affected skin; in cases of cholera and typhoid fever, from the intestinal canal; in cases of diphtheria, from the nose and throat; likewise, in cases of any eruptive fever, the general exhalations of the sick. The caution which is necessary with regard to such matters must of course extend to whatever is imbued with them; so that bedding, clothing, towels and other articles, which have been in use by the sick, do not become sources of mischief.[51]

The opening sentence highlights the ambiguity associated with defining what was and was not "infective" in the early 1860s. Simon articulated "infective" in the sense conveyed by zymotic disease theory; namely, the diffusion of disease poisons emanating from dead tissue. Irrespective of how these poisons came about, it was their ability to permeate, penetrate, and cling—"imbue"—to the constituents of Victorian domestic space that concerned Simon.[52]

The guidelines that accompanied Simon's memorandum were remarkably specific. For the interior of houses, local authorities were advised to whitewash ceilings and walls with quicklime. Woodwork should be cleansed with soap and water, and then washed with a solution of chloride of lime. More noxious (and by implication, more effective) measures could be implemented in an empty, closed-up room by the use of sulfuric acid gas or chlorine gas for several hours. (Interestingly for subsequent developments, this process was also referred to as "disinfection" rather than "fumigation.") Linens were to be washed and boiled or soaked in a solution of either chloride of lime or Condy's fluid. Meanwhile, woolens, bedding, and clothing had to be either washed or exposed to a temperature of 210–50°F in a heat chamber for two or more hours. I will return to this last directive later.

Simon's 1861 memorandum was a remarkable feat in the sense that it ubiquitized risk and spatially intensified it at the same time. Any and all infective bodies, in the most intimate of domestic spaces, were legitimate targets for disinfection that was applied both to the atmosphere (through fumigation) and to material surfaces. In addition, initial steps had now been taken to transcribe as a state activity disinfecting practices that were more commonly associated with the management of the sickroom in the private domestic sphere.

Legislative authorization of these tactics came soon enough. The 1866 Sanitary Act enshrined the right of a local authority to disinfect property whenever a qualified medical practitioner sent in a certificate requesting it to do so. This was an important accommodation of private medical authority that preempted GPs' role as notifiers of infectious disease, as discussed in chapter 2. The act also permitted local authorities to build a "proper place" for the disinfection of household items. The intention of the 1866 act was underlined when Simon issued a memorandum in 1869 on the prevention of scarlet fever that unequivocally located patients' infectiousness in their fluid and solid oral and nasal discharges, breath, and the flakes and grains of dry skin that were shed after the early days of the disease. These emanations landed all about the sufferer's immediate environment and attached "more or less to all objects in the room."[53] Infection stubbornly lingered for an indefinite period in the most innocuous places, such as clothes, bed furniture, and all manner of household objects.[54]

The Sanitary Act was permissive—a classic case of the liberal state wanting to govern neither too much nor too little. Undoubtedly some local authorities used it to increase their disinfecting capacity.[55] Simon told the Royal Sanitary Commission (also in 1869) that local government should be forced to provide disinfecting facilities under the operation of a skilled officer.[56] In his judgment, all districts should have a permanent hospital to isolate the infected and should operate disinfecting apparatus. As we saw in chapter 3, isolation as a technique of liberal government did not go without challenge, because it forcibly redrew the sociocultural boundaries of domesticated health care and therapeutics, especially for children. Similar sentiments were expressed by Simon when he admitted candidly that legally mandated disinfection would "doubtless . . . interfere with certain hitherto permitted freedoms."[57]

Public health officials were acutely aware of this problem. Francis Bond, medical officer of health in Gloucestershire, thought about disinfection as a question of duties and rights, a contradiction of freedom that riddled Victorian liberalism:

> Looked at from the largest point of view, it is the right of society to protect itself from the incursion of infectious disease by such measures as can be shown to be necessary and practicable for this purpose, even though these measures may in some degree trench upon the liberty or personal interests of its individual members. Correlatively it will, therefore, be the duty of each member of society to give such assistance to the authorized public representatives of the community as may be required in order to make the general protection as efficient as possible. On the other hand, each individual member of society has the right to expect that, if he sacrifices his own liberty and interests to the extent above referred to, the public representatives of the community shall be compelled to afford him all the protection which is in their power against the attack of infectious disease.[58]

Bookending the 1860s, Simon's two memoranda represented a rematerialization of infection as much through the lens of domesticity as that of medical science. Microscopic grains of skin and dried mucus were granted a physical status that was neither intangibly miasmatic nor constituent of other solid human wastes that could be easily flushed away. Sanitary connectedness—that is, the linkage of homes to water supplies and sewer networks—offered a limited remedy for these dangerously obdurate, adhesive substances. Though modes of chemical disinfection offered the prospect of destruction (a prospect that later was revealed to be largely unfounded), this particular iteration of infective materiality was decidedly *not* ameliorable through existing infrastructural systems—sewers and drains—that were designed to function autonomously.

## Disinfection: Self-Regulated and Easily Managed

Disinfection activity was given fresh impetus once provincial authorities appointed medical officers of health from 1872, and once the 1875 Public Health Act consolidated and mandated disinfection-related legislation. By the end of that decade, many large cities disinfected an impressive number of household items. Manchester and Oldham disinfected about 5,000 and 6,000 articles per year, respectively.[59] Birmingham disinfected more than 30,000 items during the smallpox epidemic of 1883. Freakish though this number was at the time, the trend was definitely upward. By the mid-1890s Birmingham and Nottingham routinely disinfected more than 20,000 articles (figs. 5.1 and 5.2). Bristol, Liverpool, Manchester, Oldham, and Sheffield in the provinces, and Kensington and Whitechapel in London, built similar disinfecting capacities.[60] Disinfection in these cities was spurred by Sections 5 and 6 of the 1890 Infectious Disease (Prevention) Act, which gave increased powers to councils to disinfect bedding.[61]

Remarkable though some of these figures are, it would be wrong to imagine that activity in cities with enormous financial resources represents what was happening everywhere else.[62] A government survey of more than 1,600 sanitary districts in 1892 revealed that over half of the population (55 percent) was not served by disinfection facilities (table 5.1).[63] Urban districts had better coverage than rural ones, yet 40 percent of town dwellers still could not expect their local authority to disinfect their household belongings. When Sir Charles Cameron (Dublin's MOH) canvassed eighty provincial and metropolitan urban districts at the around this same time, he concluded that disinfection was imperfectly performed in many English towns.[64] Even in the hinterlands of extremely active cities, little or nothing was being done. Sanitary districts governing 36 percent of Nottinghamshire's urban population owned no disinfecting apparatus, and the urban districts of Lancashire and the West Riding of Yorkshire fared little better (table 5.2). Coverage in the countryside was extremely uneven.[65] Neither Leicestershire's nor Nottinghamshire's rural population—totaling almost two hundred thousand people—were served by disinfecting facilities.

Despite the supposed centrality of disinfection to the English system of infectious disease surveillance, government administrators exhibited little enthusiasm for systematically collating information to monitor enforcement and standardize procedures. The information in tables 5.1 and 5.2, for example, was collected for a report that was overwhelmingly concerned with hospital provision. Information about disinfection was logged alongside another sixty-four columns of data that predominantly recorded isolation capacity.

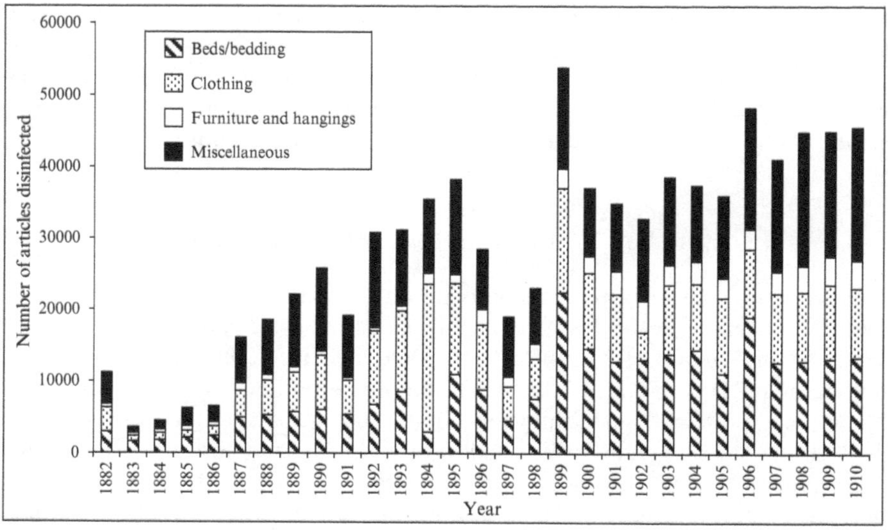


Figure 5.1. Number of articles disinfected, Nottingham, 1882–1910. Borough of Nottingham, *Annual Health Reports*.

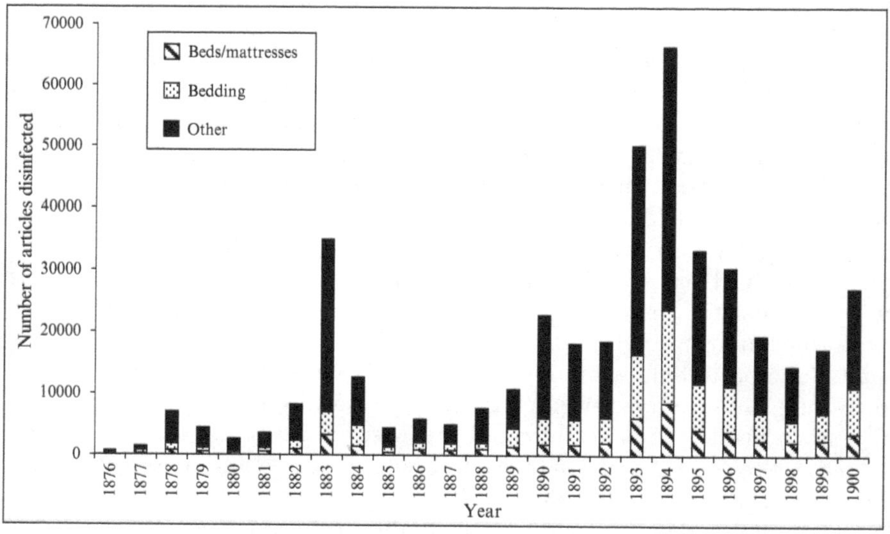


Figure 5.2. Number of articles disinfected, Birmingham, 1876–1900. City of Birmingham, *Annual Health Reports*.

As with many other forms of public health activity, disinfection practice was left in the hands of localities and was heavily circumscribed across large swaths of the country. Some of the big cities apart, it was not carried out in a particularly methodical way, as some historians have assumed. Many possible factors

Table 5.1. Population covered by disinfection methods in rural and urban sanitary districts, provincial England and Wales, 1892

| | Rural | | Urban | | Total | |
|---|---|---|---|---|---|---|
| Method | 1891 Population (thousands) | Percent | 1891 Population (thousands) | Percent | 1891 Population (thousands) | Percent |
| Fumigation | 190 | 2.4 | 433 | 2.7 | 623 | 2.6 |
| Dry air | 447 | 5.6 | 2,626 | 16.1 | 3,073 | 12.7 |
| Moist air[a] | 0 | 0.0 | 39 | 0.2 | 39 | 0.2 |
| Steam | 314 | 4.0 | 6,311 | 38.8 | 6,626 | 27.4 |
| Other | 0 | 0.0 | 31 | 0.2 | 31 | 0.1 |
| Unknown[b] | 191 | 2.4 | 349 | 2.1 | 539 | 2.2 |
| None | 6,782 | 85.6 | 6,496 | 39.9 | 13,279 | 54.8 |
| Total | 7,924 | 100.0 | 16,285 | 100.0 | 24,210 | 100.0 |

*Source*: House of Commons Parliamentary Papers, 1895, *Return of Provision for Isolation Hospitals* (cd. 28).

[a] Usually involved placing a pan of water in a dry-air chamber.

[b] Indicates the definite occurrence of some form of disinfection, but either the statistical return does not sufficiently determine the method used (e.g., "an oven," Trowbridge USD, Wiltshire) or details about the system listed (e.g., Dr. Schollick's patent used in Kingston USD, Surrey) could not be traced.

account for this patchiness. The legislation allowed for a high degree of flexibility, and, as we saw in chapter 2, some districts' politicians and medical officers were more creative and proactive than others.[66] The adoption of infectious disease notification stimulated more disinfecting work and often prompted a local authority to invest in disinfection facilities.[67] Provision of an isolation hospital in a remote location was an advantage. Disinfecting apparatus could be situated conveniently in hospitals (indeed, isolation hospitals created their own voracious demand for disinfection). To illustrate, Solihull Rural Sanitary District (RSD) in Warwickshire had a twenty-six-bed isolation hospital equipped with a steam disinfector. The aggregation of infected things at a hospital was unlikely to arouse local opposition given the prior aggregation of infected bodies.[68]

Variable levels of financial investment determined the strength of personnel and the alacrity with which technology was adopted. The disinfection enterprise was run like a military operation in places like Leeds, Liverpool, and Manchester, where the number of employees ran well into double figures. But investment in most other districts was far less conspicuous and a meager staff often had to make do with outdated equipment, fewer vans for transporting articles, and an altogether less rigorous approach.[69] Efficacy was partially dependent on the personal qualities and foibles of the staff employed, as was the case in other realms of the inspectorial state.[70]

Table 5.2. Provision of disinfection apparatus in rural and urban sanitary districts in five English counties, 1892

| County | District type (number) | Total population 1891 (thousands) | Population covered by disinfection: Number (thousands) | Percent[a] |
|---|---|---|---|---|
| Lancashire | RSD (22) | 316 | 56 | 17.6 |
| | USD (131) | 3,670 | 2,548 | 69.4 |
| Leicestershire | RSD (10) | 138 | 0 | 00.0 |
| | USD (10) | 230 | 193 | 83.7 |
| Nottinghamshire | RSD (7) | 153 | 0 | 00.0 |
| | USD (16) | 352 | 224 | 63.8 |
| Warwickshire | RSD (12) | 158 | 55 | 34.9 |
| | USD (11) | 687 | 662 | 96.4 |
| Yorkshire West Riding | RSD (27) | 367 | 99 | 27.1 |
| | USD (142) | 2,062 | 1,447 | 70.2 |
| Total, five counties | RSD (78) | 1,132 | 210 | 18.6 |
| | USD (310) | 7,00 | 5,074 | 72.5 |

*Source:* House of Commons Parliamentary Papers, 1895, *Return of Provision for Isolation Hospitals* (cd. 28).

[a] This refers to the percentage of these districts' total populations that was covered by a local authority's disinfection facilities.

Some local authorities did not help their cause by charging for disinfection, though this was discontinued either when it was found to deter the general public or when it proved difficult to recover expenses.[71] Resistance to the removal of articles for disinfection was occasionally reported, especially when it became more commonplace after the introduction of disease notification.[72] But such instances were few and far between, as confirmed by the oral historian of working-class health culture of this period, Lucinda McCray Beier.[73] According to Nottingham's health committee, the reduction in the number of disinfected items after the initial spurt in 1882 had nothing to do with any sort of resistance; rather, householders had heeded advice to remove furniture from the sickroom at the beginning of an episode of infectious illness.[74] Of course, this also makes interpretation of data about the amount of disinfection hazardous: for example, a decrease in activity might be due to municipal laxity on the one hand, or greater vigilance of sickroom rituals by the general public on the other. Nor does the comment of Nottingham's health committee about greater householder awareness in the early 1880s explain why it developed such a remarkable thirst for disinfection in later decades (fig. 5.1).

Equally significant for the acceptance of disinfection was that technologies were designed and deployed to minimize intrusion into the running of the household. A remarkable transformation in the apparatus of disinfection took place from the 1860s to the end of the century. Disinfection took on freedom's mantle, becoming self-regulating, highly risk-averse, and unobtrusive. That disinfection assumed these characteristics at all is attributable to the resolution of a fundamental question that public health practitioners repeatedly asked themselves: can disinfection be carried out on personal property while leaving that property undamaged?

The search for a practical solution to this dilemma was a restless negotiation between the socially contingent nature of public health practice, laboratory experimentation, and the problematic implementation of science in the field. Limiting damage to household items was an important consideration in the popularization of disinfection, as the *Daily News* pointed out to its readers in the mid-1880s:

> In our great towns and cities where the clothes and garments of the poor require cleansing from germs it is evident that if the work of disinfection is to prove of economical and satisfactory nature it must provide for the saving of the materials and for their restoration in uninjured form to their owners. . . . Efficient disinfection, especially of the clothes of the sick poor, should be a feature of the municipal arrangements in every city.[75]

Economy and efficiency—the twin demands of the market for unhindered labor, and of the budget-conscious ratepayer for value for money—made the safety of disinfection a political necessity.

A third political consideration, of course, was the material and practical worth of possessions to the household—"the clothes of the sick poor" mentioned above. Some working-class families were known to stow away their better clothing to avoid the disinfector's grasp.[76] More significantly, the material possessions of the poor, including clothes, had speculative value, since they could be taken to the pawnbroker in times of desperate need (times that were often the end of every week for many families).[77] But in addition to all sorts of clothing, a wide range of household articles were disinfected, and, as Beier has pointed out, the destruction of useful possessions was not only wasteful; their replacement was a financial burden.[78] Table 5.3 breaks out some of the Nottingham data from the early 1880s that was summarized in figure 5.1. The data in this table were only made possible by the form of contract that householders commonly entered into with health departments. Before removal to the disinfecting facility, householders checked their assembled possessions against a preprinted inventory that was filled out by the disinfector. After disinfection, the operator of the machine at the disinfection station checked the inventory before the disinfected articles were dispatched in the van. The householder signed off the inventory when the articles were safely returned in an undamaged state.[79]

This series of visual and paper-based checks and balances gave individuals and households a material existence beyond private space. As a mobile documentary technology that had to be verified by the householder, the inventory allowed for the retrieval of that existence. The contract laid out a conduit of

Table 5.3. Disinfection of household items, Nottingham, 1882–87

| Item | 1882 | 1883 | 1884 | 1885 | 1886 | 1887 | 5-year mean |
|---|---|---|---|---|---|---|---|
| Beds | 323 | 202 | 208 | 248 | 301 | 754 | 339 |
| Mattresses | 381 | 273 | 244 | 420 | 378 | 874 | 428 |
| Bolsters | 221 | 128 | 127 | 193 | 232 | 509 | 235 |
| Pillows | 697 | 363 | 370 | 494 | 514 | 1,119 | 593 |
| Blankets | 705 | 483 | 624 | 501 | 608 | 921 | 640 |
| Sheets | 174 | 67 | 60 | 116 | 185 | 307 | 152 |
| Quilts | 434 | 98 | 134 | 182 | 193 | 472 | 252 |
| Bedding total | 2,935 | 1,614 | 1,767 | 2,154 | 2,411 | 4,956 | 2,639 |
| Dresses | 392 | 100 | 97 | 156 | 146 | 364 | 209 |
| Jackets | 194 | 73 | 90 | 124 | 106 | 339 | 154 |
| Flannels | 232 | 84 | 79 | 55 | 134 | 430 | 169 |
| Coats | 448 | 73 | 53 | 96 | 171 | 315 | 193 |
| Vests | 319 | 45 | 31 | 113 | 113 | 191 | 135 |
| Trousers | 350 | 61 | 71 | 81 | 122 | 217 | 150 |
| Dressing gowns | 34 | 20 | 18 | 14 | 22 | 41 | 25 |
| Skirts | 426 | 114 | 95 | 111 | 144 | 501 | 232 |
| Stockings | 639 | 130 | 374 | 75 | 150 | 748 | 353 |
| Bonnets | 0 | 6 | 4 | 1 | 37 | 110 | 26 |
| Hats | 111 | 17 | 34 | 32 | 50 | 161 | 68 |
| Shawls | 177 | 48 | 79 | 86 | 121 | 257 | 128 |
| Clothing total | 3,322 | 771 | 1,025 | 944 | 1,316 | 3,674 | 1,842 |
| Carpets | 236 | 145 | 195 | 374 | 364 | 615 | 322 |
| Curtains | 82 | 118 | 122 | 133 | 88 | 224 | 128 |
| Cushions | 62 | 25 | 61 | 69 | 71 | 143 | 72 |
| Rugs | 62 | 28 | 35 | 37 | 17 | 38 | 36 |
| Mats | 60 | 55 | 72 | 60 | 22 | 44 | 52 |
| Hassocks | 7 | 9 | 7 | 14 | 10 | 27 | 12 |
| Furniture/ hangings total | 509 | 380 | 492 | 687 | 572 | 1,091 | 622 |
| Books | 17 | 148 | 15 | 36 | 77 | 98 | 65 |
| Wrappers | 29 | 29 | 30 | 26 | 33 | 97 | 41 |
| Sundries | 4,337 | 588 | 1,082 | 2,316 | 2,037 | 6,078 | 2,740 |
| Miscellaneous total | 4,383 | 765 | 1,127 | 2,378 | 2,147 | 6,273 | 2,846 |
| | 11,149 | 3,530 | 4,411 | 6,163 | 6,446 | 15,994 | 7,949 |

*Source:* Nottinghamshire Archives, CA/HE/2/1/1, Borough of Nottingham, *Annual Reports on the Health of Nottingham, 1882–7.*

publicity that ran directly into and out of the interior space of the home, thus destabilizing any given notion of what was, and could ever be, "private." In this sense, the visit of the disinfection crew was no less of a public shame than a trip to the pawnbroker.[80] The inventory also protected both the householder and the health department, since it was a testament to the worth of the possessions to the household, however small and insignificant those items might have been to an outside observer. It was also a tacit admission that the disinfecting process could be damaging.

The problem of material damage was associated with another knotty question for public health practitioners: what *is* the most effective method of disinfection? The answer to this was far from clear-cut, and there was no single defining moment in which the parameters of a successful disinfecting process were agreed upon. Scientific uncertainty about the properties of various disinfecting methods was indivisible from sociopolitical concerns about the removal and destruction of infective debris from the homes and belongings of the working classes.[81] Even with the advent of a reliable test for a substance's disinfecting power in the early twentieth century, this uncertainty did not go away.[82]

Although chemical agents had been shown to arrest putrefaction and treat sewage, they could not be used on many household items for obvious caustic reasons. At the beginning of the Victorian period, very little was known for sure about the disinfecting properties of one alternative, heat. The complete incineration of personal property was one way of using heat to disinfect, but too drastic; it was costly to property owners and a clear deterrent to public acceptance.[83] Many articles of clothing could be washed and then boiled in water, but this too was not a viable option for many items in Victorian homes that offered safe haven to infection, such as heavy blankets, mattresses, rugs, carpets, curtains, furs, books, and certain items of clothing. Excessive atmospheric heat also had many drawbacks when applied to items such as these. It could either scorch or parch textiles, rendering them brittle and weak. Stains might fix. Adhesives, waxes, and varnishes could melt. Heat sometimes altered the color and gloss of dyed goods. Woolen materials would shrink and felt. The key, then, was to find an affordable method of heat disinfection that could be used on as many materials as possible and that was powerful enough to destroy the most resistant infectious agents. The effort to find a solution spanned more than half a century, and the search had begun well before local government became seriously interested in disinfecting household property.

The first scientific experiments on disinfection with heat were carried out with vaccine lymph in the 1830s by the physician, chemical manufacturer, and distinguished Manchester citizen William Henry.[84] Henry's explorations initially were prompted in the 1820s, when Manchester's merchant community became anxious that plague fomites were being imported inside bales of Egyptian raw cotton, but he soon abandoned these preliminary inquiries. Henry's interest in disinfection was revived in the face of the potentially devastating arrival of cholera in the early 1830s. His hypothetical reasoning about the disinfecting potential of heat drew on both natural history and chemistry, circles of thought that overlapped in Manchester's early nineteenth-century scientific community. Influential to Henry's thinking was Alexander Russell's *Natural History of Aleppo*, which described how the progress of plague was halted in the hottest months of July. Equally helpful to his ideas were experimental observations that showed simple gases were unchanged unless temperatures were raised above 212°F, and that many organic and inorganic compounds could be converted into different substances upon exposure to heat.

Since it was entirely beyond his "power to try the agency of heat on those contagions which propagate the formidable diseases," Henry explored the closest tangible material he could get his hands on: smallpox vaccine lymph. Vaccine lymph did contain cowpox, but Henry's experiments provided no more than an analogous inference for the action of heat. He had some of his Mancunian medical acquaintances vaccinate healthy children: one arm with fresh vaccine lymph, and the other arm with vaccine lymph that had been heated. These trials (a term used by Henry himself) demonstrated that the lymph was rendered completely inert by exposure to a temperature of 140°F. The trial results were coupled with a set of experiments that showed items of clothing made from cotton, silk, wool, and fur were unharmed after exposure to a temperature of 180°F for three hours. He concluded that 212°F was the minimum temperature required to disinfect items of clothing by heat.

Directing his lymph-contagion analogy toward the impending cholera threat, Henry recommended the construction of dry-heat chambers at seaports. Such an apparatus—it is unclear whether it was ever built—would sit in a wall so that the operator could make no mistake keeping infected and disinfected articles separate (fig. 5.3). The two-inch space between the inner and outer cast-iron cases was heated with steam generated by a coal boiler. A tap at the top of the chamber allowed air and uncondensed steam to escape, while a pipe carried off any "undecomposed infectious effluvia" to the flue. Henry did not describe any means of thermostatic control, and the internal temperature of the chamber could only be measured by inserting a thermometer through a hole in one of the doors.[85] Henry himself thought 250°F might be a safe temperature for the preservation of textiles and furs, but this upper bound was only later affirmed outside the laboratory through extensive trial-and-error use of heat chambers in hospitals (to disinfect patients' clothes) and workhouses (to delouse pauper clothes) in the 1850s.[86] Thus amended, Henry's recommendations carried through to the 1860s and clearly formed the basis of Simon's guidelines in 1861 that were discussed above.

As far as I am aware, no further experiments on the disinfecting capabilities of heat were carried out in England until 1870–71, when another Manchester-based chemist, Frederick Crace-Calvert, showed that some forms of "protoplasmic" or "germ" life (what Crace-Calvert called "black vibrios" observed in putrid meat fluid) could survive exposure to temperatures in excess of 300°F.[87] Crace-Calvert had been part of Manchester's scientific community since the mid-1840s and was a well-established manufacturer of carbolic acid and other disinfecting products.[88] Nevertheless, the potential significance of his laboratory contribution to disinfection practice was downplayed by the City of London's medical officer of health and public analyst Henry Letheby, who deferred to the conclusions of the Académie

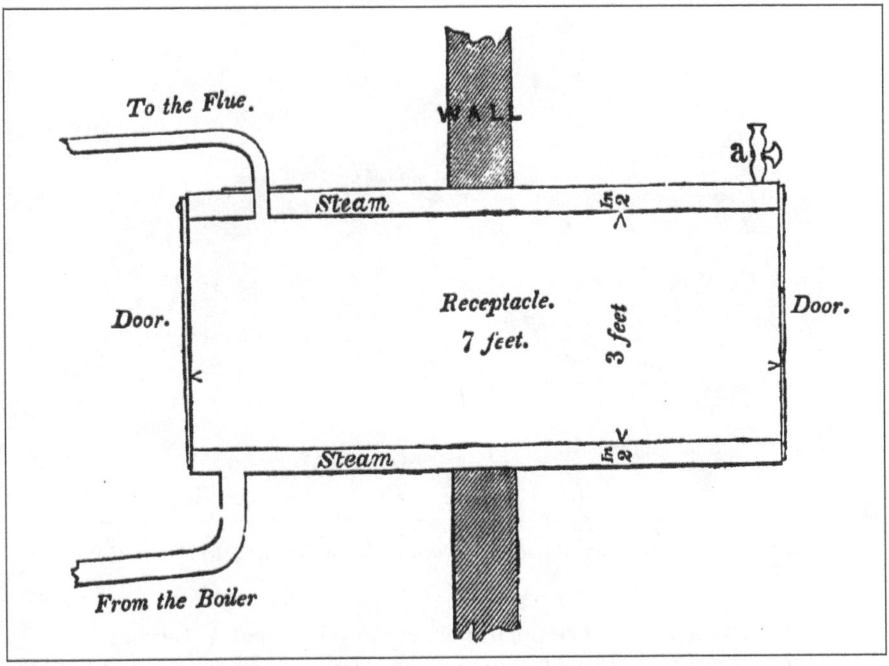


Figure 5.3. William Henry's heat disinfecting apparatus. Henry, "Letter from Dr. Henry," 206. Reproduced by permission from Taylor & Francis.

des Sciences in Paris following the infamous spontaneous generation controversy in 1864. It was from this controversy that Pasteur's version of germ theory emerged victorious.[89] In an extensive article in the *Lancet* in 1873, Letheby recapitulated the Académie's pertinent conclusions: "None of the lower organisms or their germs would resist in air a temperature of 130°C (= 266° Fahr.), and in liquid a temperature of 110°C (= 230° Fahr.)," adding that "in most cases in fact, a temperature of 180° Fahr. is sufficient to destroy infusorial life."[90] Letheby was otherwise extremely reverential toward Crace-Calvert's writings on chemical disinfectants. However, in his capacity as City of London medical officer he had used dry heat on almost two thousand articles during the recent smallpox epidemic and was convinced that 240–50°F was sufficient to kill "common contagia," regardless of that temperature's lack of impact on Crace-Calvert's mysterious black vibrio.

Letheby's comments came at a time when a number of dry-heat disinfectors were hitting the market.[91] George Fraser demonstrated his newly patented dry-heat disinfector for clothing at the Medical Officers of Health Association in London in 1870. The disinfector was designed as a brick oven, heated from underneath by a coke fire. The iron carriage used to transport the clothes was driven directly into the disinfecting chamber, meaning that employees did not need to handle infected clothing and the carriage itself was disinfected during the disinfecting process (fig. 5.4).[92]

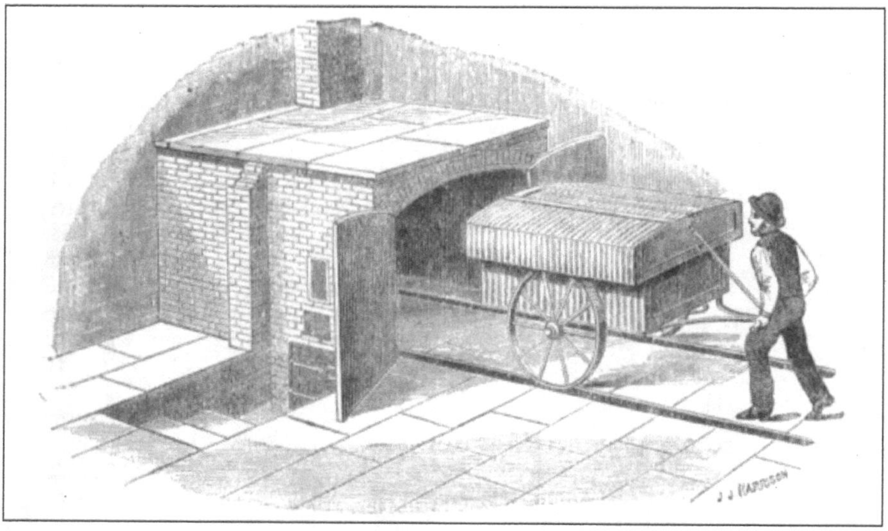

Figure 5.4. Fraser's disinfecting apparatus. Priestley, "Disinfectors and Disinfectants," 19.

Fraser's became the most popular machine in London and elsewhere, particularly when a portable version was introduced. There was no shortage of alternatives. Most of the other machines, like Thomas Bradford's, were constructed to further minimize the risk of infection to the operator by requiring that the disinfection building be partitioned into "infected" and "disinfected" spaces, as per William Henry's design back in the early 1830s (fig. 5.5). But with a potentially massive demand for the disinfection of thousands of items during epidemics, these machines came under intense scrutiny and were shown to have fundamental flaws. Exhaustive tests carried out in the 1880s with accurate pyrometers showed that the machines' thermometers rarely provided a precise reading of the temperature inside the chamber. To some extent that was an academic problem, since almost all of the machines failed to maintain an equal temperature throughout the chamber anyway. Meanwhile, the hot dry air could not penetrate bulky items such as mattresses. These deficiencies frustrated practitioners, because the maintenance of a consistent temperature over a number of hours required the skill and attention of a conscientious operator. To counter the possibility of human error, it was desirable that the disinfecting apparatus "should be self-regulating and self-registering . . . and, therefore, be easily managed."[93]

One dry-heat device that partially addressed these issues was invented by William Ransom, physician to the Nottingham General Hospital. Ransom turned his attention to disinfection after two of his children died from scarlet fever. In 1870 he designed a self-regulating gas-heated disinfecting stove for clothing and bedding. It was easier to keep a uniform temperature in such appliances because the temperature was regulated by the pressure of the gas. Ransom's prototype was located at the hospital, and one of its attractions was that the hospital

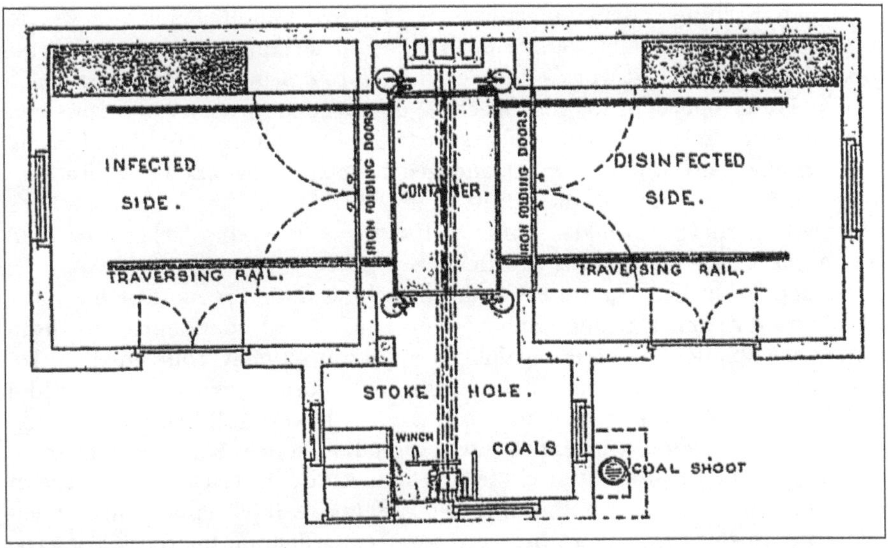


Figure 5.5. Bradford's Patent "Safety" steam disinfecting apparatus. Parsons, "Report on Disinfection by Heat," following page 272.

nurses were able to operate it after only brief instruction, thus dispensing altogether with the services and expense of an experienced stoker or engineer.[94]

These core principles of self-regulation and ease of management were maintained as steam disinfection gradually replaced dry heat in the 1880s. Historians have suggested that steam disinfection was only adopted after Robert Koch and his colleagues at the Imperial Office of Hygiene demonstrated its superiority to chemicals and hot air, research that was published in 1881.[95] Contemporary accounts would seem to affirm this view. Here, for example, is Leicester's medical officer of health Joseph Priestley describing how German laboratory work was unproblematically translated into English public health practice: "An improvement [to the hot-air, dry-heat method] was suggested in the form of moist heat or steam, which was experimentally proved by Koch and others to be a more powerful germicide than dry heat. The practical work of the bacteriologist was accepted, and steam under pressure was accordingly used by Mr. Washington Lyon in his patent Steam Disinfector."[96]

In fact, Washington Lyon's disinfector was in use *before* Koch's research was published. Lyon was a partner in a London firm of fabric bleachers, cleaners, and calenderers.[97] In his capacity as chair of the local sanitary committee, in 1867 Lyon provided the general public with free chemical disinfectants during a cholera outbreak. He became more interested in the disinfection process in the late 1870s when his firm was asked by a steamship company to rid its ships of vermin allegedly brought aboard by immigrants. This led to a patent in 1880 for a steam disinfector used at the Lyon's Old Kent Road premises and on the Metropolitan Asylum Board's smallpox hospital ship, the *Endymion*.

Lyon's machine was manufactured by Manlove, Alliott, Fryer and Co. in Nottingham, a well-established company that made municipal refuse destructors. The machine had wheels and could be carted around by just one horse (unlike Fraser's portable dry-heat machine that needed two horses). It consisted of an inner chamber and an outer jacket (fig. 5.6). Articles were placed in the hermetically sealed inner chamber, and steam pressure was raised to 20 lbs./in.$^2$ to give an internal temperature of 270°F. After disinfection, the inner chamber's steam was discharged, while steam at 30 lbs./in.$^2$ in the outer jacket prevented condensation and the spoiling of articles.

Heated steam had been used in the bleaching trade for most of the nineteenth century, but it is unclear how Lyon could be so confident of its disinfecting capabilities.[98] These capabilities were indisputably confirmed by Dr. Franklin Parsons, who conducted a series of important experiments for the Local Government Board in 1884. Parsons's results were still being cited thirty years later and found a receptive international audience. For example, when the prospect of an invasion of cholera prompted the American Public Health Association to set up a committee on disinfectants, its 1886 report relied extensively on Parsons's work. Parsons's three-way experimental matrix of bacteria, disinfection method, and materials established a sort of sliding scale for disinfecting efficiency.[99] Using both laboratory methods and operational disinfecting machines in situ, he assessed the impact of dry heat, boiling water, current steam, and steam under pressure on anthrax, swine fever (it was believed the mode of transmission of swine fever replicated that of scarlet fever and smallpox in humans), and tuberculosis. In the laboratory, steam heated to 212°F destroyed all these bacilli within five minutes. However, because infective matter penetrates and resides deep in the fillings of pillows and mattresses, Parsons also tested which forms of heat most successfully disinfected various materials with the least damage.

Disinfection with steam under pressure came out on top.[100] It had many advantages over dry heat. It did not take as long to reach an optimum temperature that was also uniformly distributed throughout the chamber. Time compression was important for municipalities contemplating large-scale disinfection operations because it saved on costs, increased throughput, and thus reduced potential friction with the general public. In the two years 1887–88, the hot-air apparatus in Nottingham worked around the clock, and, remarkably, its fire was not extinguished for nearly two years. The medical officer of health estimated that a disinfector using steam under pressure could manage in thirty minutes what took the dry-heat machine four hours.[101] For mattresses and bedding in particular, a quick turnaround catered to the needs of poor families who, in many cases, possessed only one bed. Dry heat required a higher temperature to penetrate bulky items, which partly explained why steam could be used on a wider range of materials without destroying them (leather was an exception).[102]

Lyon's portable and fixed machines were used widely from the mid-1880s, but other manufacturers entered the fray, including Benham and Sons from London, Salford's Thomas Bradford, and Goddard's from Nottingham (the last

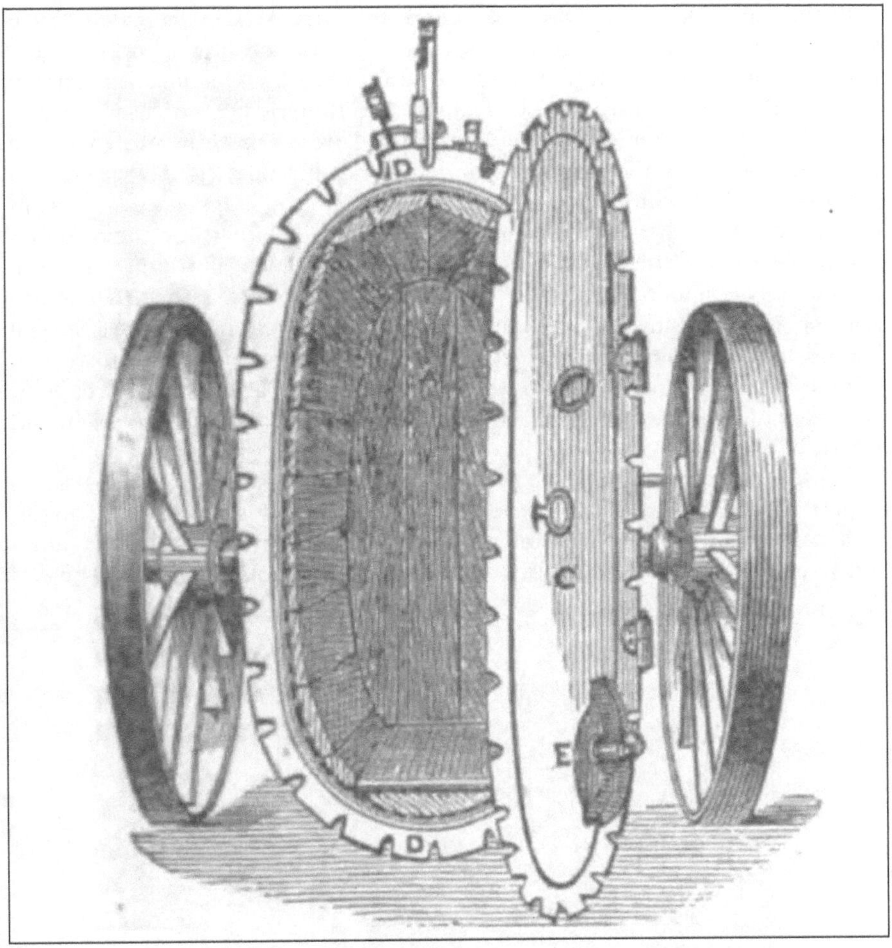

Figure 5.6. The Washington Lyon portable steam disinfector. "Disinfecting by Steam," 159.

became embroiled in a patent dispute with Washington Lyon, which Lyon eventually won).[103] These machines differed in many respects. For example, the heating chambers included elliptical, cylindrical, and box shapes. Competition heightened the threshold of innovation, and instrumentation continually was being introduced to either diminish the degree of human supervision that was required, make the technology legible to an operator with minimal training, or improve the throughput of the disinfecting process. Two gauge dials indicated the correspondence of temperature and pressure readings, for example. Lyon also introduced a vacuum at the beginning of the disinfection process (to hasten the heating of the chamber) and at the end (to shorten the drying time).[104]

In the mid-1890s, John Thresh, an entrepreneurial MOH from Chelmsford, began to use steam generated from a measured solution of calcium chloride, which had a boiling point above that of water (225°F). This meant it was no longer necessary to control the steam above atmospheric pressure as with other machines.[105] A wheel on the top at the front of Thresh's machine turned a valve that either admitted the steam or shunted it into the flue (fig. 5.7). The danger posed by the accumulation of steam under pressure disappeared because in Thresh's machine the stream was always free to escape either into the chamber or directly into the flue. Thus, close supervision was practically done away with, and the only skill an operator needed was the ability to turn a wheel. The effectiveness of Thresh's disinfector was rubber-stamped by the *Lancet's* 1896 Special Commission on Disinfection, which almost fell over itself in a rush to recommend it, on the grounds of its proven ability to destroy bacteria, its affordability, its remarkable speed (a disinfection cycle between forty and sixty minutes), and its ease of use.[106]

These qualities really were the point of the transformation of municipal disinfection of household goods from the 1860s, when the materiality of infection was repackaged as a threat to Victorian domestic life. Understanding the creation and re-creation of the disinfection chamber and its mobile extensions makes

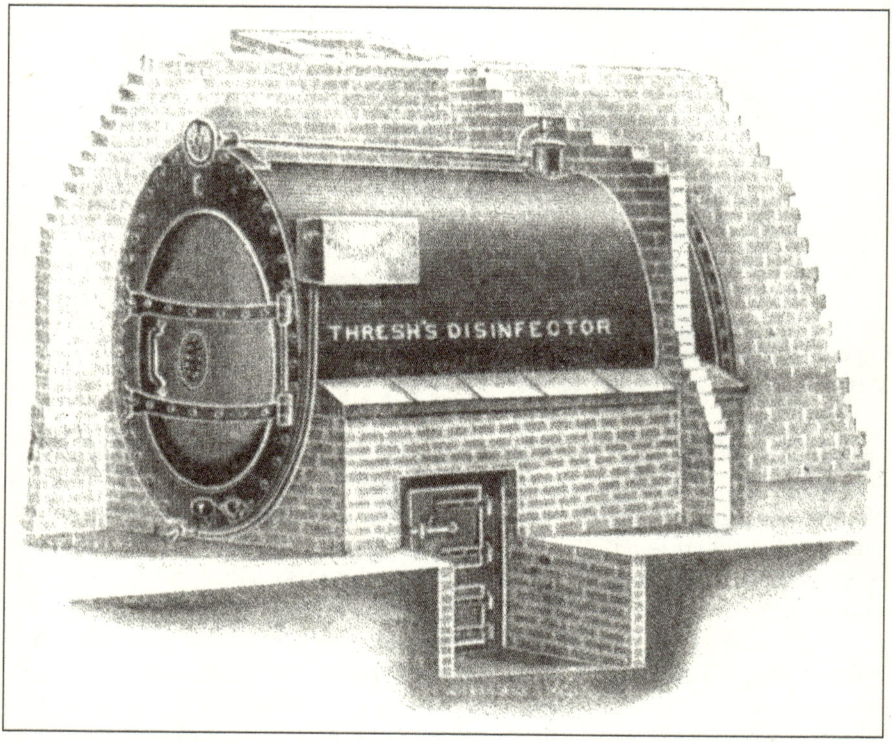


Figure 5.7. Thresh's steam disinfector. Barwise, "Disinfection by Steam," 197.

the public's lack of disdain for disinfection far more comprehensible than do explanations that blithely emphasize increasing familiarity with the procedure and the mystical power of medical science to explicate the action of germs. Ease of use, portability, and the effective means of destruction were predicated on the political recognition that basic household items were financially and socially valuable to poor families, particularly amid a burgeoning culture of domesticity.

## Social Relations in the Domesticated Laboratory

Washing floors and walls with a liquid solution of carbolic acid or chloride of lime was recognized in public health circles as the most effective chemical disinfectant. But these chemicals were impractical to use in domestic space given that they damaged surfaces and objects and caused great discomfort to those using them. A troubling indicator of this was that the sponges used to wipe disinfectants on walls turned brittle and disintegrated.[107] As such, the most common way to disinfect a room was through fumigation with vaporized chemicals such as sulfur, chlorine, carbolic acid, and iodine.[108] The two supposed and long-held objects of fumigation were disinfection of the air and disinfection of surfaces of the room, including furnishings. Fumigation was being openly questioned—indeed ridiculed—in some quarters by the early 1870s.[109] It was discredited further by Robert Koch, who demonstrated that sulfur dioxide had a very limited ability to destroy bacteria in a gastight gasket.[110]

Composing a reliable picture of house disinfection activity across mid-Victorian Britain is extremely difficult—so difficult, in fact, that it is almost impossible to evaluate the credibility of Peter Baldwin's contention that disinfection became more "systematic" after the 1860s. As mentioned above, there was no routine collection of information by central government. Consistent data that reveal trends over time are hard to extract from disparate sources; certainly there is no such data reaching back to the 1860s. A survey about the workings of the 1855 Metropolis Local Management Act partially revealed the extent of house disinfection in London between 1856 and 1870: St. Marylebone disinfected 817 homes in this period; St. Luke's 149; Poplar 679. In the early 1880s, Manchester disinfected around 600 houses and more than 2,000 rooms every year; corresponding numbers for Oldham were 450 and 1,300.[111] Though not completely meaningless, it is tricky to infer a great deal from these statistics without knowing the precise local context in which the disinfections were carried out, how many homes were deemed to be at risk, and what was meant by "disinfection" from one place to another.

Disinfection activity in Birmingham, for example, shadowed the rise and fall of infectious disease notification. During the period of voluntary notification (1878–89), the homes of all known infectious patients were disinfected (fig. 5.8). It is unclear whether this continued after 1889 because the health department began reporting the number of notifications for individual people rather than the number of homes in which infection occurred. However, disinfections

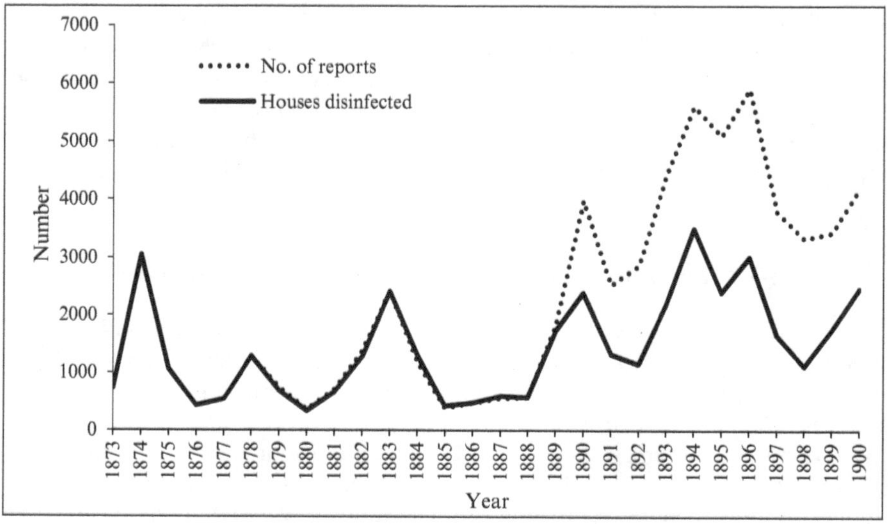


Figure 5.8. Reports of infectious disease and disinfection of houses, Birmingham, 1873–1900. Birmingham Medical Officer of Health *Annual Reports, 1873–1900.* From 1889, the number of reports are the total of all notified cases of individuals. Before that date, reports are the number of houses from which infectious cases were reported.

do still follow the underlying peaks and troughs of notifications after 1889, so it is possible that the post-1889 notifications simply count multiple cases in the same households.

In most places up to 1900, house "disinfection" usually involved fumigation, which was carried out regardless of the disease notified. A series of important experiments in the early 1890s, yet again in Manchester, confirmed that all forms of fumigation were ineffective against the most lethal of diseases, tuberculosis. These experiments were initiated by Arthur Ransome, who brought together a group of doctors to his home in the leafy south Manchester suburb of Bowden in Cheshire.[112] Medical staff from Manchester's Hospital for Consumption (which was near Ransome's home), pathologists Dr. Julius Dreschfeld and Sheridan Delépine of the Owens College Pathological Laboratory, and Manchester's medical officer of health John Tatham gathered to discuss how to go about preventing the spread of tuberculosis in the city and to test the efficacy of disinfection in what they called Manchester's "tuberculously-infected houses."[113]

The experimental procedures began when hospital cases were reported to Tatham (there was no tuberculosis notification at this point, a topic addressed in chapter 6). Tatham then directed his staff to fumigate the houses of any of these patients who were in the advanced stages of tuberculosis, or whose sputum contained tuberculosis bacilli.[114] Meanwhile, Delépine cultivated pure bacilli (human and avian) and bacilli from the sputum of the hospital patients. In the initial experiments, these bacilli were cultured onto strips of sterilized wallpaper, but later on ordinary paper was used. Glass capsules containing these papers were then handed to the municipal disinfecting team, which then exposed the samples to euchlorine vapors for two hours (euchlorine is produced when hydrochloric acid is poured onto potassium chlorate). The fumigated strips of paper then made their way back to the laboratory and were used to inoculate rabbits and guinea pigs. The animals were also inoculated with various other cultivations that had remained in the laboratory untouched, sterilized by heat, dried in the air and exposed to light, or dried in the dark. Delépine assessed the degree of tubercular infection in the animals' lymphatic glands. Euchlorine failed to disinfect the six strips of wallpaper that had been infected with pure cultivations of human tuberculosis bacilli. Subsequent experiments with other chemical agents confirmed that fumigation with sulfuric acid and chlorine also was "practically useless," doubtless a very worrying finding to the very many MOHs who still used it.[115]

Ransome's and Delépine's negative experimental results caused them to change how they referred to the vaporization of chemicals: the process called "disinfection" in 1893 became "fumigation" in 1895. The *Lancet* took to mocking the "so-called disinfection by sulphur fumes," as "little better than a superstitious rite or incantation."[116] Fumigation's ailing reputation was further damaged by Delépine's demonstration of the disinfecting properties of sunlight, yet another confirmation of Koch's laboratory research.[117] On the one hand, cultures that were left to languish in a dark laboratory took months to dry. On the other hand, none of ten animals inoculated with human tuberculosis that had been exposed to sunlight developed the disease (even with as little as one day of exposure containing nine hours of sunlight; another three animals that had been inoculated with human tuberculosis that had been exposed to sunlight were not under observation long enough).

Delépine and Ransome showed that beneath a bed, behind a table, or under a chair, tuberculosis could survive for up to 130 days if left unhindered in these murky abodes.[118] Ventilation possessed no disinfecting properties per se. It was an imprecise and inadequate process of infection removal and only remained on the prophylactic table because opening windows and doors increased the chance that bacilli would be expelled from the confines of domestic space altogether, or at the very least swept into a confrontation with sunlight. Meanwhile, multiple experiments in laboratories across Europe from the late 1870s revealed that sunlight was fatal to bacteria.[119] Arthur Downes and Thomas Blunt's observation in 1877 that direct sunlight inhibited the growth of microorganisms in test tubes containing Pasteur solution is still revered as "one of the most influential discoveries in all of photobiology."[120] Koch's own cultures of the tubercle bacillus were killed within five to seven days of exposure to diffuse daylight.[121] Ransome's and Delépine's findings that techniques of fumigation and chemical application either were completely ineffectual as destroyers of germs or irreparably damaged property raised a vital question for public health: how could technology compensate for the woeful lack of sunlight in the bacilli-ridden homes of the working class.

The answer to this question is obviously important. But the answer is not the only significant thing about the question. Also crucial is *how* the search for an answer was conducted, because this tells us a lot about the relationship between scientific knowledge and the practice of public health. Remember that in Delépine's and Ransome's experiments, glass capsules containing the diseased samples of wallpaper passed through several pairs of hands on their journey from and back to the laboratory. They were possibly exposed to sunlight on this voyage. This circulation of experimental materials between clinical, laboratory, and domestic spaces compromised the viability of the experimental results and revealed the nitty-gritty inconveniences of integrating laboratory procedures into public health. This was a serious issue for Delépine, because his laboratory was deeply embedded in the day-to-day work of public health. By the late 1890s, he and his coworkers performed bacteriological analyses for more than sixty sanitary authorities across the north of England.[122]

The Manchester tuberculosis experiments commingled materials, knowledge, and practice from three contrasting spaces that were dependent on one another. The hospital agglomerated a diverse array of infected bodies on which the domestic risk of tuberculosis was inscribed. These institutionalized bodies guided researchers to the tuberculous homes that were dotted across the city. From the hospital also came the infected material, sputum, that populated the laboratory's glass capsules. The homes themselves, vacated by patients but not their families, were accorded status as an experimental space and were, after all, the whole point of the laboratory investigations. For its part, the laboratory provided a confirmed diagnosis of cases in the hospital. The laboratory's use of wallpaper as the medium for testing the action of disinfectants on bacteria was politically symbolic.[123] By eschewing the more commonly used silk, linen, or cotton thread, wallpaper indicated that the science of the laboratory was part of a much larger instrumental process in which public health authority sought effective policies of *domestic* hygienic regulation. As such, the command of scientific knowledge was associated not only with what was understood about the biological and chemical properties of infections and disinfectants, but also with the unknowns and instabilities of domestic space.

The clinic, the laboratory, and the home—this entangled arrangement demonstrates that the authority of knowledge in the Manchester disinfection studies was remarkably diffuse in the early 1890s. From this point on, however, Delépine's disinfecting experiments were carried out in a space carved out of his laboratory that he likened to an "ordinary living room."[124] The logic of the laboratory's way of knowing dictated this maneuver since experiments with different disinfectants had to be rendered directly comparable. Bacteriologists insisted that experimental results were the only safe guide to the action of a fumigant, but amid the constant circulation of tubercule bacilli cultures in the early 1890s, the laboratory was unable to control the material heterogeneity of working-class homes. Legitimate areas of analytic concern included the efficacy of the fumigant, the amount of chemical to use, the length of time needed to kill bacteria, and the most appropriate arrangement of a room's contents during the fumigation process. To demonstrate the efficacy of different modes of disinfection outside formal experimental space, "the sick-room must become a scientific laboratory."[125]

Public health practitioners countered that laboratory conditions failed to capture the authenticity of the domestic settings in which they worked. The material world of the home was diverse and complex, despite the best efforts of disinfecting teams to stabilize it by covering up fireplaces and by filling in gaps in windows, doorways, and floorboards with cotton, cloth strips, or sticky brown paper.[126] This was a skilled and labor-intensive job, time-consuming and impractical, particularly in the many dilapidated or badly constructed houses found in working-class districts.[127] The likelihood that disinfection personnel could convert all the sickrooms they visited into laboratory-like spaces was remote indeed.

According to Delépine, his domesticated laboratory space very nearly replicated the conditions necessary to disinfect houses efficiently. "The door fits well," he wrote, "so that the room can be closed more perfectly perhaps than an ordinary living room would."[128] This was his only reservation about the comparability of the two spaces. Not unlike fumigation itself, his assertion was something of a smokescreen. The disinfecting room had a concrete floor; there were no windows, no fireplace; and the walls were made from whitewashed brick without coverings (which was somewhat ironic given the initial use of wallpaper to culture tuberculosis in the experiments). Any resemblance to the average working-class living room was chimeric.

Delépine's spatial tactic partially shifted the focus of authority toward the laboratory and away from the clinic and the home. The production of a domesticated space within the laboratory was a means of stabilizing the laboratory and its activities more generally. The laboratory's enhanced level of "control" over disinfection in Manchester did not come about simply because experiments undertaken there were more "scientific" than those carried out in the sickroom. Such a claim would have been meaningless without the spatial ploy to accompany it. The pursuit of knowledge stripped of all its nonscientific meaning was by no means the sole logic of the bacteriological laboratory. Rather, Delépine worked within and through the existing values and norms of social relations that accorded primacy to domestic space. The domesticated laboratory, however unrepresentative of a real living space, nevertheless was a spatial expression counter to the uncertainty of science and the contingent nature of public health laboratory research.[129]

Looking closely at the illustration of the domesticated laboratory, we can see that Delépine used the disinfecting room to test the efficacy of the new formaldehyde-burning lamps (which are drawn to scalar excess in the original, reproduced here in fig. 5.9). These lamps briefly revived the reputation of fumigation in the mid-1890s.[130] However, Samuel Rideal pointed out that spraying formaldehyde in water solution—popularly known as formalin—was much more efficient than vaporization.[131] Rideal, an emergent national expert on disinfection after the publication of his textbook *Disinfection and Disinfectants* in 1895, advocated the use of formalin spray. Formaldehyde vaporization was eclipsed, while formalin found a place alongside carbolic acid and corrosive sublimate as a popular chemical spray of choice.[132] The latter chemicals had been extensively

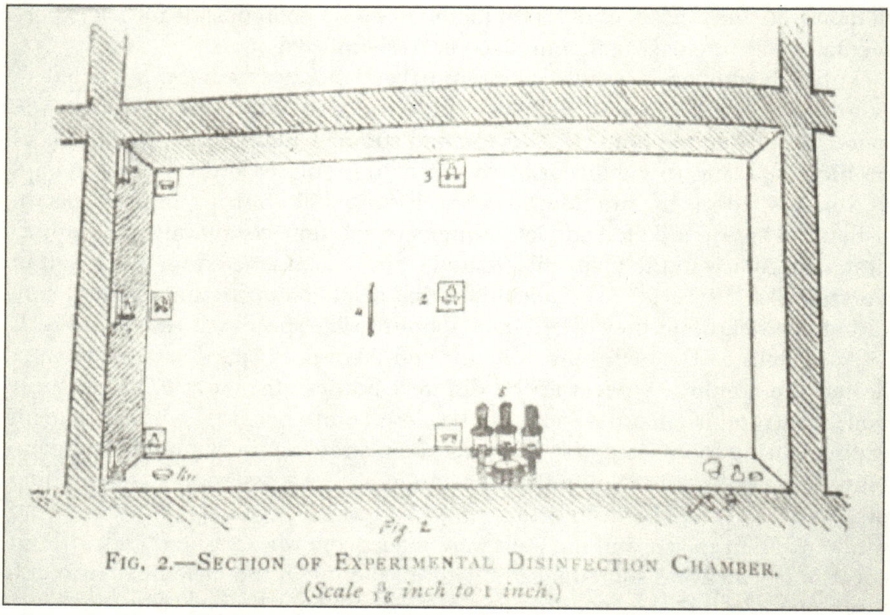


Figure 5.9. Section of the experimental disinfection chamber at the pathological laboratory, Owens College, Manchester. The illustration is drawn as though the viewer is on the threshold, looking through the door. The numbers represent the locations of (1–3) wall brackets at various heights used to hold the various test objects, (4) thermometer, and (5) Formogenic lamp (drawn at a scale larger than that of the room itself) placed on the floor. Delépine, "Some Experiments," 530.

deployed in Paris in the early 1890s, but they were risky substances for disinfectors to use.[133] Anecdotal reports in Britain indicated eye irritation, vomiting, and bronchial trouble that, given the availability of less noxious disinfectants, militated against its use.[134]

Compared to fumes, spray adhered to surfaces consistently; and unlike scrubbing and washing with chloride of lime, it was not abrasive. Moreover, in an atmosphere saturated with spray, the minute drops of formalin evaporated in situ much more slowly than did liquid solutions, especially when glycerin was added to the spray mix.[135] This particular quality gave the disinfectant more time to do its work. However, unlike steam disinfection, which according to the third edition of Pearmain et al.'s *Applied Bacteriology* was "the only process of which the efficiency is independent of the operator," the knowledge, skill, and conscientiousness of the house disinfector "put a fixed limit to the efficacy of any process of house disinfection. . . . Persons without sufficient training will fail to perform the work thoroughly, however good may be their intentions. . . . A person to whom house disinfection is entrusted should realize in their proper perspective the principles on which his art is based."[136] Dexterity, judgment, and devotion constituted the "art" of disinfecting a house with spray. Among other things, the competent and diligent disinfector was required to discern where in the house "microscopic organisms may have been borne and have alighted," view with suspicion any and all objects contaminated by air that had been in contact with the patient, ritualize the protection or removal of his own clothing, and rub down extremely dirty walls with fresh breadcrumbs as part of the preparation for the spray. The spray had to be applied at an appropriate velocity. Projected too slowly, the drops failed to penetrate surface striations. The conical jet of spray had to cover the objects evenly: set it too fine and the droplets landed too far apart; set it too coarse and they coalesced into streaks.

Preference for spraying prompted the invention of pumping machines that were cheap, easy to use, portable, and performed the job rapidly. The main criterion for portability was carriage on a bicycle, the usual mode of transport for sanitary disinfectors, especially outside large towns. In the early 1900s, W. Leslie Mackenzie, medical inspector to the Local Government Board for Scotland, designed a brass spray-pump weighing five pounds that was connected to a length of bicycle inner tube—garden hose was too heavy and bulky to pack (fig. 5.10a). Variations included a heavier model (just under six pounds) that required fewer pump strokes than the lighter version. Also the sprayer's single nozzle—normally used with horticultural pumps to spray delicate plants—could be switched out for a three-nozzle T-shaped crosspiece when treating large walls in halls, hospitals, and schools (fig. 5.10b).[137] The use of a nozzle wand meant that the disinfector did not have to reach or even see his target because it was easy to waft the wand under beds, behind furniture, and into dark corners.

The Thresh Disinfector Company scaled down Mackenzie's invention to 18 in. by 6 in. and to half its original weight.[138] Other alternatives included a bellows-style foot pump produced by Reynolds and Branson in Leeds that retailed for £2 10s., an amount well within the reach of even the most cash-strapped rural district.[139] A tank made by L. Lumley and Co. used compressed air, obviating the need for pumping altogether. It cost £3 3s. and could either be strapped to the back of the operator or placed in the center of a room. Crucially, this model sprayed about 1,500 cubic feet in five minutes, and the tank held enough solution for twenty minutes' operation. Thus, a single house could be disinfected in one short visit, and the pump could be refilled in the disinfector's truck between jobs.[140] Other pump makers, such as Equifex, made much of the fact that the pump's directionality and specificity rendered unnecessary the evacuation of a property's inhabitants during the disinfection procedure, a marked advance on fumigation (fig. 5.11).[141]

The introduction of formalin spray downgraded the application of chemicals and the use of fumigation, but it did not wipe them out altogether, so to speak. Oral evidence from working-class people in Lancashire attests to the fact that some medical officers of health (or town doctors, as they were known colloquially) persisted with sulfur fumigation well into the twentieth century, despite repeated admissions that it was useless and caused great inconvenience to householders.[142] Its durability partly was facilitated by sceptics themselves. Even Franklin Parsons and the authors of well-known public health manuals

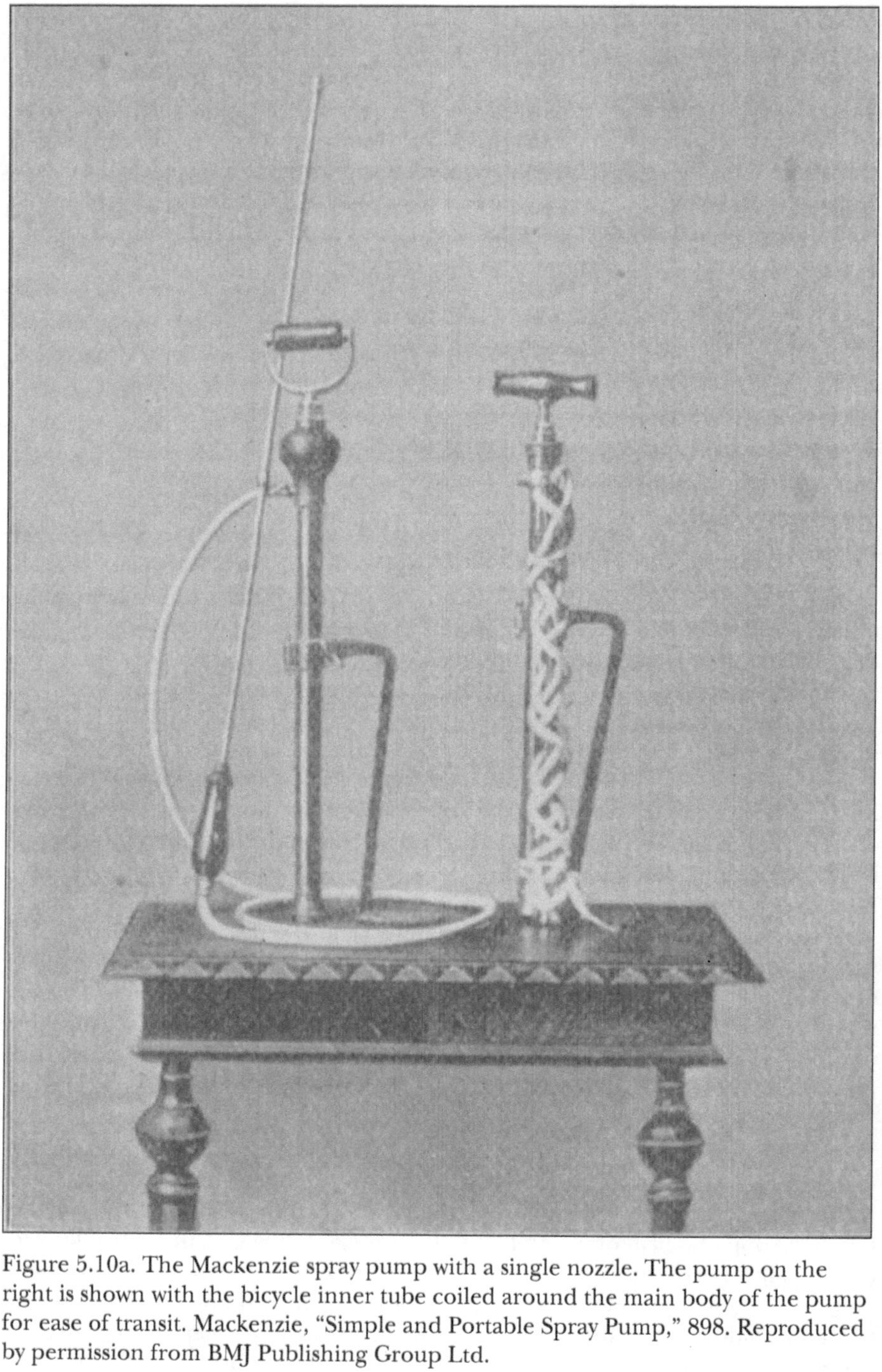

Figure 5.10a. The Mackenzie spray pump with a single nozzle. The pump on the right is shown with the bicycle inner tube coiled around the main body of the pump for ease of transit. Mackenzie, "Simple and Portable Spray Pump," 898. Reproduced by permission from BMJ Publishing Group Ltd.

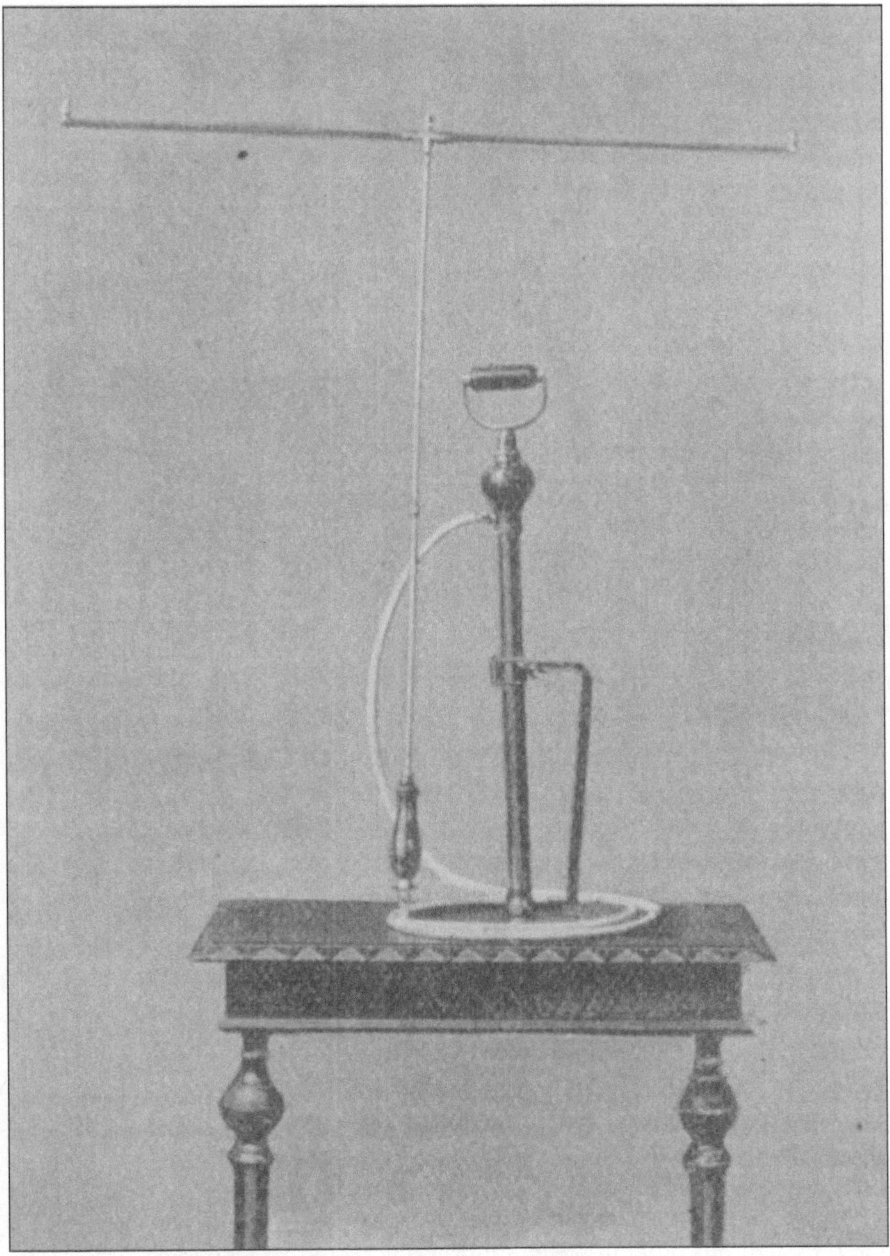

Figure 5.10b. The Mackenzie spray pump with a t-shaped three-nozzle crosspiece attachment. Mackenzie, “Simple and Portable Spray Pump,” 899. Reproduced by permission from BMJ Publishing Group Ltd.

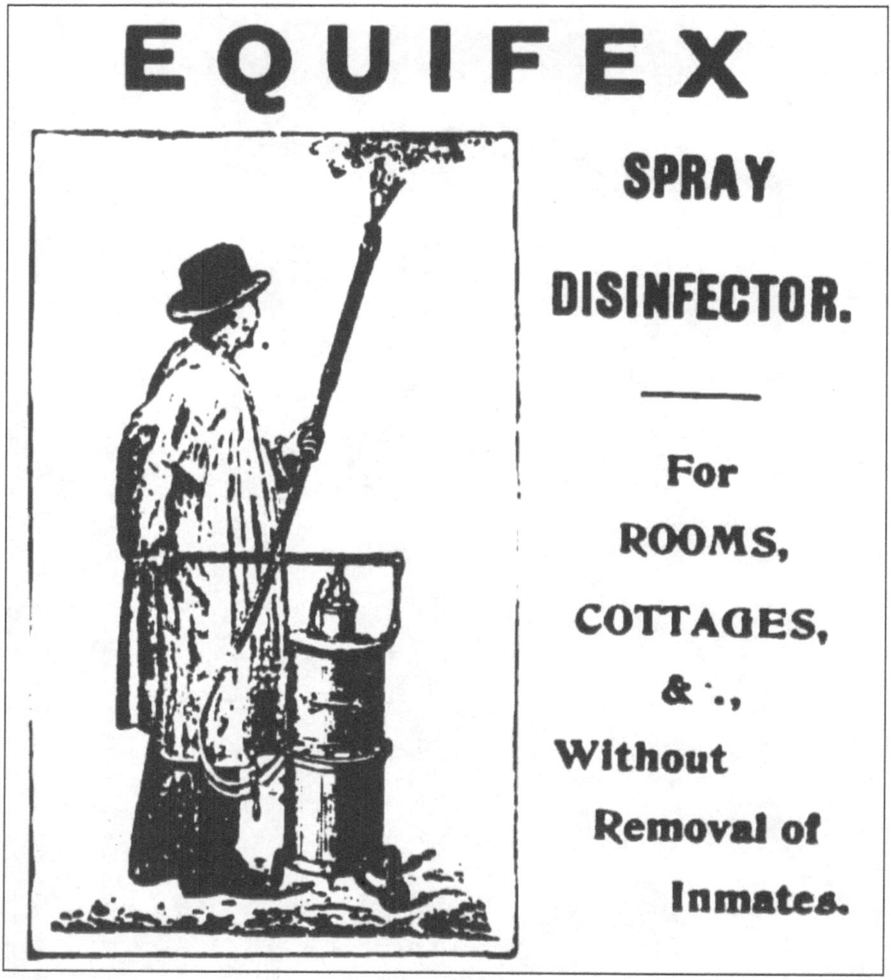
EQUIFEX
SPRAY
DISINFECTOR.
For
ROOMS,
COTTAGES,
& .,
Without
Removal of
Inmates.

Figure 5.11. Advertisement for Equifex spray disinfector. *County and Municipal Record* 1, no. 23 (1901), iii.

continued to dispense advice on how to carry out fumigation, in the minuscule hope that it might kill off the least-resistant organisms.[143] The unbearable stink of sulfur fumigation (windows had to be kept open for at least twenty-four hours afterward) also helped account for its longevity—apparently the "compelling power" of the smell convinced some householders that it must be doing some good, though this opinion was not universally shared.[144] One wag's fumigation adage lauded its indirect benefit, since "it created such a smell that people had to open their windows and so get good ventilation."[145]

The complex array of new modes of disinfection and the persistence of long-practiced interventions goes to show the oversimplification of Peter Baldwin's observation that reformers who were interested in domestic hygiene "moved easily from a concern with sewer gas to germs during the nineteenth century, employing much the same tactics to cleanse homes regardless of the noxious influence, whether miasma or microbe."[146] The "move" was far from easy, and the tactics were, in fact, transformed. When the likes of John Simon and Alfred Carpenter remade the materiality of infection in the third quarter of the nineteenth century, they did so in a discursive environment where the shifting meaning of home and domesticity grappled with the equally insecure Victorian sense of self. For example, the production of laboratory knowledge about chemicals, steam, and the heat-resistant properties of disease-causing organisms carried political meaning because instead of ignoring the complex and unstable social relations of material goods and the living arrangements of domestic spaces, the practices of the laboratory acknowledged and embraced them.

It is incontestable that disinfection invaded domesticity and privacy. But to interpret it purely as an intrusive tactic fails to acknowledge the Victorian impulsion toward the publicity and spectacle of domesticity that reconstituted the norms of liberal subjectivity. Drawing up an inventory of household items for disinfection was a powerful illustration of this. As such, disinfection practice was incorporated into the general reflexivity of domestic life from the 1860s. There is ample evidence that the British working classes made great efforts to keep their home surroundings clean with disinfectants and other hygienic products.[147] Nonetheless, disinfection became a key public health indicator of failed domestic virtue and the family's inability to secure, or difficulty in maintaining, a safe home environment.

Furthermore, the acceptance of disinfection did not occur simply because the public was increasingly familiar with it; nor was it accepted because the explanatory power of medical science made disinfection appear to be a rational intervention. These were certainly significant factors, but equally important was the liberalization of disinfection, the myriad ways in which technologies of neutralization and destruction became comparatively easy to regulate, self-managing, portable, inconspicuous, and critically, much less harmful to working-class people's belongings. Indeed, in the early 1900s the proficiency with which a local government was able to carry out disinfection became the yardstick by which it was granted ever more access to the home through tuberculosis notification.

Chapter Six

# *Rules for Home Living*

## *Tuberculosis and the Consumption of Self-Help*

By the early twentieth century, the aspirations for disinfection that had been expressed by John Simon and others in the 1860s had, to some extent, been realized. A "modern" and scientifically up-to-date program of municipal disinfection in the early 1900s combined formalin spray for houses and steam disinfection for articles and clothes. When using these processes in conjunction with technology that reduced operator error and increased capacity, sanitary authorities—certainly in the big industrial cities, but also in some rural areas that owned mobile apparatus—were as confident as they ever had been that some measure of command could be had over the infectious debris that lurked in working-class homes.

The Manchester experiments with tuberculosis disinfection in the 1890s that were described in the previous chapter were symptomatic of a widespread discussion over how to control a disease that did not readily fit into the "infectious" category and a bacterium whose virulence was uncertain.[1] Although infectivity was asserted in the wake of Koch's discovery of the tuberculosis bacillus, multiple views continued to be held about the proximate causes of tuberculosis and why mortality rates were falling. Michael Worboys stratifies five groups of opinion. "Insanitationists" believed general sanitary improvements were responsible. "Infectionists" emphasized the control of person-to-person spread. "Hygienists" looked to behaviors and lifestyle changes. "Diasthesians" sought to remove people with inherited susceptibilities. For "tubercularisationists," the development of acquired, herd immunity helped explain reductions in the disease.[2]

This typology is extremely useful for disentangling the strands of argument wrapped up in explanations of tuberculosis incidence and prevalence, though it has to be acknowledged that some individuals held opinions about tuberculosis that cut across these groups, or moved between groups over time. And although Worboys notes that these opinions emerged chronologically, they did not "replace one another in a sequential way." Worboys also points out that "the views of all the groups were linked to specific TB control policies."[3] One thing the different groups did have in common, however, was the belief that a policy for the notification of the tuberculosis patient was fundamental to the success of intervention. The Insanitationists in the 1880s, the Infectionists in the 1890s, and the Hygienists in the 1900s were all in favor of notification and disinfection for tuberculosis.

As chapter 2 showed, compulsory notification for infectious diseases was given national status through parliamentary acts in 1889 and 1899. We have seen that notification commonly resulted in a period of hospitalization for the patient. However, the prospect of a long period of sequestration for adult tuberculosis sufferers meant that central government refused to grant notification indiscriminately. In this chapter, I explore the ways in which local health authorities and tuberculosis activists brought tuberculosis patients under their care in the face of this reluctance from central government. Possibly the most important moment came in 1912 when the notification of tuberculosis was made compulsory at the national level.[4] As with infectious disease notification before it, this legislation came about through prior experimentation in the localities; but advocates had to make a whole new set of arguments about the advantages that tuberculosis notification would bring. Tuberculosis notification had to be disassociated from hospitalization, and corollary emphasis had to be placed on the usefulness of education and effective disinfection in the home of the patient.

At the turn of the twentieth century, this discourse naturalized the home as a locus of therapy. It is interesting that the home had to be reasserted as a space of healing. Hospitals, workhouse infirmaries, lunatic asylums, and pertinently in this case, tuberculosis sanatoria were increasingly seen as the most appropriate sites of health care for many kinds of patients. Of course, a lot of sick people were still cared for at home, but the steady rise of institutionalization in the nineteenth century destabilized this tradition. As we saw in chapter 2, this destabilization framed some of the libertarian opposition to infectious disease notification, which was seen as gateway legislation to coercion and forcible removal. Nevertheless, a focus on the home also highlighted that certain aspects of domestic materiality, organization, and social relations presented a risk to the health of tuberculosis patients and their relatives. For a disease with such high levels of mortality and morbidity in the adult population, the potential return on the mitigation of these domestic risks was very attractive to public health officials. In contrast to prevailing ideas about the institutional sequestration of patients with other infectious diseases, the home needed to be thought of and reproduced as a space in which interventions for tuberculosis could be imagined and implemented.[5] This can be interpreted as the emergence of a "preventive therapy" for tuberculosis.[6]

Given that so few sufferers of tuberculosis were ever likely to gain admittance to a sanatorium,[7] the domestic inculcation of both preventive and curative behaviors was paramount. If home-based interventions were to have any impact, however, as many patients as possible had to be reached. Notification offered the tool to achieve this. Partly because of the chronic nature of the disease and partly because of the limited provision of beds in sanatoria, patients had to find ways to live with tuberculosis on a daily basis. I look at two aspects of the material life of the consumptive to illustrate the domestication of therapy. First, self-help manuals promoted a technology of the self founded largely on the principles of sanatorium therapy but that was necessarily reconfigured to reflect the social relations of domestic space. Second, I draw upon the promotional literature of the *British Journal of Tuberculosis* (*BJTB*) to assess the ways in which consumer goods were marketed to the domiciled tuberculosis sufferer. It is suggested that a common tubercular "language" of material consumption was fashioned in order to normalize the accumulation of possessions for use in the home. These arguments are made in relation to recent historical research on material culture and identity at the turn of the twentieth century, which has stressed the cultivation of individuality and that the right sort of possessions appropriately arranged in domestic space signified well-regulated morality.

## The Voluntary Notification of Tuberculosis

Arthur Newsholme quite rightly gets credit for pushing through the first scheme of voluntary tuberculosis notification in Brighton in 1899.[8] Newsholme advanced tuberculosis notification in Brighton with extreme caution, as part of a comprehensive program of measures against the disease. An invitation to Brighton's GPs to notify phthisis in April 1900 was preceded in September 1899 with notification of working-class patients only, and before that in January 1899 with notification just of charitable and pauper patients. With each step, Newsholme had to convince his council of the viability of the scheme and gradually allay the fears of local GPs, fears that essentially repeated their misgivings about infectious disease notification in the preceding decades. Developments elsewhere also helped prepare the way for national legislation. As early as 1893, Oldham's MOH James Niven unsuccessfully attempted to get the town council to adopt voluntary tuberculosis notification.[9] In September 1899, having become MOH for Manchester, Niven instigated the official reporting of tuberculosis cases from the city's public institutions.[10] Manchester GPs were asked to notify tuberculosis in 1900.[11] Voluntary notification was adopted in Plymouth in 1900 at the recommendation of the Devon and Cornwall branch of the National Association for the Prevention of Consumption.[12] Bath, Bolton, Cardiff, Exeter, Liverpool, Norwich, Scarborough, Sheffield, Stockport, and Warrington quickly followed suit.[13] A total of twenty-seven voluntary respiratory tuberculosis notification schemes were in place by 1903.[14]

The momentum and rationale for these voluntary schemes came from the promotion of home-based education and treatment rather than the desire to isolate sufferers in institutions.[15] Activities in the northwest were particularly significant in this regard. From 1886 the Manchester and Salford Sanitary Association distributed educational leaflets specifically targeting phthisis.[16] Oldham householders received similar leaflets about sputum and milk in 1888 and 1892. Niven, Oldham's MOH at the time, claimed this as a local authority "first."[17] In July 1892, Arthur Ransome prompted the northwest branch of the Society of Medical Officers of Health (SMOH) to adopt a memorandum "As to the Prevention of Phthisis or Consumption," which enshrined Ransome's view at the time that the disease was not "directly" infective via close human contact but was transmitted through exposure to dried sputum particles that became airborne (as described in chapter 5, this idea helped justify the disinfection experiments in Manchester). The memo listed thirteen measures dealing with the safe disposal of expectoration, appropriate fixtures and fittings in the home that did not give infected dust a safe haven, and the need for thorough disinfection of belongings and homes.[18] These measures were, in fact, very similar to those spelled out in the educational leaflets given to the working classes by the MSSA in the early 1890s.[19] An additional list of "general precautions" included avoidance of breastfeeding by consumptive mothers, boiling milk, thorough cooking of meat, and proper ventilation of dwellings. The memorandum was circulated to all local sanitary authorities and sent to the council of the SMOH in London.[20]

The trajectory of this memorandum was inextricably caught up with the question of notification. In March 1893, the SMOH invited Niven (who by then was Manchester's MOH and president of the northwest branch of SMOH) to London to present the memo in person.[21] Niven grasped the opportunity to move a series of resolutions relating to the prevention of tuberculosis. The first was that sanitary authorities should give a copy of the memorandum, or some form of it, to all medical men and consumptive patients. The second called for tuberculosis to be made a compulsorily notifiable disease under the 1889 Infectious Disease (Notification) Act. The third proposed that local taxes should be used to provide isolation facilities for tubercular patients. A fourth resolution sought to bring tuberculosis in cattle under the Contagious Diseases (Animals) Act.[22] One gets the distinct impression that Niven's audience—which included prominent MOHs such as Shirley F. Murphy, Arthur Newsholme, Edward Seaton, and John F. J. Sykes—were taken aback. Niven had treated the group to something of a broadside that, in the words of Murphy, had brought them "face to face with a large subject."[23] Niven himself felt compelled to say that his recommendations were not made "in an aggressive spirit." Queasy at the idea of rubber-stamping Niven's resolutions then and there, the Society of Medical Officers of Health deferred discussion until its national meeting in Newcastle later in the year.

Between the London meeting in March and the August conference in Newcastle, Niven's paper was published in *Public Health*, which at the time was edited by Newsholme. The logical but far-reaching implications of naming phthisis as a "dangerous infectious disease" under the terms of the Notification Acts caused alarm. Well-respected members of the public health profession such as Louis Parkes, MOH for Chelsea, expressed reservations about the role of local authorities in implementing a "whole fabric of measures" that would be injurious to the patient. To provide rate-supported hospitals for tuberculosis would leave victims "in lonely isolation, unvisited, untended by friends and relations, debarred from their occupations and the means of earning a livelihood."[24] Nottingham's MOH, Philip Boobbyer, said it was the "exaggerated appreciation of the risk of infection" that had led some public health authorities to advocate a set of home-based measures that were tantamount to solitary confinement and that he thought were "both inhuman and useless."[25] James Russell, MOH for Glasgow, was scathing about the potential restrictions on the patient: "The announcement of the sad diagnosis is to be signalled and proclaimed to the world by a domestic ceremony of purification, conducted by the high priests of the sanitary department."[26] Domestic solitude was not the only problem. Parkes was uncomfortable about sanitary authorities' having the power to prosecute a consumptive "under nearly half-a-dozen sections of Acts of Parliament if he [the patient] ventured to pursue the ordinary course of daily life." He wondered whether Niven and the others who advocated compulsion had even considered this contingency or if they thought it likely that the LGB would sanction a measure that would interfere so much with the public's rights and liberties.[27]

In any event, Newsholme put forward two specific recommendations about phthisis prevention to the Newcastle meeting of the SMOH. In one, the northwest branch's memorandum was adopted as an "excellent basis" for precautionary action. The other proposal, also adopted, was to promote the *voluntary* notification of consumption from public institutions and from GPs. Compulsion was deemed a premature move, and Niven's other requests regarding isolation hospitals and tuberculous cattle were not even mentioned in Newcastle.[28]

As described above, it was another six years before Newsholme himself persuaded Brighton's sanitary authority to pursue voluntary notification, and wherever it was implemented it met with limited success. In most places voluntary notification failed to bring the vast majority of cases to a local health authority's attention. The schemes were not uniform in their requirements. In Cardiff and Liverpool, for example, GPs were encouraged to notify only if they felt the intervention of the local health authority was useful. In part, GPs' reluctance lay in the lack of tact and discretion shown by sanitary inspectors.[29] In 1905 barely a quarter of Scarborough's forty phthisis deaths had been notified voluntarily. The town's MOH held that this low rate was due to existing prejudice against routine disinfection after a phthisis death. Of the forty deaths, five of the surviving families refused to take any information at all from the health authority on precautions they should take to prevent phthisis in the future. An additional twenty-one families rejected the offer of disinfection, nine acquiesced to disinfection after the death, while only five families had agreed to it before the patient had passed away (one assumes these last five were among those cases notified). If Scarborough's experience is anything like a reliable indicator of what was happening elsewhere, it is clear that the shame and indignity harbored by the families of tuberculosis victims seriously hampered the efforts of the public health department.[30]

By attracting unwelcome publicity to sufferers, voluntary notification left GPs vulnerable to legal action from a patient whose livelihood was injured because of it. Although there seems to be little evidence that voluntary notification schemes did anything overtly "coercive" to tuberculous patients, on balance this was a valid concern because a GP's actions were not protected by legislation when notification was voluntary. However unintentional and unanticipated, if detrimental consequences ensued—the patient's loss of employment, for example—the doctor could not plead that he had been compelled to notify by law. These sorts of concerns had to be neutralized before tuberculosis notification could become effective.

## From Voluntarism to Compulsion

Sheffield was one of the first cities to adopt voluntary notification, in 1899. The city's MOH, John Robertson, wanted compulsory notification so that he could pay attention to "the special environments which ought to be attacked."[31] The unique industrial makeup of Sheffield lent urgency to the tuberculosis discourse. Narratives of tuberculosis mortality in the city were preoccupied with "industrial phthisis," a result of the metal grinding, file cutting, and cutlery manufacture that was central to the city's economy. Robertson called attention to the excess phthisis mortality of Sheffield men over the age of thirty-five compared to those in the rest of the country and in other urban areas. Within the city itself, men died at twice the rate of women.[32] It was thought that about 20 percent of Sheffield's male phthisis deaths were directly attributable to these occupations. Yet, older women (that is, fifty-five years of age and over) in Sheffield also had elevated tuberculosis mortality rates compared to elsewhere. It was believed that this was the result of husbands contracting the disease at around the age of forty and then infecting their wives, whose symptoms then manifested at a later age.[33]

Robertson made his first move to secure notification in autumn 1902. In October he requested that the town clerk, Henry Sayer, include two clauses in upcoming parliamentary legislation: one for compulsory notification, and the other for power to prosecute consumptives who did not burn or destroy the contents of their spit-bottle with germicide provided by the council.[34] In the first iteration of the Sheffield Corporation Bill that emerged in 1903, the council included both of these proposals, and it intended to include phthisis under the Infectious Diseases (Notification) Acts. In February 1903, the corporation's parliamentary agents tried to excise these clauses;[35] in the previous year Halifax Corporation had a similar clause struck out of that town's bill.[36] Robertson later conceded the point about the destruction of sputum, but he was ready to challenge the LGB's block on local authorities that wanted to make consumption compulsorily notifiable. The LGB argued that many notified cases would be in the early stages of the disease and would have many years of life in prospect. Since these people needed to earn a livelihood for themselves and perhaps also for their family, it was not reasonable to put phthisis on the same footing as "ordinary" infectious diseases such as scarlet fever and diphtheria, because the inevitable conclusion of compulsory notification in these diseases was hospitalization.[37] Robertson argued that tuberculosis sufferers should be exempted from public health legislation that made them liable to hospital removal, to prosecution for exposing others to risk, and in the event of death, to restrictions on burial.[38]

The LGB summoned Robertson and Sayer to London for a meeting on May 11, 1903.[39] In attendance were the LGB's assistant secretary, John Lithiby; its parliamentary agent, Mr. Herbert E. Boyce; and one of its assistant medical officers, Dr. Theodore Thomson, a former medical officer of health for Sheffield.[40] The result was that the LGB redrafted the clause to exempt notified phthisis sufferers from other public health legislation that would hospitalize them and restrict their movements. The board also stipulated that the provisions were granted on a trial basis for five years.[41]

When Sheffield's bill came before the House of Commons Committee on June 23 and 24, Robertson testified for Sheffield, as did Arthur Hall, who was professor of pathology at the University College and a physician at the Sheffield Royal Hospital. Although it is unclear whether the city had arranged by this point to pay Hall's department to examine specimens of sputum from notified cases (which is what eventually transpired), Hall doubtless realized it was in his professional interest to promote the measure.[42] Indeed, historian Steve Sturdy has written that the income from such bacteriological work was crucial for the financial stability of the medical school, since it underwrote teaching laboratories, a professorship, and other staff in the Pathology Department.[43] Sheffield tried to bolster its case by inviting both Newsholme and Niven to give evidence, though only Newsholme turned up. Boyce and Thomson spoke on behalf of the LGB. Since the Sheffield Corporation and the LGB had pretty much thrashed out their differences by this stage, all that remained to be seen was whether the force of these testimonies would convince the House of Commons Committee.

Sheffield's strategy emphasized four key points.[44] First, that voluntary notification only revealed a limited number of cases, probably about 50–60 percent of the total in the city. This was an inadequate proportion for effective prevention.[45] Second, that interference with the future livelihood of the tuberculous patient was out of the question.[46] The corporation and the LGB had inserted a paragraph that stated, "No provisions contained in any general or local Act of Parliament relating to infectious disease shall apply to tuberculosis of the lung."[47] Basically, this vindicated the views of Louis Parkes and others from a decade earlier who had registered their objection to the inevitable designation of phthisis as "dangerous" under the terms of Infectious Diseases (Notification) Acts. As such, the committee was satisfied that notification would not stop consumptives "from doing their work."[48] Indeed, the LGB was now sponsoring the clause because it had been convinced that the measure as framed would not be detrimental to the individual. This also meant that the corporation had to downplay the possibility that patients would be removed to sanatoria.[49]

The third tactic made it clear that the public did not see notification as problematic. According to Arthur Hall, the dread of consumption among the poor exceeded the dread of notification. He had "known people come up to the laboratories on their own account without consulting their medical men at all, bringing up specimens of their sputum to ask if they are suffering from consumption, and if it can be examined; and in that case they are perfectly aware that by doing so they are putting themselves into full touch with the health authorities."[50]

Robertson estimated that about twenty people had made an effort to thank him for the educational information his office had provided after notification and how "they were pleased at having some chance of saving their relatives."[51]

This leads to the fourth important aspect of Sheffield's case: the domesticated nature of the actions taken after notification. There were two elements to this: domiciliary education and disinfection. The corporation's policy was to give intensive education to the patient in the home. Robertson's position was that public lectures and blanket leafleting of the community were too diffuse to have a lasting impact:

> However much the country is roused to the danger that lurks in the person of every consumptive, who does not know (or who does not carry out) the necessary precautions, I am certain that in a few years interest will flag. . . . In Manchester, during the past twelve years, more has been done in the way of popular lectures, the distribution of leaflets, &c, than in any other city, and yet the result so far has been almost inappreciable.[52]

Arthur Hall concurred: changing people's habits through the distribution of literature was a very slow process.[53] In the word of the bill's draftsman, Mr. Gerald Fitzgerald, compulsory notification would put the working classes in contact with a "competent" adviser and supervisor. Fitzgerald did not have the patient's physician in mind; competence, here, came in the form of the sanitary authority.[54] Essentially, however, the proposals about education offered nothing different than what was already available under voluntary notification schemes in Sheffield and other cities where patients and their caregivers received advice, in the domestic setting, about isolation, ventilation, disinfection, and the disposal of sputum.

The insufficiency of disinfection facilities had been *the* main sticking point for the Local Government Board when other authorities had applied for compulsory notification. Sheffield made it apparent that it possessed the wherewithal to carry out domestic disinfection. Under voluntary tuberculosis notification, the health department disinfected five hundred dwellings of consumptives each year, "always," according to Robertson, "with the willing assent of the householder."[55] Both Boyce and Thomson for the LGB took great pains to make it clear that in the future any local authority applying for powers similar to those sought by Sheffield would need to have proper disinfecting apparatus, adequate staff, and an efficient administration to deal with the workload.[56] Interestingly, Thomson framed the issue of disinfection in the language of freedom and citizenship. Disinfection was the tangible benefit the public had every right to expect if their taxes were being used to pay physicians to notify. This benefit could not be conferred "unless you have staff and appliances sufficient to deal with the problem," said Thomson. "There is, in a case like this, as in very many other sanitary provisions, some interference with the liberty and possibly the comfort of the subject. I should not care to see a power given which conveyed that danger unless some adequate amount of benefit was to be obtained in return."[57]

Thomson warned that each case should be judged on its merits; there was no disinfecting standard to measure all towns against because each town was unique. Obviously Sheffield met the LGB's standard. Thomson's previous association with Sheffield probably did the city's cause no harm. As mentioned above, he was MOH there between 1887 and 1891. The Infectious Diseases (Notification) Act had been adopted during his tenure, and he was in that post when Sheffield's disinfecting station opened on June 7, 1888.[58] While in Sheffield, Thomson witnessed the annual number of houses disinfected in the city leap from around 30 in the mid-1880s to an average of more than 1,000 by the early 1890s.[59]

So, a combination of factors convinced the House of Commons Committee to grant Sheffield compulsory tuberculosis notification for a trial period of seven years.[60] The correspondence of local and national government officials and the survival of the parliamentary evidence in the Sheffield case reveal how public health business was performed (the testimonies were not always transcribed by the Police and Sanitary Committee). The Sheffield contingent was lucky that Thomson had empathy with its case and that it was able to exploit this. But the power of the city's arguments came from intense negotiations prior to the House of Commons hearing and the assembly of a stellar cast of characters to give evidence. The importance given over to domestic interventions should not be underestimated. The Sheffield delegation were keen to underline the utility of disinfecting homes and belongings, while stressing that access to domestic space was vital if educational efforts were to have an impact.

Given the lengths to which the health authority in Sheffield went to underscore its commitment to domesticated therapy, it is somewhat startling to read the words of Robertson's immediate successor as MOH, Harold Scurfield, who wrote in his 1904 annual report that "it is not to be expected that the full benefit of the new provisions will be obtained until something is done in the way of providing hospital accommodation for the badly housed cases . . . and sanatorium treatment for the early and curable cases."[61] Scurfield started to use data from visits to notified cases to explore the issue of domestic transmission and conditions in the home, thus reinforcing the idea that domestic space posed a risk that had to be addressed. In particular, information from five hundred cases visited between 1907 and 1911 demonstrated the particular vulnerability of women: "infection in the home affects the woman more than the man. The wife nurses the husband when ill; the husband does not nurse the wife." Sharing sleeping accommodations did not help matters.[62] It became clear that the vast majority of patients could not pay for sanatorium treatment. Some working men offset costs by membership in a Friendly Society, yet almost half of all male patients and 84 percent of women with phthisis had no means whatsoever to pay for sanatorium treatment.[63] These figures were clear evidence for the argument that there could not be much extension of sanatorium treatment without some system of invalidity insurance that provided benefits not only to working men but also to their dependents.[64]

## Self-Help and Therapeutic Space

Health authorities who sought compulsory notification were opening up the possibility for a comprehensive scheme of what might be termed a "preventive therapy" of the home; the model for that therapy came from the sanatorium. The number of private, public, and voluntary sanatoria mushroomed from the late nineteenth century. Funding developed along three lines. Private sanatoria arrived in Britain in the early 1890s, and by the turn of the century more than twenty of them contained over four hundred beds. Many public sanatoria were funded by local Poor Law authorities, which is not surprising given the burden of tuberculosis morbidity in workhouse infirmaries. Voluntary provision was a third route. Some charitable institutions began to organize some form of sanatorium provision, usually as an addition to an existing consumption hospital. Elsewhere, either the National Association for the Prevention of Consumption established sanatoria or local fund-raising efforts directed by a well-known medical figure kick-started provision. Initially a relatively small proportion of people who had tuberculosis were treated in sanatoria. Michael Worboys has estimated there were only 1,500 sanatoria in-patient stays in 1900. In 1913 this had increased eightfold to 12,000 stays, but still represented no more than 4 percent of all victims; or, if we accept that sanatoria reached their intended population of "early" cases, about 20 percent of 60,000 sufferers nationwide.[65]

The "sanatorium benefit" included in the National Insurance Act of 1911 stimulated yet more provision.[66] From this date to 1920, the number of beds available for tuberculosis patients (excluding the Poor Law system) increased by about a factor of five to almost 16,000 beds.[67] The term "sanatorium benefit" is somewhat misleading, because it also provided funds for care beyond the walls of sanatoria, including home treatment. Most notably, local authorities were required to provide a tuberculosis dispensary that served as a diagnostic center. A tuberculosis officer and a team of nurses determined the most suitable treatment on a case-by-case basis, working in conjunction with the patient's GP.[68] These cases included the dependents of insured individuals, another aspect of the National Insurance scheme that was unique to the "sanatorium benefit." Dispensary treatment rocketed accordingly. There were 64 tuberculosis dispensaries in 1911; by 1920 there were 398.[69]

Debate about the effectiveness of home treatment seems to have intensified in the aftermath of the 1911 act. Some commentators, such as Oscar Holden, a tuberculosis officer with experience in Birmingham and Southampton, warned that the continuing risk of infection by advanced cases living at home was a serious danger to the wider community.[70] Some were skeptical about the lack of moral support available at home; anxious parents, relatives, and friends made for bad advisers, and it was impossible for them to be alert to all sorts of imprudent acts by the patient that might endanger themselves and their families.[71] Others were convinced that many cases of tuberculosis could be successfully managed and cured at home, particularly with the additional level of monitoring offered by the dispensary system.[72] Despite fairly vehement support for both sides, there was no clear and convincing evidence about the advantages of either approach. An uneasy consensus emerged that sanatorium treatment was most suitable for early cases that were actively infectious, whereas home treatment was more appropriate for noninfective cases and advanced cases that were infective.[73]

Sanatoria mattered not so much because of their impact on tuberculosis mortality but because of their strict treatment regime.[74] While precise details varied from institution to institution, some combination of wholesome diet, exercise, graduated labor, and plentiful fresh air was a common route to "cure."[75] The involvement of the adult patient in deciding the parameters of his or her sanatorium treatment was important. Sanatoria staff tailored treatments to provide the patient with an individualized regime that the patient could manage him- or herself. Contemporaries believed that sanatoria and the open-air movement had the potential to "revolutionise social, municipal and national life."[76] Historian Michael Worboys has gone so far as to suggest that the sanatoria-based "attempt at 'cultural control' was of equal, if not greater, significance than the better-known Edwardian campaigns about motherhood and physical degeneration; indeed it may be artificial to separate them."[77]

More recently, Flurin Condrau questioned the suitability of categorizing the sanatorium as a "total institution." He argued that historians have written about the sanatorium as a "façade behind which discipline, order and militaristic concepts of hygiene were used to control working-class sufferers."[78] Condrau's concern was to reintegrate patient agency into sanatorium narratives and to reorient inquiry toward the precise meaning of clinical effectiveness in a historical context. I wish to extend this aspect of Condrau's thesis by focusing on domestic preventive therapy for tuberculosis patients—the blueprint for which was drawn up in the sanatorium. By considering how the home-based consumptive patient was expected to care for him- or herself, it becomes clear just how crude the concept of "control" really is; a more subtle interpretation is required that considers questions about auto-regulation and governance of the self. In addition, when thinking about the diffusion of tubercular therapeutic space from the sanatorium to the home, serious attention needs to be devoted to the ways in which that diffusion took place. How was this governance of the self realized? What aspects of tuberculosis therapy were prioritized? What technologies were deployed to achieve a clinically effective outcome?[79]

One method was the promotion of hygienic discipline through tuberculosis education, which was popularized from the 1880s.[80] Before the rise of the sanatorium, the inculcation of both preventive and curative behaviors in domestic space was adopted as a credible tactic because so few nonpauper tuberculosis sufferers were ever likely to be admitted to local institutions. As we have seen, publicly and privately funded leaflet campaigns for tuberculosis emerged in Britain in the mid-1880s, initially in northwest England (notably Oldham and Manchester).[81] Transgressions of a well-ordered domestic space were identified, and appropriate forms of self-regulation were codified: keep your home clean, people were told; ventilate it too; destroy your sputum; disinfect furniture; maintain an unblocked chimney; practice open-air living; and stay away from close and crowded rooms, especially concert halls, theaters, and pubs. This is all familiar historical ground. Yet, just like the Sheffield delegation to the House of Commons, public health administrators—who, Gerry Kearns has demonstrated, were increasingly drawn toward more individualistic modes of explaining and tackling disease—bemoaned this dissipated technique of didactic intervention.[82] Even with the free provision of spittoons, waxed tissues, and other tools of bacillary containment, lifestyles and behaviors were simply too slow to change, if at all.[83]

To some extent, self-help manuals bridged the limits to public health education and were eagerly embraced as an effective means of communicating the most up-to-date and appropriate forms of tuberculosis therapies. As a genre, medical self-help books have an extremely long tradition.[84] Those that began to appear for consumptives at the beginning of the twentieth century were little different than many other medical self-help manuals that had gone before them in that they provided a fallback mechanism for poor patients who were either unable or unwilling to avail themselves of medical attendance.[85] However, they were also directed at patients who had undergone a period of sanatorium treatment and, it was presumed, wanted to maintain the institutional treatment in a domestic setting. These texts were the product of a particular historical moment when sanatorium treatment was gaining credence as the most appropriate mode of therapy but access to that treatment was limited either by availability or by the political reluctance to hospitalize thousands of patients.

Three British self-help manuals were aimed specifically at patients. The authors of these texts all agreed that a sanatorium stay was time well spent, but their opinions were shaded by the provision and accessibility of sanatoria at the time of writing.[86] In 1906 Henry Warren Crowe's *Consumption: Treatment at Home and Rules for Living* targeted patients who had not passed through a sanatorium. Crowe observed that the "day in which public institutions will afford services to all consumptives is far off."[87] However, when the first editions of Noel Bardswell's *Advice for Consumptives* (1910) and Henry Hyslop Thomson's *Consumption, Its Prevention and Home Treatment* (1911) hit the market, the National Insurance Act was about to bring that day somewhat nearer. Both Bardswell and Thomson were medical superintendents of a sanatorium, but Bardswell's book was aimed specifically at maintaining the regime of sanatorium treatment that he assumed his reader had already undergone.[88] This fitted with the views of some tuberculosis activists, one of whom argued that "the lessons taught at the sanatorium are comparatively easy to enforce, and the after-care of sanatorium patients is child's play compared to the home-visiting required for the consumptive out-patients of our London hospitals."[89] Thomson made no such assumption.[90] Depending on the financial resources available to each patient, Thomson recognized a range of therapeutic alternatives, including long-distance health-seeking travel, a walk to the tuberculosis dispensary at the end of the street, or staying at home. Thomson's guide attempted to cater to all-comers, but regardless of where and how treatment was taken, he insisted that the home was the fundamental "battleground" of cure and prevention.[91]

Essentially, the regime of home treatment replicated as far as possible that of the sanatorium. In terms of direct surveillance, the main point of difference was that medical staff could no longer monitor the patient; patients had to perform that monitoring function themselves. The key to success, then, was the patient's self-knowledge about, and control over, his or her body and domestic surroundings. Bodily regulation was achieved by the regularity and repetition of physical conditioning: exercise, rest, and diet were scrutinized as patients were asked to undertake vigilant surveillance of their own temperature and weight. Patients were expected to eat, sleep, and rest at prescribed times of the day and even to breathe in precise ways.[92] The solitariness of the domesticated regime teetered on the tedious: "How monotonous! How unvarying!" admitted Crowe, "but ask yourself this . . . to what length will I go to save my life?"[93] Very boring lengths was the answer; but boredom was the inevitable by-product of successful self-regulation, as implied by Thomson: "The more closely one day conforms to another, and the more strictly the patient adheres to the routine of treatment, from day to day, and from week to week, the more beneficial and effective will the result be."[94]

Opinion was divided over the significance of body temperature.[95] Bardswell wrote that temperature readings were essential in the early stages of treatment but much less so during convalescence. He was witheringly skeptical about the competence of the average person to administer a thermometer properly and advised that "the fewer observations taken the better," ruing the fact that "many would be better if they had never learnt how to use it."[96] It was, nevertheless, standard practice in some sanatoria to have patients take their own temperature rectally. Crowe and Thomson expressed no reservations over the ability of the layperson to interpret the thermometer.[97] The ebb and flow of rest and exercise that was so vital to the control of fever depended entirely on the mercury level, and Thomson's manual included an illustration of a thermometer, marking the temperatures at which he advised rest and exercise (fig. 6.1). Crowe warned that "your every act depends on the reading of the thermometer."[98] He advocated taking four temperature readings per day; Thomson advised three.

Weight gain was a crucial indicator of recovery, though Bardswell was less distracted by body weight than the others: "say once every two or four weeks" was his comparatively insouciant opinion on the frequency with which patients should jump onto their scales.[99] Like Bardswell, Thomson directed biweekly measurements, and he included height/weight tables for each sex so that consumptives might know what he meant when he spoke of "normal" men and women.[100] Meanwhile, Crowe advised that weight should be recorded once each week and recommended the "Standard" scales, which cost a sovereign.[101]

So, body temperature synchronized home treatment, while body weight gauged the patient's progress. These physical markers replicated the markers that were used in sanatoria. The repeated actions of taking temperature and weight, and then recording them, mimicked the routine of life in the sanatorium. But this process of recording the readings is significant for other reasons. Both Thomson and Crowe guided the patient on how to fill in a temperature

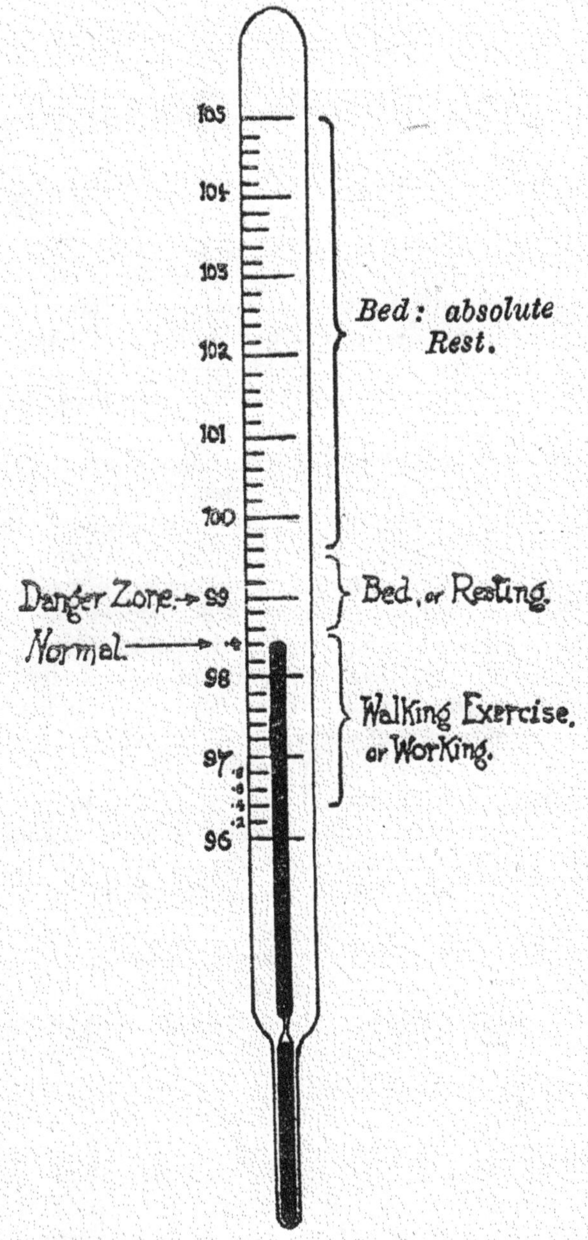


DIAGRAM OF CLINICAL THERMOMETER.

Figure 6.1. Diagram of clinical thermometer showing "normal" and "danger zone" temperatures and directives for domiciled consumptive patient. Thomson, *Tuberculosis* (1928), 51. Reproduced by permission from Oxford University Press.

chart. Thomson reproduced illustrated examples of what a fever curve might look like at different stages of the disease, given a specific body weight. Crowe, meanwhile, showed his readers the temperature chart of a "normal" man. (Unsurprisingly, given his skepticism about patients' ability to take their own temperature, Bardswell provided no such charts.) Comparing these printed reproductions is instructive. Crowe's chart has a naturalistic appearance. Some of the lines meet the dots; some do not. The crosses have different stroke widths. The chart is annotated with handwriting. Even though Crowe's chart regresses to a "normal" standard, it lacks the standardized appearance of Thomson's curve types. In other words, Crowe's chart looks like it could have been filled in by a patient. Crowe's book also included loose-leaf blank charts for the patient to fill in.[102] Each chart provided space for two weeks' worth of temperature measurements (figs. 6.2 and 6.3).

Voker Hess and J. Andrew Mendelsohn have shown how paper technologies shaped clinical practice between the mid-eighteenth and mid-nineteenth centuries. Registers and preprinted forms, they argue, "linked rather than separated the increasingly differentiated fields of medicine in the hospital. . . . Generic pre-printed formatting served recording of knowledge in very different spaces of knowledge." Standardized inscription practices compressed space, so that "on paper, the distance even from outpatients to the pathologists was short." If we think of these tuberculosis self-help manuals not just as repositories of democratized therapeutic knowledge, but also as documentary technologies, we can see that they did very similar sorts of work. But rather than linking spaces *within* a hospital, they linked the practices of the hospital to the home.[103]

The fever chart, created by Carl Wunderlich in Germany in the 1860s, condensed the long traditions of recording and transcribing for clinical purposes. The fever chart reified continuous observation; it collated the "patient's entire illness as a unit of knowledge"; and it extracted one feature of an illness narrative to stand in for the heterogeneous whole. For tubercular patients using these self-help manuals and thus "trained" in the art of reading and recording their own bodily signs, the curve was a truth-telling, reflexive tool created by their own hand. It became the unfolding (quite literally) narrative of their illness.

The chart provided an objective narrative that could be shared with the family doctor, opened up, and spread out on the bed covers. Ostensibly, the role given to GPs in these self-help texts was to manage the home-based consumptive. The fever chart became documentary proof that between visits from the GP the patient was able to "intelligently order and supervise his whole method of living."[104] Through the acquaintance of repeated visits, the family doctor could integrate the fever curve with the patient's "circumstances, occupation, and home conditions." As such, Thomson warned his readers about the perils of moving from doctor to doctor and the value of sticking with the same physician.[105] This in itself reinforced the value of stability, constancy, and regularity through which character was formed. It is worth emphasizing, then, that GPs served in more than a surveillance capacity. Equally as wedded to the individualistic mode of medicine as were the sanatorium hygienists, family doctors were

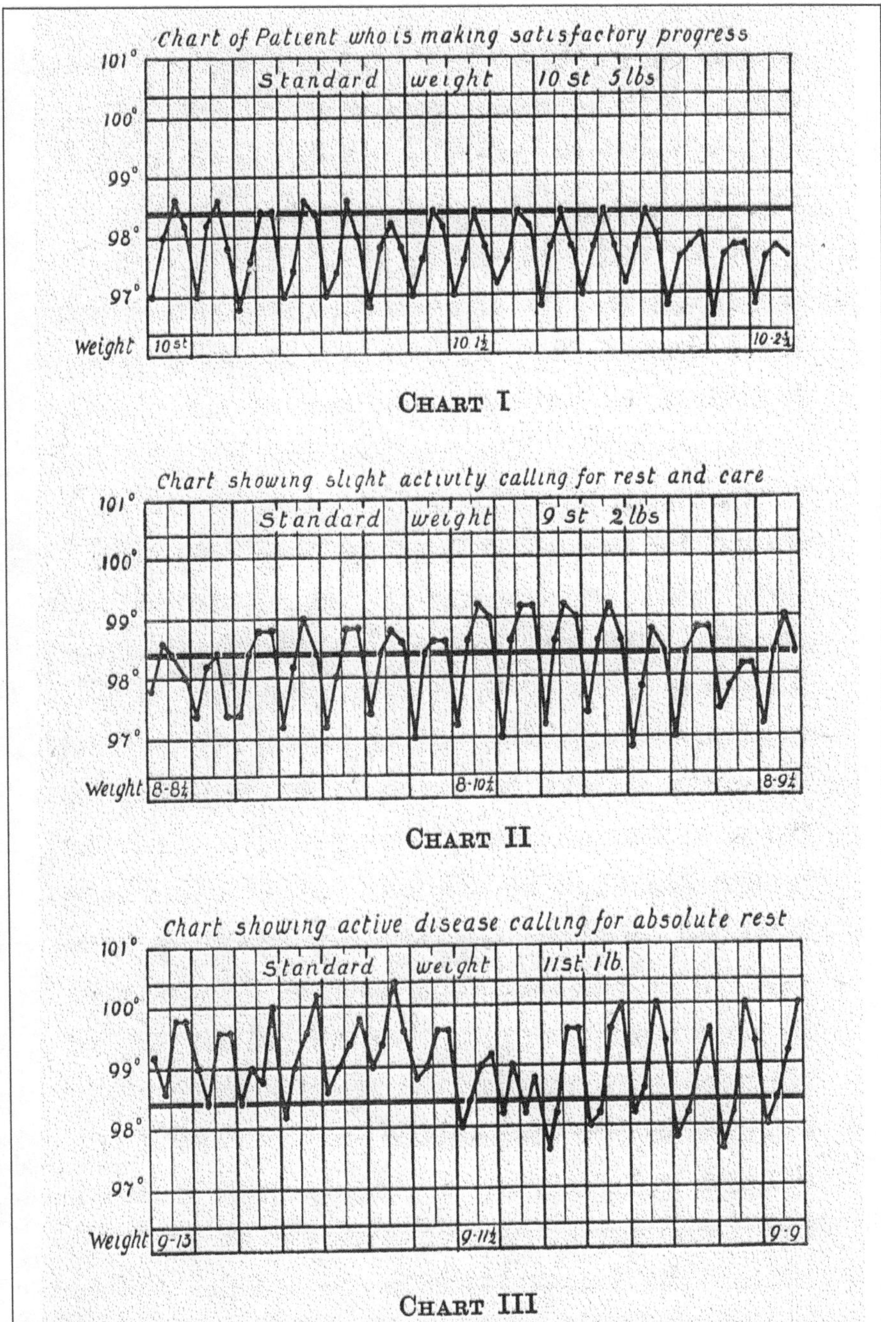


Figure 6.2. Chart I of a patient who is making satisfactory progress; chart II showing slight activity calling for rest and care; and chart III showing active disease calling for absolute rest. Thomson, *Tuberculosis* (1928), 49. Reproduced by permission from Oxford University Press.

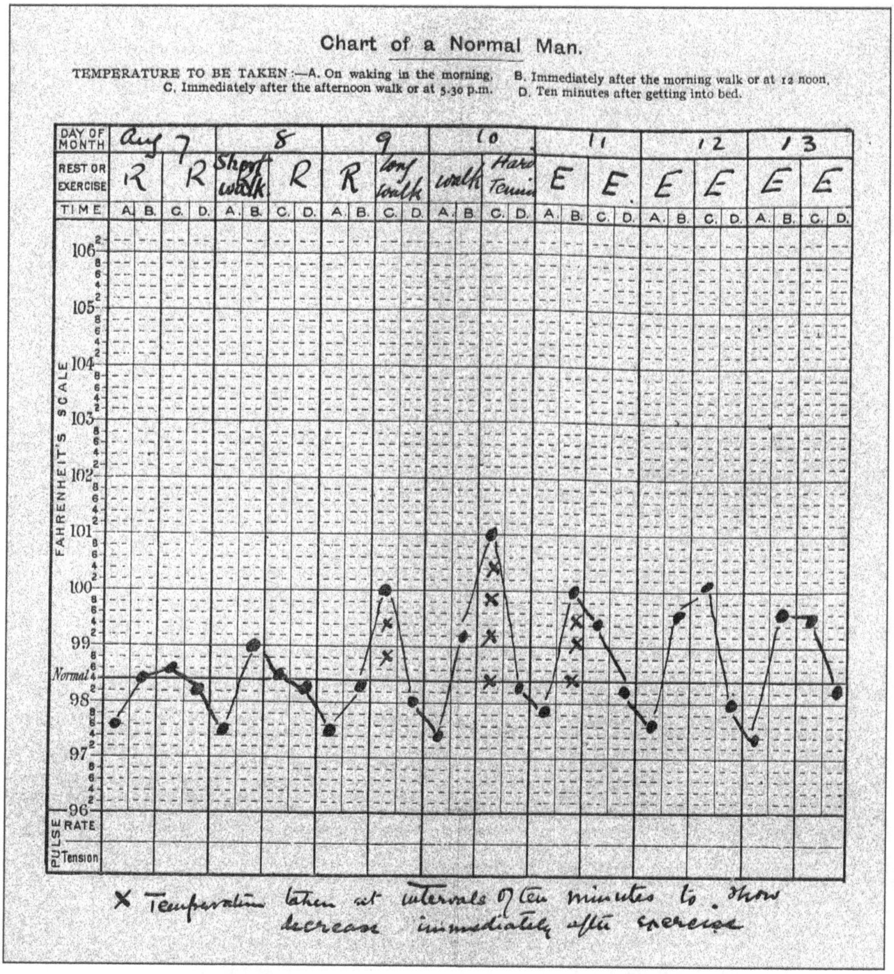


Figure 6.3. Chart of a normal man. Crowe, *Consumption*, following page 32.

well placed to act as missionaries for the sanatorium regime. Not least, they had privileged access to domestic space. Crowe wanted GPs to give his manual directly to their consumptive patients (which had the added advantage of saving time for a hardworking doctor).[106] Affordably priced at just 1s., it was by no means an unrealistic hope that GPs would deliver the sanatorium regime directly into the hands of sufferers. Reinforcing the partnership of patient and practitioner, blank pages were deliberately bound into the back of Crowe's manual so the doctor could write down supplemental instructions.[107]

Experts expressed differences about many aspects of the therapeutic regime, differences that depended partly on the stage of the disease and partly on the individual patient; no two patients were the same.[108] Disagreements over detail were overridden by the commonalities and the deeper purpose of some activities. For Bardswell, an evening walk in the park helped stave off the temptation to fritter away money down at the pub. Self-responsibility and strength of character was the key to the conclusion of a successful course of home treatment, be that complete cure or, more realistically, a prolonged period of capacity for work and the enjoyment of life.[109] Bardswell wrote:

> Character or temperament, as in all other things, is a very large factor in success. The irresponsible, the undisciplined, and the despondent have nothing like the same chance of recovery as the cautious, the level-headed optimist, and the man of purpose. It is well for the patient to recognise frankly, from the first, that the fight for life and health is to be a hard one, with the odds against him. . . . The odds can be levelled up by learning the principles by which consumption may be cured, and resolutely adhering to them. . . . The happy-go-lucky consumptive, though perhaps the shorter-lived, is a happier man than the discontented hypochondriac. He is certainly the more contented companion. The mid-course between these two extremes should be aimed at.[110]

These interrelated points about individual responsibility, self-help, and determination were constantly reiterated. Thomson spoke of "personal effort," "intelligent effort," "constant effort," "unswerving allegiance to the rules," and "personal endeavour": "in many cases, the consumptive holds in his hands the power of treating and curing himself. . . . [He] must intelligently order and supervise his whole method of living."[111] Bardswell was sure that there would be "little setbacks" and acknowledged the regime involved "much troublesome care and self sacrifice."[112] But the most successful patients, wrote Crowe, will be "those who can form a resolution and steadfastly carry it out, and who are sufficiently master of their own surroundings."[113]

As well as developing bodily consciousness, patients had to comprehend the domestic conditions that caused their "deviation from the normal healthy standard" and mediated the risk of infection.[114] It is clear that these authors believed that long-standing public health campaigns against poor ventilation, uncleanliness, and inappropriate furnishings had made but a small dent in the public consciousness: there was still much "ignorance and mistaken views as to what constitutes a healthy home."[115] Awareness of the minutia of domestic life was exalted. For example, Crowe wanted consumptives to study the direction of drafts through the house so that they might know where to position their bodies to take the greatest advantage.[116] No detail was "too trivial" if the patient was to become "familiar with everything relating to himself and his surroundings."[117] The constituents of domestic space—beds, furniture, windows, floor coverings, people—were construed as problematic and risk laden. Interactions with other family members represented an obstacle to the patient's progress. Of course, one of the main benefits of sanatorium treatment in the eyes of its promoters was isolation from meddlesome family and friends, a condition that proved extremely difficult to replicate in the crowded domestic sphere.[118] As with other infectious diseases, the patient was expected to take sole occupancy of a separate room in the house whenever possible.[119] Even still, complete segregation was practically impossible, particularly for working men and women and housewives who moved in and around the house out of necessity.[120]

This feature of home treatment worried the writers of self-help manuals not only because the patient might continue to infect other family members, but also because the family had a potentially corrupt influence on the stringent therapeutic regime.[121] Consequently, the patient's routine was aimed at restricting the likelihood of contact. Consumptives with active disease "should never be kissed on the lips."[122] Retiring early to bed not only delivered much-needed rest, but it also "removed the temptation to join the family circle in sitting up till a late hour."[123] Reinforcing advice readily handed out by sanitary authorities, Crowe recommended disinfection and the disposal of spit, since it was the "bounden duty" of the patient to control his or her expectorations and not be a source of infection to others.[124]

## A Material Culture of Consumption

The emphasis on discipline, self-control, and the suppression of intimacy and irresponsibility reflects the persistence of interventions centered on character formation that had their high-water mark in the late Victorian period.[125] This helps explain what made the slide from the "rules of health" (as they were known in the sanatorium) to "rules for living" (as they were called in the title of Crowe's manual) practically imperceptible. As Bardswell put it: "The best way . . . of escaping consumption, is to live as if trying to cure it." This was guidance for all, not just for the diseased.[126] Some commentators thought that consumptives had certain psychological traits that made them vulnerable to lapses of the sort that the likes of Crowe, Thomson, and Bardswell feared. For example, in 1907 an anonymous correspondent of the *British Journal of Tuberculosis* observed:

> An attempt has been made to show that consumptives have certain more or less psychological characteristics. Be this as it may, it is generally admitted that suitable amusements and reasonable forms of work must be found for tuberculosis patients, whether treated in their own homes or in sanatoria, if intellectual deterioration and moral decadence is to be prevented. In too many cases bodily healing is now secured only with the loss of that which makes life the most worth the saving.[127]

At a time of intense national anxiety about the degeneration of the British race, it is hard to imagine a more intoxicating rhetorical mix than psychological weakness, intellectual deterioration, moral decadence, and tuberculosis—which, after all, was popularly known as a "wasting" disease. Yet, it is almost laughable that in this instance, the message was conveyed while extolling the virtues of the recently invented substance plasticine, which was portrayed as a "delightful form of instructive amusement suited to [tuberculosis] patients of almost every age and position" (fig. 6.4).[128]

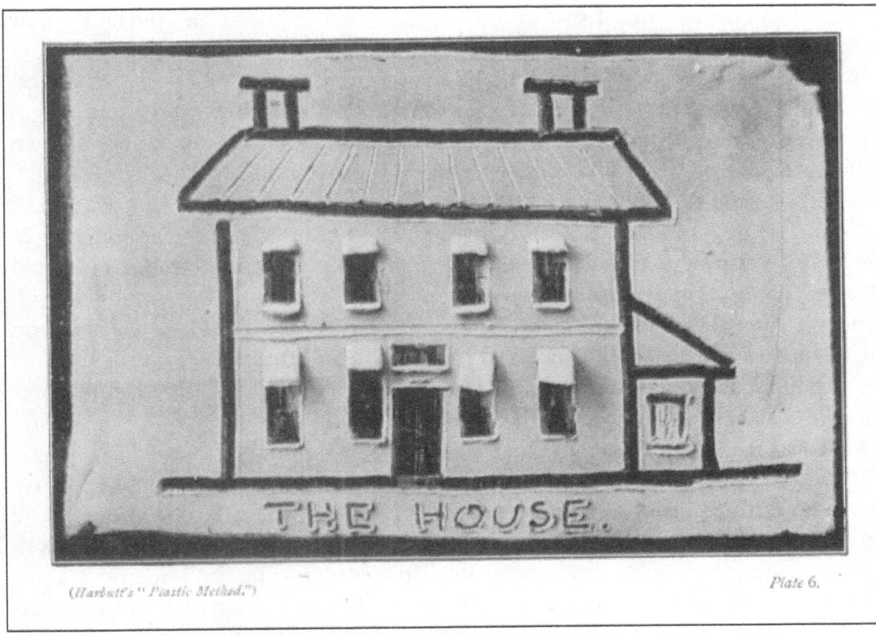


Figure 6.4. The House. Harbutt, *Harbutt's Plastic Method*, 51.

How are materiality, public health, and domestic space connected? In her book *Household Gods*, Deborah Cohen describes the complex, shifting relationship between domestic space and possessions, and what it signified about notions of the self at the turn of the twentieth century. She argues that from the 1890s in particular, "personality" and the domestic interior were deeply entwined. Whereas the moral self had embodied "character," personality denoted an "earned distinctiveness" that was put on display and enacted in the home.[129] Some of the intricacies and subtleties of this transition from character to personality can be teased out by looking at the consumer culture surrounding tuberculosis.[130]

One obvious starting point is the medical and public health journals that carried direct advertising in order to supplement subscription income, sustain print runs, and increase circulation. Indeed, at the end of the nineteenth century, advertising constituted the largest revenue stream for prestigious medical journals.[131] By this date, direct advertising pages in most newspapers and professional journals gave the impression of a multitude of commodities jostling for space and attention. Advertisements were individually bordered and designed in an attempt to distinguish one product from all the others on a congested page.

As with other publications, however, the *British Journal of Tuberculosis* also provided editorial information about commercial products that its editors thought might be of interest to its readers. There is no direct evidence to substantiate this claim, but it seems likely that the "Preparations and Appliances" section of the journal involved a form of indirect advertising known as "puffing" (now commonly termed "advertorials"); that is, the inclusion of an editorial item promoting the virtues of a product for which a payment was made by the advertiser. In the newspaper trade, a puff piece commanded a higher rate than a regular advertisement because it carried the imprimatur of the newspaper itself. In contrast to the pages of direct advertising at the front and back of the journal, "Preparations and Appliances" was set in the journal's preferred typeface and column format. It looked no different than the main articles in the journal. In the *BJTB*'s running order, it frequently appeared between the book reviews and "Notes," a segment that informed readers of conferences they might attend, research they should keep up with, health resorts that could be visited, and tuberculosis institutions that needed patients.[132] In other words, "Preparations and Appliances" was no more than a sequential component in the journal's procession of tuberculosis commodification, an example of the way in which the power of private capital became institutionally entrenched.

Products appearing in "Preparations and Appliances" were given an easy promotional ride. Assertions claiming that a product "only needs to be known to be extensively used,"[133] or that it "should gain an entrance to every home,"[134] were just as common as the journal's assurances that commodities had been tried and tested extensively before receiving recommendation.[135] It is not known what filtering criteria (if any) were used to include or exclude particular commodities. The author(s) praising these products were not identified; such anonymity applied a veneer of objectivity. Manufacturers' artwork was reproduced faithfully, and the promotional language was never critical.

Readers were either directed to retail outlets where these goods could be purchased or provided with the name and address of the manufacturer to buy directly from them. The journal's (probable) middle-class British audience of tuberculosis activists, doctors, and patients was undoubtedly familiar with some form of "purchasing at distance," either in response to advertisements in newspapers and magazines or through mail-order catalogues that were touted by agents.[136] This type of consumer behavior was boosted by the institution of the Royal Mail's parcel post in 1883. Just two years earlier, the introduction of postal orders had given people without access to a checkbook a secure means of sending money. By World War I, £57 million worth of postal orders were issued and the General Post Office delivered more than 130 million packages each year. Much of this traffic was driven by the mail-order business.[137] Writers at the *BJTB* and elsewhere who came up with copy about commodities inserted themselves into this burgeoning mail-order trade, acting more or less like those catalogue agents who were working steadily in communities across the country.[138] Though plying their powers of persuasion from a distance and in print, these writers compiled and showcased inventories of potentially useful products and cajoled readers into contacting a manufacturer or retailer for further details, if not enticing them into an impulse purchase.

The motors of this consumer culture were rising incomes, the expansion of the middle classes—which, by 1901, represented 25 percent of the national population—and the ready availability of goods through mass production.[139] The purchasing power of both the working and middle classes increased, but the latter spent a smaller proportion of their incomes on housing and necessities such as food and heat. When middle-class disposable income was expended on filling homes with possessions, the explosion of acquisitive behavior abraded Victorian notions of religious restraint, particularly given the indelible influence of domestic space over individual character. One solution to this dilemma, argues Cohen, was to bestow upon possessions moral qualities. Household goods conferred domestic propriety and decency. Appropriate, well-designed furnishings raised the moral tone, whereas inappropriate fixtures and fittings indicated a kind of deception or ugliness that should not be tolerated: "By redefining consumption as a moral act, and the home as a foretaste of the heaven to come, the British middle classes sought to square material abundance with spiritual good."[140] The right sort of possessions and their appropriate arrangement in domestic space denoted morality, spirituality, distinctiveness, and personality.[141]

I do not claim that the *BJTB*'s puff pieces tell us very much, if anything at all, about the motives and actions of consumers. Rather, I suggest that "Preparations and Appliances" was an interstice where a common tubercular "language" of material consumption was fashioned. This language could be understood by sanatorium officials, public health activists, family doctors, patients, and patient caregivers alike; not because this sort of language was specific to the world of tuberculosis activism but because it was ubiquitous.[142] The journal's readers were educated on how to visualize the domiciled tuberculosis patient. The things on show helped solidify the idea of the home-based patient and preventive therapy. The journal's pages reveled in a "technology of possession" that sought to integrate tuberculosis patients into a contemporary consumer culture that everyone could recognize (if not partake of equally).[143]

In the early twentieth century, then, plasticine was just one of hundreds of items that appeared in the *British Journal of Tuberculosis*'s "Preparations and Appliances." A bewildering multitude of commodities were determined as "requisites" of both the sanatoria *and* the "hygienic" home. Some of these objects explicitly unified the medical regimen of these discrete spaces. One example is the "Presto Thermometer," which purportedly overcame the deficiencies of most models "in common use," that were slow acting, indistinctly marked, and difficult to adjust, if not defective altogether. The Presto model had a scale range of 12°C (94°C to 106°C) instead of the customary range of 16°C or 20°C, with more generously spaced fractional divisions. The markings above the normal temperature were indicated in red.[144] Another example was a bed screen and shelter that was shown at the first Ideal Home Exhibition in 1908. For patients practicing the open-air life, this screen protected them from the wind, drafts, and direct sunlight, as well providing privacy; the screen would be appreciated "in hospitals, sanatoria, as well as in the home."[145] Crucially, these devices sought to simplify the mechanics of sanatorium therapy: easily readable, manageable dimensions, and readily maneuverable.

This could also be said of equipment that explicitly inculcated hygienic norms. The "Beb" Bath, for example, could be used for a body wash in the bedroom or in the single ward room of the sanatorium. Moreover, it was an affordable way of becoming clean, since it was on sale "at the specially low price of 13s 6d for the working classes."[146] The design of a telescopic, portable douche potentially was a "veritable boon" for travelers and those who were lucky enough to be still active in the workplace.[147] Portable disinfection spray pumps and cleaning equipment delivered the "gospel of germs" into the home, though not necessarily within the financial reach of many more households than was previously the case.[148] Lightweight, with directional nozzles and long handles, these appliances could reach every surface and penetrate the darkest nooks and crannies, mirroring the sort of technology that was being adopted by the municipal disinfecting teams of health departments. Also promoting domestic cleanliness were a boot cleaner and a boot dryer that were advertised for keeping out of the home the inconvenient muddiness of the open-air life. The former cleaned off dirt to prevent it entering the house; the latter meant that even during wet weather leather footwear could be dried out between daily walks.[149] When the *BJTB* observed that "at last it would seem that homes may be kept free from dust all the year round," it confirmed that the mass production of mechanical cleaning technologies had finally realized Alfred Carpenter's dreams about removing the "debris of everyday living."[150]

Many commodities invited the home-based tuberculosis patient to become involved in middle-class leisure pursuits. Telescopic reading stands, bed rests, and foot rests were presented as an entryway into the market of luxury goods that multiplied the comforts of modern life. The Kumfee was "an ingenious addition to the comforts of life which will be appreciated by invalids, luxury-lovers, and weary workers . . . [that] appeals to both healthy and sick, and it is certainly an economizer of energy and an increaser of comfort."[151] It doubled as a leg rest and fire screen (fig. 6.5). The Dumbnurse was "the greatest comfort and convenience to patients, invalids, and, perhaps we might add, healthy luxury-lovers."[152] For the bed-ridden, the Dumbnurse was a table, a backrest, and a reading stand (fig. 6.6). Similarly, the "Axis" portable bed table could be used for personal hygiene rituals such as washing and shaving, the serving of meals, and was a writing, card, or work table.[153] Multifunctionality equaled sophistication equaled luxury. Sophisticated, too, were electrical appliances that converted all sorts of items into a source of warmth. "A great future for the application of electric power" was predicted. For use in sanatoria and homes, in health and in sickness, "heat can be provided for comfort or," said the *BJTB*, "for healing under strict regulation and without danger."[154] The novelty of these products was sometimes conveyed by their names. Manufacturers used portmanteau words—the blending of two words to create a new one, such as ReferReader and Dumbnurse—and new spellings of old words (such as Kumfee) to create product interest.

The products described here represent only a very small selection of what was on offer. Patients, physicians, and tuberculosis activists were constantly

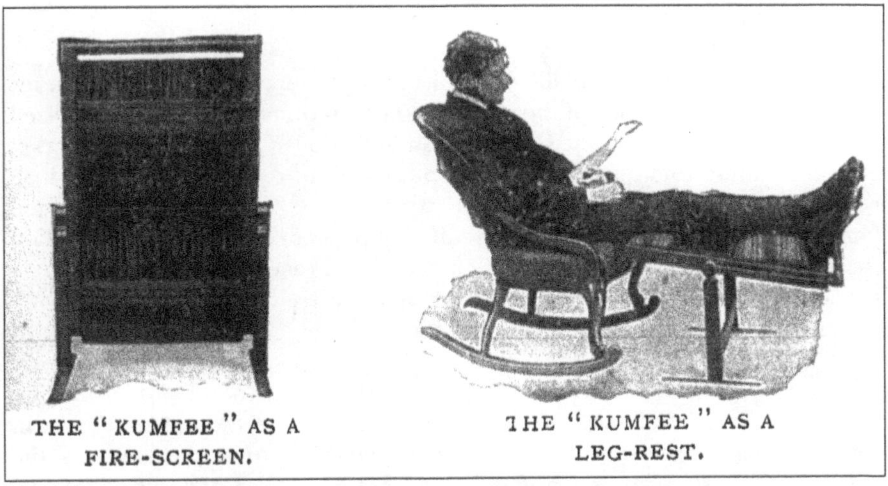
THE "KUMFEE" AS A FIRE-SCREEN.
THE "KUMFEE" AS A LEG-REST.

Figure 6.5. The Kumfee. "Kumfee," 211. Reproduced by permission from Elsevier.

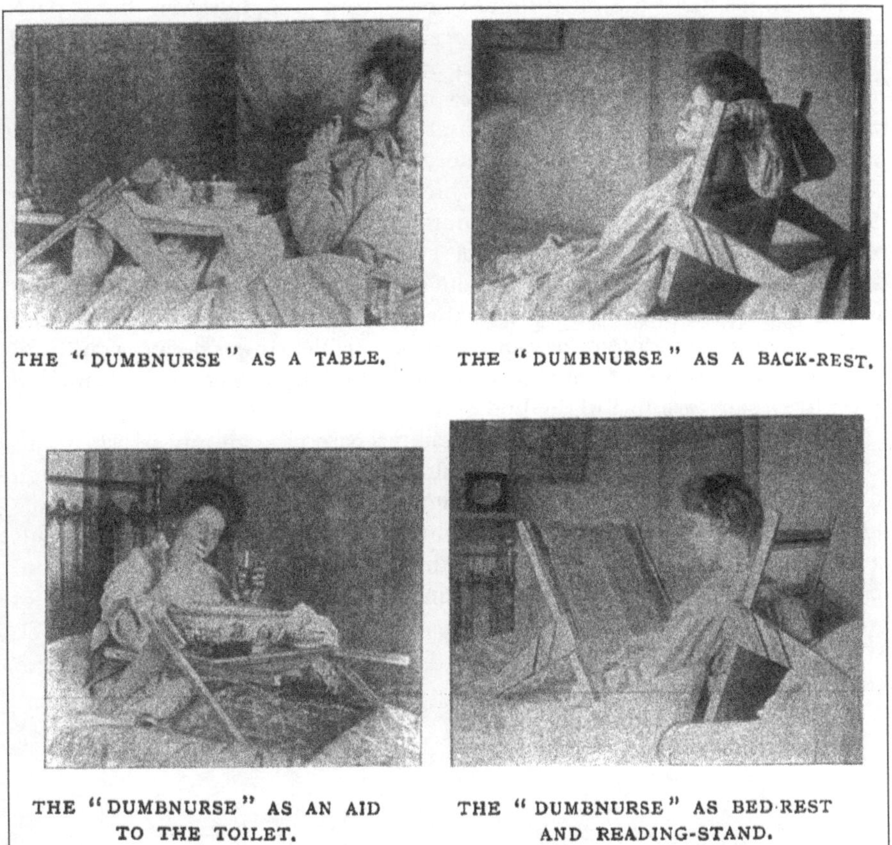


Figure 6.6. The Dumbnurse. "Dumbnurse," 192. Reproduced by permission from Elsevier.

apprised of opportunities to ally themselves with the materiality of modern living. The putative presence of these commodities in domestic spaces normalized tubercular life for home-based patients. Simultaneously tapping a *mass* market and succumbing to a fetishized novelty produced an expression of individuality that typifies the so-called "quest for personality."[155] Yet, these domesticated items were also imbued with a moral value that resonated with the long-standing Victorian attitude toward strength of character and rectitude. Just like the manuals written by Crowe, Thomson, and Bardswell, these commodities were nothing less than tools for a technology of the self.

The *British Journal of Tuberculosis* pointed out that all of these "numerous new inventions greatly facilitate the rational management of the sick and assist in the protection of the sound."[156] This claim neatly captures the idea that the melding of sanatorium and home spaces created a kind of preventive therapy that combined elements of public health prevention with a strict regimen for individual patients. It should not be forgotten, however, that experts also sought to transmit ideas about prevention-as-therapy in terms of moral behavior. The suppression of intimacy and avoidance of public houses made practical sense because it reduced exposure to infection.[157] But hygienists consistently reiterated the deeper moral purpose of these recommendations. Intemperance was, according to Thomson, "indirectly the chief predisposing cause by reason of the conditions of life to which it gives rise. The children of the drunkard are badly clothed, indifferently fed and poorly housed, and readily fall prey to the ravages of tuberculosis."[158] As such, the materiality of the consumptive life did not just denote spiritual worthiness; all things—from a reading stand to plasticine—potentially could promote homely pastimes and be a stimulating antidote to morally corrupt activities. It was deeply significant from the hygienist's point of view that these commodities could be marketed to both the sanatorium and the home.

The formal power structures of the state prepared the ground on which this sort of domiciliary regulation of tuberculosis patients gained traction. Through the implementation of compulsory notification, disinfection, educational schemes, dispensary management, and the home-based surveillance of patients and contacts, national and local government negotiated the legitimation and naturalization of the home as a site of intervention; the home was a space of both risk and opportunity.

# Conclusion

*Intrusive Interventions* opened with a focus on citizenship. It closes with the same. The year is 1908. The place is the inaugural issue of the *Sociological Review*, edited by Leonard Trelawney Hobhouse, a leading proponent of social liberalism. We have already met the writer, Dr. (later Sir) W. Leslie Mackenzie, from the Scottish Local Government Board. Mackenzie was the innovator who attached a bicycle inner tube and a T-shaped crosspiece to a disinfecting spray pump, thus making it "liberal."

The theme for Mackenzie's paper was "The Family and the City: Their Functional Relations."[1] Explicating the tenets of a new liberalism, Mackenzie stressed the interdependence of the family and urban space. In a quite remarkable disquisition, he explored the idea that modern city life decimated the traditional role of the family, which was "the infant school of ethics . . . a social molecule . . . to provide nurture for the child."[2] In a passage reminiscent of Benjamin Ward Richardson's *Hygeia*, Mackenzie argued that the ultimate object of the city was to preserve the family: there "must be streets to move by, space to give air and light, water to make cleaning and cleanliness possible, drains to remove soil, artificial light to reduce the dangers of darkness, and the thousand other mechanisms organic to the city." The technological components of the liberal city were no less "organic" than the families that lived in it.

George Buchanan had called in 1876 for "Citizenship in Sanitary Work" through a type of voluntary participation that cast responsibility on individuals but rewarded them with the right to self-government. Little more than thirty years later, Mackenzie extolled the virtues of city administration in the early twentieth century that had been "created by multitudes of men, out of millions of individual impulses and ideas [and] is capable of becoming the imaginative expression of every one man's mind, the instrument of every one man's will."[3] Despite the breathtaking ignorance and carelessness of parents, the potentiality of the city worked to resist the decay of responsibility. When a father sent his son to elementary school, it was not "an alien association," but "the office he himself has created, the organ of culture originating at the home but outgrowing the home in largeness of effect and in efficiency." Similarly, the isolation hospital was "an institution he himself has created just for this contingency and, handing over his child for the time, he has him taken into safe keeping."[4]

Infectious disease control had changed a lot in the forty years or so following the Royal Sanitary Commission at the end of the 1860s, and only partly because the diseases themselves came to be scientifically and popularly understood as "infectious" and amenable to "control." From practically a standing start, isolation hospitals became a common sight in the urban landscape (or, to be more precise, on the edges of it). Roving teams of municipal disinfectors competed with fever ambulances for street space. And young working-class children not only went to school as a matter of course; they were also routinely sent home from it for health reasons. As shown in chapter 1, this transformation was underpinned by a spatial imaginary propelled by the Victorian state's impulse to map the population that it governed. While the state never could quite know where and in whom all sickness was located, chapter 2 demonstrated that infectious disease notification proved to be a kind of gateway legislation that made the ailments of the poor visible to the state and opened the door to a set of intrusive interventions. Isolation, removal to hospital, disinfection, and contact tracing were piecemeal and contested processes that depended on the contingencies and contexts of local political circumstances. What I have tried to show, however, is that each of these interventions sought to unravel the perceived dangers and potentialities of the home and family life, thus maintaining public health's interest in domestic space that can be traced back to its emergence as a formal realm of state activity in the early nineteenth century. This focus on the domestic was sustained by the creation and reproduction of other spaces—hospitals, disinfection chambers, classrooms, laboratories—that were physically discrete but conceptually and materially connected to the home through processes that sought to govern through the family. As shown in chapter 6 on tuberculosis, the home itself was an integral component in the spatialization of public health.

Like George Buchanan three decades earlier, Mackenzie chose infectious disease notification to illustrate how the conditions of English citizenship had been transformed in the process:

> Look to the actual father and mother of a child suddenly smitten with an infectious disease. In a moment, they think of the doctor; then they take his advice. The doctor notifies the case to the municipality, whose officers, in a few minutes, are in attendance. Observations are made; records are taken; a nurse and an ambulance appear and in half an hour the child, under the care of two trained women and a surgeon, lies carefully watched in a dainty cot. Perhaps, within the hour, an operation to save his life has been completed and the immediate urgency is over.[5]

Given Mackenzie's political viewpoint, we should not be surprised that this paragraph glosses over so much that it borders on a shameless caricature. This book has documented, for example, how the whole process described by Mackenzie, from the initial recognition of the disease to the completion of "an operation"—a tracheotomy perhaps—was neither a uniformly common experience across the country, nor one free from resentment and opposition from the people who were drawn into it.[6] Nevertheless, Mackenzie was aware of the conflicting emotions that infectious disease surveillance provoked in working-class parents—which have since been well documented by historians[7]—ranging from the fear of municipal official power to an overwhelming sense of relief when a child returned from hospital, apparently restored to health.

Mackenzie argued that the education and public health systems delivered services to families that they were in no position to provide for themselves. In the case of disease surveillance, the fear of infection that a parent experienced "only revealed the inadequacy of the home to carry through the salvation of the child. Under stress of fear, the parent creates or discovers a new mechanism and thereafter he is ready always to use it. The home is saved from an impossible duty and the death-rate goes down."[8] Unlike the opponents of notification and isolation who appear in chapters 2 and 3, it was obvious to Mackenzie that the family was strengthened by welfare and social services, even though these techniques of disease management destabilized the familial locus of care. As with much else in the exercise of liberal freedom, however, there was an internal contradiction. In removing sick children from the care of the family (which, in the quote above, Mackenzie revealingly conflates with the "home"), the state was, in effect, asserting that parents were nothing more than social trustees for the child. One of the many obligations of parenthood was to learn "that the child belongs not exclusively to them, but, through them, to the society they live in."[9] If nothing else, this claim demonstrates how, as an interconnected set of management techniques, disease notification, mandatory removal to isolation hospital, contact tracing, and the disinfection of homes were an influential and controversial collection of tools that had the power to shape human subjectivity. The persuasiveness of scientific authority and the influence of didactic means of public education were necessary, but not sufficient, conditions for this. As disruptive as these interventions proved, they were made more palatable to the general population through an appreciation of scientific uncertainty and the socially contingent nature of technological change, which rearranged them into liberal mediations rather than coercive admonishments.

The compelling task, then, was *how* to realize a social contract between the family and the government under the altered states of education and public health. The terrain of citizenship was perpetually negotiable and constantly in flux, but Mackenzie himself had few concrete solutions other than to trust that the city itself would offer unending opportunities for parents and families to re-create themselves:

> The hopes and the fears that, in a system of city development, the family will be absorbed and superseded by some monstrous growth that destroys personality, sterilises ambition, and leaves every personal duty to someone else, are ungrounded in fact and incoherent in theory. . . . [The parent] is ever finding new revelations of what the potentialities are, new ways of increasing his own and their [children's] efficiency, new stimuli to active citizenship, new invitations to greater personal effort. All this, it is true, we find only now and then, in moments of social enthusiasm, at local elections, or when some great war

> excites the people; but none the less it is a reality and has in it the promise of great developments.[10]

Here, it is interesting to read what Mackenzie had to say about tuberculosis notification, which, as we have seen, was under trial in Sheffield in 1908. As the medical member of the Scottish Local Government Board, Mackenzie was closely involved with the decision to allow local authorities to put phthisis on the list of notifiable diseases in Scotland in 1906. By 1910, 50 percent of the Scottish population was covered by tuberculosis notification, and Mackenzie was working hard at the board to ensure that a sanatorium, a dispensary, and visiting nurses were available to everyone who wanted them. He also approved of house disinfection, isolation, and any other means by which individual patients were situated in an immediate environment that improved their chances of increasing personal resistance to infection and reducing complications: "the quickest way to get at the house," he wrote, "is to deal with the patient in the house."[11]

The account of tuberculosis control offered in chapter 6 provides an example of the sort of reconfigured citizenship that Mackenzie hoped for. By resiting and rescaling therapies from the sanatorium to the home, tuberculosis sufferers and their families were presented with "new stimuli to active citizenship" and the rules for living did indeed issue them with "new invitations to greater personal effort." Moreover, Mackenzie may well have approved that the broken bond between the family and the state that he so feared was in the restorative hands not only of doctors, health visitors, and crucially, self-treating patients, but also of that other mainstay of liberalism, the free market.

# *Notes*

## Introduction

1. Buchanan, "Sanitary Work"; Buchanan, "Citizenship in Sanitary Work"; Editorial, *Lancet* 108 (November 18, 1876): 722–25.

2. Hardy, "Buchanan, Sir George." Buchanan eventually took up the position of chief medical officer at the LGB in 1879 and was knighted in 1892. For an outstanding analysis of his work on yellow fever in Swansea in 1865 conducted for the Medical Office of the Privy Council, see Coleman, *Yellow Fever in the North*, chap. 6.

3. For more details see Rosenkrantz, *Public Health and the State*, 65–66.

4. Waddington, *Bovine Scourge*.

5. Buchanan, "Citizenship in Sanitary Work," 389–92.

6. Ibid., 396.

7. Sigsworth and Worboys, "Public's View of Public Health."

8. Buchanan, "Citizenship in Sanitary Work," 399.

9. Ibid., 399–400.

10. Buchanan's concept of citizenship relates particularly well to the idea of "social" citizenship put forward by T. H. Marshall in the mid-twentieth century. The relationship between citizenship and health has attracted increasing interest from historians in recent years. Most of this attention has been focused on the production and maintenance of a healthy population in the twentieth century through primary health care, physical fitness, health education, and army propaganda. See the essays in Huisman and Oosterhuis, *Health and Citizenship*. Other examples include Beach, "Potential for Participation"; De Haan, "Vigorous, Pure and Vulnerable"; and Welshman, "Child Health."

11. Hall, McClelland, and Rendall, *Defining the Victorian Nation*, 58–62. For the ways in which nationhood and national belonging were crucial to state formation in the nineteenth century and before, see Corrigan and Sayer, *Great Arch*, chap. 6.

12. McClelland, "England's Greatness, the Working Man," 116.

13. Durbach, *Bodily Matters*.

14. McClelland and Rose, "Citizenship and Empire," 277.

15. Pugh, "Limits of Liberalism," 7; Biagini, *Liberty, Retrenchment, and Reform*, 274–75, 286–87.

16. Armstrong, "Rise of Surveillance Medicine"; Fairchild et al., *Searching Eyes*.

17. Newsom Kerr, "'Perambulating Fever Nests.'"

18. Biagini, "Liberalism and Direct Democracy," 42.

19. Mandler, *Liberty and Authority.*

20. Foucault, "Governmentality"; Foucault, "Subject and Power"; Dean, "Social Structure of Many Souls"; Joyce, *Rule of Freedom*; Rose, *Powers of Freedom.*

21. Gunn, "From Hegemony to Governmentality"; Clarke, "Programmatic Statements and Dull Empiricism." Similarly, geographer Matthew Gandy has pointed out that such studies present "a highly generalized interpretation of a medley of different developments: the differential experience of the modern city is obscured by an abstract account of the governmental strategies of political liberalism." Gandy, "Bacteriological City," 20–21.

22. Hennock, *Fit and Proper Persons.*

23. Worboys, "Practice," 112.

24. Foucault, *Security, Territory, Population,* 207; Cadnam, "How (Not) to Be Governed."

25. Brunton, *Politics of Vaccination*; Howell, *Geographies of Regulation.*

26. Porter and Porter, "Enforcement of Health."

27. Biagini, *Citizenship and Community,* 3.

28. Hardy, "Cholera"; Baldwin, *Contagion and the State,* 151; Maglen, *English System.*

29. Rosen, *History of Public Health*; Wohl, *Endangered Lives.*

30. Worboys, *Spreading Germs.*

31. Mooney, "Public Health versus Private Practice."

32. Hardy, *Epidemic Streets.*

33. Porter and Porter, "Enforcement of Health."

34. Barnes, *Great Stink of Paris.* Barnes discusses isolation, disinfection, and public health interventions in schools in one chapter that is tellingly titled "Putting Germ Theory into Practice."

35. Mooney, "Public Health versus Private Practice."

36. Thacker, "Historical Development," 1. This is the definition most commonly used by the US Centers for Disease Control and Prevention.

37. Fairchild et al., *Searching Eyes*; Bayer and Fairchild, "Public Health."

38. Niemi, *Public Health,* 160. Niemi concentrates primarily on infant welfare and the relationship between housing and tuberculosis.

39. Otter, *Victorian Eye,* 110.

40. Newsholme, "Notification of Sickness."

41. Marks, "Until the Sun of Science."

42. One can also argue, as David Armstrong has done, that the naming of disease became spatialized in the Victorian period, since diagnostic practice involved pinpointing an underlying lesion that was, in his words, a new way for "the volume of the human body to be mapped": Armstrong, "Rise of Surveillance Medicine," 394–95. See also Mooney, "Diagnostic Spaces."

43. Morus, "Illuminating the Victorians," 160. Historians of science have tended to incorporate geographical modes of inquiry more readily than historians of medicine: Powell, "Geographies of Science."

44. Armstrong, "Public Health Spaces."

45. Harvey, *Cosmopolitanism,* 141.

46. Lefebvre, *Production of Space,* 234–54.

47. Harvey, *Cosmopolitanism,* 135–36.

48. Ibid., 137–38.

49. Massey, *For Space*, 107; emphases in the original. "Relational Politics of the Spatial" is the title of pt. 5 in *For Space*.

50. King, "Scale Politics of Emerging Diseases"; Ali and Keil, "Public Health and Political Economy."

51. See Livingstone, *Putting Science in Its Place*, and the essays in Dyck and Fletcher, *Locating Health*.

52. Jessop, Brenner, and Jones, "Theorizing Sociospatial Relations."

53. Biernacki and Jordan, "Place of Space." Mooney and Reinarz, "Hospital and Asylum Visiting."

54. See also Allen, *Lost Geographies of Power*.

55. Friendly Societies were mutual associations set up by groups of individuals (e.g., in the same trade) to provide services to their members, particularly sickness insurance.

56. Kearns and Reid-Henry, "Vital Geographies."

57. City of Birmingham Archives and Heritage (hereafter cited as BAH), Birmingham City Council Health Committee, Alfred Hill, *Report on the Health of the City of Birmingham for the Year 1891*.

58. Manchester City Council Archives and Local History, 614.0942.S8, John Tatham, *Annual Report on the Health of Salford for the Year 1886*.

59. An important recent collection of essays has begun to address the lack of work on workhouse hospitals: Reinarz and Schwarz, *Medicine and the Workhouse*.

60. Beier, *For Their Own Good*, 195.

61. For comparison with the Parisian case of "*le foyer*," see Aisenberg, *Contagion*.

62. Barnes, *Great Stink of Paris*, chap. 4.

63. Carpenter, "Address on Domestic Health," 1008; see also Cleere, "Victorian Dust Traps," 139.

64. Marcus, *Apartment Stories*, 115.

65. Davidoff et al., *Family Story*, 83.

66. Bachelard, *Poetics of Space*; Douglas, "Idea of Home"; Tuan, "View of Geography"; Tuan, *Space and Place*, chap. 10 ("Intimate Experiences of Place").

67. For a recent summary of the state of interdisciplinary research on home, house, and household, see Mezei and Briganti, *Domestic Space Reader*.

68. In "Home Sweet Home," Mark Jackson deals specifically with the relationship of the home to health, noting how it can be a physical place of habitation, a psychological or emotional space, and a political and ideological construct subject to medical intervention.

69. Griffin, Delap, and Wills, "Introduction"; Wahrman, *Imagining the Middle Class*, 298–408.

70. Hammerton, *Cruelty and Companionship*, 74–75.

71. Davidoff and Hall, *Family Fortunes*.

72. As Patrick Joyce has recently claimed, we need to move away from accounts that treat the state and "'cultural' things like families" as separate. Joyce, *State of Freedom*, 26–27.

73. Bashford, *Purity and Pollution*; Gilbert, *Citizen's Body*; Hamlin, *Public Health and Social Justice*; Poovey, *Making a Social Body*.

74. Bryden and Floyd, *Domestic Space*; Davidoff and Hall, *Family Fortunes*; Tosh, *Man's Place*.

75. Marcus, *Apartment Stories*, 7.
76. Hendrick, *Child Welfare*, 283.
77. Pooley, "All We Parents Want," 545.
78. Vincent, *Poor Citizens*, 8–9.
79. Davidoff et al., *Family Story*; Hammerton, *Cruelty and Companionship*, chap. 5.
80. Donzelot, *Policing of Families.*

## Chapter One

1. Brand, *Doctors and the State*, 60–64; Wohl, *Endangered Lives*, 140; Hardy, *Epidemic Streets*; Mooney, "Public Health versus Private Practice."

2. Barnes, *Great Stink of Paris*, 3; Baldwin, *Contagion and the State*, 151; Worboys, *Spreading Germs*, chap. 7; Pelling, *Cholera, Fever and English Medicine*, chap. 6.

3. Dennis, *Cities in Modernity*; Morris, "Governance."

4. Scott, *Seeing like a State*, 91; see also Joyce, *Rule of Freedom*, 103–5.

5. Curtis, "Surveying the Social," 93. This formulation draws on Foucault, *Discipline and Punish*; Foucault, *Birth of Biopolitics*; Deleuze and Guattari, *What Is Philosophy?*

6. Poovey, *Making a Social Body*, 32.

7. Osborne and Rose, "Governing Cities," 742.

8. Hannah, *Governmentality*, 17–25.

9. Rose, *Powers of Freedom*; Joyce, *Rule of Freedom*; see also Desrosières, *Politics of Large Numbers*, 16. The prevalence, multiple forms, and ambiguity of the Victorian culture of detachment are dealt with more broadly in Anderson, *Powers of Distance.*

10. Hacking, *Historical Ontology*, 107.

11. Osborne and Rose, "Governing Cities," 747.

12. Frankel, *States of Inquiry*, 3–4.

13. Crook, "Putting Matter"; Wohl, *Endangered Lives*, 72; Adams, *Architecture in the Family Way*, chap. 2; Porter, "Medical Futures," 314; Platt, "From Hygeia."

14. Edwin Chadwick himself had hinted to Richardson that a mortality rate of five per thousand was possible given unlimited resources and planning freedoms. Richardson, *Hygeia.*

15. Osborne and Rose, "Governing Cities," 747; Rockey, "From Vision to Reality," 95.

16. Otter, *Victorian Eye*, 63; see also Joyce, *Rule of Freedom.*

17. Richardson, *Hygeia*, 38–41.

18. Ibid., 37, 35.

19. Cassedy, "Hygeia," 220; Crook, "Putting Matter"; Platt, "From Hygeia."

20. Schweber, *Disciplining Statistics*; Szreter, "GRO"; Higgs, *Life, Death and Statistics*; Desrosières, *Politics of Large Numbers.* This chapter borrows from the ideas of Lorraine Daston and colleagues to interrogate sickness registration as a "scientific object"; see Daston, *Biographies of Scientific Objects.*

21. Rumsey, *Essays and Papers.*

22. Higgs, *Life, Death and Statistics*, 20.

23. Wohl, *Endangered Lives*, 159. Wohl mistakenly states that Rumsey was a member of the twenty-one-strong Royal Sanitary Commission, which is not the case. Rumsey and Alexander Stewart (coauthor in 1866 of *Medical and Legal Aspects of Sanitary Reform*) were dropped when the new Liberal government recomposed the

committee in 1868, reducing the number of doctors from five to one. Stewart was not even called on as a witness, though Rumsey was.

24. Goldman, *Science, Reform and Politics*, 191; Novak, "Professionalism and Bureaucracy," 450–51; Huch, "National Association." The memorial was based on a document drawn up by Rumsey in 1867. Goldman discusses the SSA's history of memorializing government on matters of state medicine (see chap. 6).

25. House of Commons Parliamentary Papers (hereafter cited as HCPP), C. 4218 (1868–69), *First Report of the Royal Sanitary Commission, with the Minutes of Evidence up to 5th August 1869* (hereafter cited as RSC *First Report*), appendix II, papers 5 and 6. For more on the SSA's reaction to the RSC's findings, see Goldman, *Science, Reform and Politics*, 191. A useful summary of the history of sickness registration is in Newsholme, "Notification and Registration of Sickness."

26. HCPP, C. 281 (1871) XXXV.1, *Second Report of the Royal Sanitary Commission* (hereafter cited as RSC *Second Report*), 1:59.

27. Lambert, *Sir John Simon*.

28. RSC *Second Report*, 1:60.

29. Deaths, of course, were registered at place of death. See Mooney, Luckin, and Tanner, "Patient Pathways"; Higgs, "Cuckoo in the Nest?"

30. RSC *Second Report*, 1:60. On "facts," see Poovey, *History of the Modern Fact*.

31. RSC *First Report*, question (hereafter "q.") 5,087.

32. Ibid., Simon q. 1,912, Christison q. 5,320, Rumsey q. 4,374; HCPP, C. 281-I C. 281-II (1871) XXXV.1, RSC *Second Report*, vol. 2, *Arrangement of Sanitary Statutes, Analysis of Evidence, Precis of Oral Evidence, Paper on Watershed Boards, and Memorandum on Duties of Medical Officers of Public Health*; and vol. 3, *Part I, Minutes of Evidence, 1869–70*, Druitt q. 9,029, Burke q. 8,836.

33. Alborn, "Calculating Profession"; Eyler, *Victorian Social Medicine*, 76; Woods, *Demography of Victorian England*, 181. Edmonds was actuary to the Legal and General Life Assurance Society.

34. Eyler, *Victorian Social Medicine*, 108–9; Edmonds, "Laws of Collective Vitality," 5; Edmonds, "Statistics of the London Hospital," 778.

35. Alborn, *Regulated Lives*, chap. 4.

36. Farr was invited onto this committee after giving evidence to the Army Sanitary Commission, on which he collaborated closely with Florence Nightingale. Farr did not much discuss sickness returns in his evidence to that Commission and confined most of his remarks to mortality. The three-man committee also included Lord Sidney Herbert and Colonel Sir Alexander Tulloch. John Eyler notes that Tulloch resented Farr's domination of the committee, Eyler, *Victorian Social Medicine*, 161–72.

37. HCPP, C. 366 (1861), XXXVII.455, *Report of the Committee on the Preparation of Army Medical Statistics, &c., and of the First Annual Report of the Statistical Branch of the Army Medical Department*, 25.

38. Ibid., 28.

39. Ibid., 28; HCPP, C. 2318 (1857–58), XVIII.1, *Report of the Commissioners Appointed to Inquire into Regulations Affecting the Sanitary Condition of the Army, the Organization of Military Hospitals, and the Treatment of the Sick and Wounded, with Evidence and Appendix*, q. 7,132.

40. HCPP, C. 2318 (1857–58), XVIII.1, *Royal Commission on the Sanitary Condition of the Army . . . with Evidence and Appendix*, qq. 7,045–46.

41. HCPP, C. 366 (1861), XXXVII.455, *Report of the Committee on the Preparation of Army Medical Statistics, &c.*, . . . , 31. It was predicted that production of a twelve-page return for the whole army (179 regiments) would occupy four clerks two working days.

42. Ibid., 83.

43. Ibid., 43.

44. Ibid., 47–48.

45. The committee for the Section on Sanitary Statistics included Drs. Neil Arnott, William Henry Duncan, Headlam Greenhow, Henry Letheby, John Simon, and Southwood Smith. Other members in the section were Chadwick, Rumsey, Edmonds, and Florence Nightingale.

46. Farr, "General Sanitary Statistics," 49.

47. Crawford, *Counting the People*, 71–72; Froggatt, "Sir William Wilde."

48. Farr, "General Sanitary Statistics," 49.

49. Ibid.

50. RSC *Second Report*, 1:60.

51. Graham, "Remarks," 288.

52. Ibid., 289.

53. RSC *First Report*, q. 6,453. See also Higgs, *Life, Death and Statistics*, 20.

54. RSC *First Report*, q. 6,482; emphasis added.

55. Graham, "Remarks," 290.

56. Lambert, *Sir John Simon*; Eyler, *Victorian Social Medicine*.

57. "Medico-Meteorological Observations." These observations were collected in Wakefield, Hawarden, Grantham, Bedford, Uckfield, Exeter, Ryde, and Guernsey.

58. Paget, *Wasted Records of Disease*.

59. Richardson, *Hygeia*, chap. 8.

60. Wallis, "Richardson, Sir Benjamin Ward."

61. Richardson claimed that the first cases of diphtheria in England came to light as a result of the reports from Canterbury in April 1857. Richardson, *Ministry of Health*, 297.

62. Richardson, *Hygeia*, 297–98, 232; Newsholme and Stevenson, "Decline of Human Fertility."

63. Marks, "Until the Sun of Science," 148, 153.

64. Ransome, "Need for Combined Medical Observation," 407–8.

65. RSC *Second Report*, 3: q. 8,836.

66. Ibid., qq. 9,029–42.

67. Dickens, "Registration of Sickness." For background on Dickens's perspective on public health, see Litsios, "Charles Dickens."

68. Dickens, "Registration of Sickness," 228.

69. "Registration of Disease," *Lancet* 94 (November 13, 1869): 680.

70. RSC *First Report*, q. 6,481; Lewis, *Suggestions for National Returns*. The publication of Poor Law sickness returns would also bring the GRO and public health reformers closer and in fact justified the RSC's proposal to include the GRO under the umbrella of a "Central Authority," which became the LGB but excluded the GRO. RSC *Second Report*, 1:61.

71. Simon, *English Sanitary Institutions*, 249–50.

72. Lambert, *Sir John Simon*, 116–17.

73. Kearns, "Town Hall and Whitehall," 104.

74. Laxton, "Fighting for Public Health," 63–64. According to the clerk of the city's sanitary committee, Newcastle-upon-Tyne had a similar dual system in the late 1860s. The board of guardians there was responsible for hospital accommodations and medical relief during a cholera epidemic, while the corporation took on these duties in other times. See RSC *First Report*, Robert Carr, qq. 2,797–98.

75. Laxton, "Fighting for Public Health," 87; Kearns, "Town Hall and Whitehall," 104.

76. Bullin, Hutchinson, and Digby, "Memorial of the Medical Officers."

77. Laxton argues that Simon "seems not to have had the character or persistence to work with these humble medical toilers." Laxton, "Fighting for Public Health," 87n114.

78. Allan, "Early Days."

79. Newsholme, "Notification and Registration of Sickness," 5.

80. Allan, "Early Days," 80–83; RSC *First Report*, q. 4,283 to Rumsey; Newsholme, "Notification and Registration of Sickness," 5.

81. Lewis, *Suggestions for National Returns*; Dudfield, "Critical Examination"; HCPP, C. 4127 (1868–69), XXXII.1, *Eleventh Report of the Medical Officer of the Privy Council, 1868*, appendix 3; Ballard, *Results of an Analysis*; Manchester and Salford Sanitary Association, *Annual Report, 1864*.

82. Ballard, *Results of an Analysis*, 37. Ballard's study might never have seen the light of day had John Simon not urged its publication.

83. Fox, "Why Should the Existing System . . . ?," 563.

84. Ballard, *Results of an Analysis*, 37.

85. Platt, *Shock Cities*, 71–74.

86. Manchester and Salford Sanitary Association, *Report of the Committee, 1859 and 1860*, 6.

87. Hewitt, "Travails of Domestic Visiting," 210–11. Hewitt disputes convincingly the notion that domestic visiting (in all its forms) overcame the social distance between classes. Many aspects of working-class culture, especially in the domain of leisure, were incongruous to middle-class evangelicals.

88. Manchester and Salford Sanitary Association, *Annual Report, November 1853 to October 1854*, appendix B. It is probable that this request was provoked by Dr. John Hatton's investigation into disease and sanitary conditions in Chorlton-upon-Medlock that was sponsored by the MSSA. Hatton was consultant surgeon to the dispensary, and his analysis used rate assessors' books, mortality registers, and cases of illness admitted by the dispensary and the Poor Law between 1847 and 1851. See Hatton, *Sanitary Condition of Chorlton-upon-Medlock*, 24.

89. Manchester and Salford Sanitary Association, *Report of the Committee, 1861*, 7; Manchester and Salford Sanitary Association, *Annual Report, 1880*; "Disease in Manchester," *Times*, November 9, 1861.

90. "Dr. Ransome and Sanitary Work in Manchester and Salford," *Manchester Guardian*, November 1, 1894.

91. In 1860 the PLMO for Salford's Greengate District, Mr. J. Teale, was a member of this subcommittee. In subsequent years it also included Mr. George Greaves, surgeon at the Chorlton Union Workhouse, as listed in *Slater's General and Classified Directory*.

92. Manchester and Salford Sanitary Association, *Annual Report, 1857–1858.*

93. Platt, *Shock Cities*, 210; Hewitt, *Emergence of Stability*, 145.

94. Hewitt, *Emergence of Stability*, 81.

95. Manchester and Salford Sanitary Association, *Report of the Committee, 1859 and 1860*, 6.

96. Manchester and Salford Sanitary Association, *Report of the Committee, 1862*, 5.

97. "Slight Increase in the Amount of Employment," *Times*, January 3, 1863; Buchanan, "Typhus at Manchester." James Kay-Shuttleworth also referred to the sickness returns in his capacity as vice chair of the Central Executive Relief Committee: Manchester and Salford Sanitary Association, *Report of the Committee, 1862*, 10; Longmate, *Hungry Mills*; Oddy, "Urban Famine."

98. Thomas Turner, Arthur Ransome, and C. H. Knight, "Typhus Fever at Manchester," *Times*, January 23, 1863; Thomas Turner, Arthur Ransome, and C. H. Knight, "Letter to the Editor," *Times*, January 29, 1863; Noble, *Fluctuations in the Death Rate.*

99. "Slight Increase in the Amount of Employment," *Times*, January 3, 1863. For more on the politics of the Cotton Famine relief operation, see Farnie, *English Cotton Industry*; and Longmate, *Hungry Mills.*

100. Manchester and Salford Sanitary Association, *Report of the Committee, 1862*, 6–8.

101. Ibid., 8–9.

102. Philipson, *Investigation of the Prevalent Diseases*, 13. As a guarantee of his colleagues' future cooperation, Philipson took the signature of each practitioner who was present at the NDMS meeting at which his proposals were accepted. Northumberland and Durham Medical Society, *Report, 1863–4*, October 29, 1863, 5.

103. RSC *First Report*, appendix II, paper 4.

104. Ibid., q. 2,777.

105. Ibid., q. 2,778.

106. Ibid., qq. 2,320–22.

107. Ibid., q. 2,361. Heron's display of ignorance—willful or otherwise—agitated the MSSA, and Rumsey disabused the commission of Heron's disinformation. Manchester and Salford Sanitary Association, *Annual Report, 1869*, 7–8; RSC *First Report*, q. 4,283.

108. Leigh, *Infectious Disease in Manchester.* Heron later advocated the notification of infectious diseases, in "Association of Municipal Corporations," *Sanitary Record* 8 (February 22, 1878): 120.

109. Hardie, "Duty of Municipal Authorities," 14–15.

110. Milroy, "Suggestions." A well-known opponent of quarantine, Milroy had been one-time editor of the *Medico-Chirurgical Review* and inspector for the General Board of Health. He later became secretary of the Epidemiological Society of London.

111. Rumsey, *Essays on State Medicine*, 241–42; Lewis, *Suggestions for National Returns.*

112. Rumsey, *Essays on State Medicine*, 105–6.

113. Dudfield, "Critical Examination," 14. The standard of medical record-keeping in the Poor Law system was roundly criticized, though documentation in the voluntary hospital system was also frowned on. For a comparison see Mooney, "Diagnostic Spaces."

114. Fox, "Why Should the Existing System . . . ?," 563–64. On the "necessaries" ordered by PLMOs, see Hodgkinson, *National Health Service*, chap. 11.

115. Fox, "Why Should the Existing System . . . ?," 566.

116. Crowther, *Workhouse System*, chap. 7. On the plus side, PLMOs were allowed private practice and potentially had access to the social world of the guardians.

117. HCPP, C. 4127 (1868–69), XXXII.1, *Eleventh Report of Medical Officer of the Privy Council, 1868.*

118. Lambert, *Sir John Simon*, 339–40, 420n55; HCPP, C. 468 (1870), LVIII.727, *Return of Numbers of Paupers on District and Workhouse Medical Officers' Relief-Books in England and Wales, 1869–70* (hereafter cited as *Return of Numbers of Paupers*).

119. For examples, see HCPP, C. 372 (1866), LXI.171, *Metropolitan Workhouse Infirmaries, &c. Copy of the Report of Dr. Edward Smith LL.B., F.R.S., Poor Law Inspector and Medical Officer to the Poor Law Board, on the Metropolitan Workhouse Infirmaries and Sick Wards* (hereafter cited as *Metropolitan Workhouse Infirmaries*); HCPP, C. 445 (1867–68), LX.203, *Return of the Number of in-Door Poor in Workhouses in England and Wales (Exclusive of the Metropolitan District) on 1st July 1867 and 1st January 1868; and, of the Number of in-Door Poor on Workhouse Medical Relief Books on 1st July 1867 and 1st January 1868; and Other Particulars*; HCPP, C. 4 (1867–68), LX.325, *Report of Dr. Edward Smith, Medical Officer to the Poor Law Board, on the Sufficiency of the Existing Arrangements for the Care and Treatment of the Sick Poor in Forty-eight Provincial Workhouses in England and Wales* (hereafter cited as *Report of Dr. Edward Smith*).

120. *Return of Numbers of Paupers*, iii. There were almost 1 million paupers in all.

121. Ibid., iv; "Registration of Diseases," *Manchester Guardian*, October 19, 1870.

122. *Return of Numbers of Paupers*, vi.

123. Ibid., iv.

124. Ibid., xxii.

125. Lambert, *Sir John Simon*, 340.

126. *Return of Numbers of Paupers*, xxii.

127. Ibid., xxiv.

128. Ibid., xxv.

129. Hurren, "Poor Law versus Public Health."

130. Rogers, *Reminiscences*; Crowther, *Workhouse System*; Flinn, "Medical Services," 63; Hodgkinson, *National Health Service*, chap. 14, 668–70.

131. *Metropolitan Workhouse Infirmaries*; *Report of Dr. Edward Smith*.

132. Driver, *Power and Pauperism*, chap. 5; Green, "Pauper Protests."

133. Ayers, *England's First State Hospitals*.

134. Frankel, *States of Inquiry*, 145–46.

135. Joyce, *Rule of Freedom*, 13, 21.

136. North, "Registration of Disease," 322.

137. Richardson, *Ministry of Health*, 278–79.

138. North, "Registration of Disease," 321.

139. Frankel, *States of Inquiry*, 3.

140. Newsholme, "Notification and Registration of Sickness"; Havelock Ellis, "Nationalisation of Health," *Time*, January 7, 1890, 690–98; "Dr. Ransome and Sanitary Work in Manchester and Salford," *Manchester Guardian*, November 1, 1894.

## Chapter Two

1. Nottinghamshire Archives (hereafter cited as NA), Open Shelves, Borough of Nottingham, Reports Presented to the Council, 1881–82, *Report of the Health Committee as to the Memorial Presented to the Council on the Notification of Infectious Disease* (hereafter cited as Nottingham *RHC, 1882*).

2. Newsholme, "Notification of Sickness."

3. Baldwin, *Contagion and the State*, 154–55; Wohl, *Endangered Lives*, 136–37.

4. Porter and Porter, "Enforcement of Health," 108; Eyler, "Scarlet Fever and Confinement."

5. HCPP, C. 194 (1892), LXVIII.105, *Return of Sanitary Districts in England and Wales Adopting Infectious Disease (Notification) Act, 1889; Infectious Disease (Prevention) Act and Public Health Acts Amendment Act, 1890; Districts with Notification System under Local Acts*, 21.

6. Wohl, *Endangered Lives*, 137.

7. Events in the southern coastal town of Brighton are described in Eyler, *Sir Arthur Newsholme*, chaps. 2 and 4; the Manchester region is dealt with briefly in Pickstone, *Medicine and Industrial Society*, 170–71; and the situation in Liverpool is discussed in Mooney, "Public Health versus Private Practice."

8. Ayers, *England's First State Hospitals.*

9. Sheard, "Reluctant Providers?"

10. HCPP, C. 3290 (1881), XXX Pt.II.1, *Tenth Annual Report of the Local Government Board 1880–81: Supplement*, Richard Thorne Thorne, "On the Use and Influence of Hospitals for Infectious Diseases" (hereafter cited as Thorne, "Use and Influence of Hospitals").

11. Examples from the vast and rich historical literature on Victorian liberalism include Bellamy, *Liberalism and Modern Society* and *Victorian Liberalism*; Collini, "Liberalism and Mill" and *Public Moralists*; Biagini, *Citizenship and Community*; Biagini and Reid, *Currents of Radicalism*; and Mandler, *Liberty and Authority.*

12. Collini, "'Character' in Victorian Political Thought."

13. Bell Taylor, "Notification of Infectious Diseases."

14. On the "game" of liberalism and the consumption of liberty as a technique of government, see Foucault, *Security, Territory, Population*, chaps. 2 and 3; and Foucault, *Birth of Biopolitics*, chaps. 1–3.

15. Valverde, "Despotism and Ethical Liberal Government," 358; Howell, *Geographies of Regulation*, 2; Beckingham, "Historical Geography of Liberty," 388–90.

16. Gunn, "From Hegemony to Governmentality," 716–17.

17. Harling, "Centrality of Locality," 218.

18. On sanitary inspection as a practice of liberal government, see Crook, "Sanitary Inspection"; and on its geography see Hamlin, "Sanitary Policing."

19. Otter, *Victorian Eye*, 127.

20. Ibid., 134.

21. Seaton's justification for notification cited at the beginning of this chapter testifies to its value for making faulty technologies visible.

22. Harling, "Powers of the Victorian State," 33. On the multiple meanings and uses of the "residuum," see Harris, "Civic Virtue and Social Darwinism."

23. Crook, "Accommodating the Outcast," 418. On vagrancy, casual labor, and lodging houses, see Jones, *Outcast London*, 88–92, chap. 11.

24. Koven, *Slumming*, chap. 1.

25. There is now an extensive literature on the CD Acts: see Walkowitz, *Prostitution and Victorian Society*; Smith, "Contagious Diseases Acts Reconsidered"; Sigsworth and Wyke, "Study of Victorian Prostitution"; Ogborn, "Law and Discipline"; Hall, "Venereal Diseases and Society"; Baldwin, *Contagion and the State*; and Hunt, *Governing Morals*. With a couple of notable exceptions, comparatively little is known about the micropolitics of commercial sex regulation in municipalities that fell outside the reach of the CD Acts. One is Howell, *Geographies of Regulation*, which considers Liverpool and Cambridge; another is Mahood, *Magdalenes*, with a focus on Glasgow.

26. Walkowitz, *Prostitution and Victorian Society*, 71.

27. McHugh, *Prostitution and Victorian Social Reform*, 63–64; Smith, "Contagious Diseases Acts Reconsidered," 204; John Simon, while medical officer at the Privy Council, insisted that the "civilian population" was not to be included under the terms of the CD Acts, arguing that this would have represented an "illegitimate extension of state authority"; see Ogborn, "Law and Discipline," 43.

28. Mort, *Dangerous Sexualities*, 87–92; see also Hunt, *Governing Morals*, chap. 5.

29. Brunton, *Politics of Vaccination*, chap. 3; Baldwin, *Contagion and the State*, 267; Lambert, "Victorian National Health Service"; MacLeod, "Law, Medicine and Public Opinion: Part I"; MacLeod, "Law, Medicine and Public Opinion: Part II."

30. Durbach, *Bodily Matters*.

31. Mill was an MP when the 1867 Vaccination Act was passed, and he did not openly oppose it.

32. HCPP, C. 408, C. 408-I (1871), XIX.1, 29, *Report of Royal Commission upon the Administration and Operation of the Contagious Diseases Acts*, J. S. Mill, q. 20,084.

33. Sanitary Act, 1866, 29 & 30 Vic., c. 40.

34. Lambert, "Victorian National Health Service."

35. Prest, *Liberty and Locality*, 210.

36. Armstrong, "Rise of Surveillance Medicine" and "Medical Surveillance of Normal Populations."

37. Hamlin, "Sanitary Policing"; Kearns, "Cholera," 104–9.

38. Dudfield, *25th Annual Report . . . Kensington, 1880*, 47.

39. Eyler, "Scarlet Fever and Confinement," 1–2; Pickstone, *Medicine and Industrial Society*, 170–71.

40. "Compulsory Information of Infectious Diseases," *Sanitary Record* 8 (1878): 25.

41. "Compulsory Notification of Infectious Disease," *Sanitary Record* 7 (1877): 287–88.

42. "Prevention of Epidemic Disease," *Liverpool Mercury*, January 27, 1877.

43. "Registration of Infectious Diseases," *Sanitary Record* 8 (February 22, 1878): 121.

44. HCPP, C. 229 (1881), II.367, *Infectious Diseases Notification: A Bill for the Better Notification of Infectious Diseases*; HCPP, C. 52 (1882), II.509, *Infectious Diseases Notification: A Bill for the Better Notification of Infectious Diseases*; HCPP, C. 100 (1883), *Infectious Diseases Notification: A Bill for the Better Notification of Infectious Diseases.* Hastings's father, Sir Charles Hastings (1794–1866), was founder of the BMA, and in the mid-1850s George was instrumental in creating the National Association for the Promotion of Social Science.

45. "Registration of Infectious Diseases," *British Medical Journal* 1000 (February 28, 1880): 340; "Registration of Infectious Diseases," *Manchester Guardian*, February 10, 1880; Dudfield, *25th Annual Report . . . Kensington, 1880*, 57.

46. Livy, "Notification of Infectious Diseases."

47. Elmy, "Local Government Board," 76; "British Medical Association and the Compulsory Notification of Infectious Diseases," *Journal of the Vigilance Association for the Defence of Personal Rights* 21 (September 15, 1882): 81–83; Goff and Levy, *Politics and Disease*; Butler, "Vigilance Committee." The VADPR grew out of the anti–Contagious Diseases Acts crusade and later became the Personal Rights Association. It is not to be confused with the National Vigilance Association, a purity movement set up in 1885 by William Stead. Though only small in membership, and having shed its initial focus on legislation injurious to women, the VADPR was important because "its executive provided as near an equivalent to a theory-debating inner circle for the most radical and agenda-setting section of the feminist elite as existed between the early 1870s and mid-1880s." Roberts, "Feminism and the State," 89. One parliamentary opponent of notification was Liberal MP for Stockport Charles Hopwood, one of Josephine Butler's spokesmen in the House of Commons; see Bristow, "Liberty and Property Defence League," 773.

48. "Memorial against Compulsory Notification," *Journal of the Vigilance Association for the Defence of Personal Rights* 27 (April 15, 1883): 39–40.

49. Dudfield, *25th Annual Report . . . Kensington, 1880*, 57.

50. "Ministerial Views on Compulsory Notification," *Journal of the Vigilance Association for the Defence of Personal Rights* 27 (April 15, 1883): 34–35.

51. Bell Taylor, "Notification of Infectious Diseases."

52. Elmy, "Compulsory Notification of Infectious Disease," 92.

53. "Nemo," "Medical and Administrative Despotism."

54. Editorial, "Notification of Infectious Diseases," *Sanitary Record*, n.s., 6 (1884): 17–18.

55. HCPP, C. 226 (1882), XII.345, *Report from the Select Committee on Police and Sanitary Regulations*, ii.

56. Rydz, *Parliamentary Agents*, 190.

57. HCPP, C. 226 (1882), XII.345, *Report from the Select Committee on Police and Sanitary Regulations*, appendix 1.

58. BMA Archives, *Parliamentary Bills Committee Minute Book* [hereafter cited as BMAPBC *MB*], *1875–87*, April 30, 1885, 169. Bolton's mayor openly acknowledged that while the inclusion of notification in its 1877 local act was not deliberately kept secret, "it did not come prominently before them [the local medical profession], and therefore we got the clause without any opposition." City of Liverpool, *Notification of Infectious Disease: Evidence Taken by the Deputations Appointed by the Health Committee* (hereafter cited as Liverpool *Evidence*) (Liverpool: Henry Greenwood, 1882), Bolton Deputation, T. Glashier, q. 4.

59. Liberty and Property Defence League, *Overlegislation in 1884*, 24–25; on the league itself see Liberty and Property Defence League, *Self-Help v. State-Help*; and Bristow, "Liberty and Property Defence League."

60. "Doctors and Local Legislation," *Saturday Review of Politics, Literature, Science and Art* 53 (June 17, 1882): 763; Elmy, "Legislation." According to Muriel Fielding, Elmy became a parliamentary agent in the early 1870s, which undoubtedly gave her

a unique insight into the workings of private bill legislation that lent authoritative weight to her writings. Fielding, "Ignota, the Unknown Woman," 155.

61. Bellamy, *Administering Central-Local Relations*, 199.

62. "Annual Meeting," *Journal of the Vigilance Association for the Defence of Personal Rights* 26 (March 15, 1883): 21–26; "Fidelis," "Sanitary and Police Clauses." Bellamy describes the SCPSR as operating a "safety valve in the face of legislative stagnation." Bellamy, *Administering Central-Local Relations*, 205–8.

63. "Local Opposition to the Private Bills," *Journal of the Vigilance Association for the Defence of Personal Rights* 18 (June 15, 1882): 58–59.

64. On the use of provisional orders see Bellamy, *Administering Central-Local Relations*, 210–14.

65. The Local Government Board's Provisional Orders Confirmation (Halifax, Leeds & Manchester) Act, 1881, 44 & 45 Vic. c. 64. Amendments to local laws for public health purposes were allowed under section 303 of the Public Health Act, 1875, 38 & 39 Vic., c. 54.

66. Bellamy, *Administering Central-Local Relations*, 208.

67. "Mr Ritchie at Sheffield," *Times*, January 31, 1888.

68. "Compulsory Information of Infectious Diseases," *Sanitary Record* 8 (1878): 25.

69. Tatham, "Compulsory Notification of Infectious Diseases," 473–76; "Destructive Liberty of the Subject," *British Architect* 31, no. 13 (March 29, 1889): 240; Russell, "Department of Health," 619, 622–23.

70. "Ladies National Association," *Sentinel* 11, no. 9 (1889): 103–4. McLaren was a well-known radical and was married to social reformer and feminist Eva McLaren.

71. Infectious Diseases (Notification) Act, 1889, 52 & 53 Vic., c. 72. The act's compulsory clauses regarding London were later consolidated under the Public Health (London) Act, 1891, 54 & 55 Vic., c. 76.

72. Half of the London vestries had petitioned the House in favor of the bill becoming law. *Hansard* Parl. Deb. (3rd ser.) (1889) 1819–20, 1825, and 1830–31.

73. "Compulsory Notification of Infectious Diseases Bill," *Sanitary Record*, n.s., 11 (1889): 58. "Infectious Diseases Notification Bill," *Saturday Review of Politics, Literature, Science and Art* 68 (August 3, 1889): 125–26; HCPP, C. 300 (1888), XV.1, *Special Report from the Select Committee on Police and Sanitary Regulations*, iii.

74. Hastings, "Inaugural Address."

75. Infectious Diseases Notification (Extension) Act, 1899, 62 & 63 Vic. c. 8.

76. Many local authorities were energetic and proactive when it came to sanitary reform in the third quarter of the nineteenth century, independent of central government interference. See, for example, Hamlin, "Muddling in Bumbledom."

77. Shepherd, *Liverpool Medical Institution*, 102–6.

78. Liverpool Medical Institution (hereafter cited as LMI), *Minutes, 43rd Session*, October 20, 1881, and Town Clerk to Reginald Harrison, October 21, 1881. Harrison was the president of the LMI at the time. With more than 180 members in the early 1880s, the LMI might be said to represent the spectrum of medical opinion of the 400 or so doctors living within ten miles of the Liverpool city center. Shepherd, *Liverpool Medical Institution*, 142.

79. LMI, *Minutes, 43rd Session*, November 3, 1881, and Circular from Edgar A. Browne, October 21, 1881; Liverpool Central Library (hereafter cited as LCL), 352

MIN/HEA II 1/34, City of Liverpool, *Health Committee Minute Book* [hereafter cited as Liverpool *HCMB*], *October, 1881 to March, 1882*, November 10 and 17, 1881.

80. Carter was lecturer at University College Liverpool and physician to Liverpool's Royal Southern Hospital. Jordan and Sharp, *Josephine Butler*, 3:175–76. On the deputation see Lowndes, "Medical Profession in Liverpool."

81. LMI, *Minutes, 43rd Session*, Dr. E. Sheldon to the President, December 1, 1881.

82. Liverpool *HCMB, October, 1881 to March, 1882*, December 1, 1881, 234–39; "Registration of Infectious Diseases," *Liverpool Mercury*, December 2, 1881.

83. Forwood apologized for the hurried nature of his action but argued that unless the council were empowered by the health committee at its September meeting, then nothing could be done for a further twelve months. "Prevalence of Typhus in Liverpool—the Notification of Disease," *Liverpool Mercury*, September 1, 1882.

84. LCL, 352 MIN/HEA II 1/36, Liverpool *HCMB, August 1882 to February 1883*, September 7, 1882, 83; "Liverpool: The Notification of Infectious Disease."

85. City of Liverpool, *Notification of Infectious Diseases: Circular Addressed by the Chairman of the Health Committee to the Mayors of the Boroughs, and the Chairmen of the Local Board Districts in which Notification of Infectious Disease is Compulsory, and the Replies Thereto* (Liverpool, 1882) (hereafter cited as Liverpool *Circular*).

86. Liverpool *Evidence*; Liverpool *HCMB, August 1882 to February 1883*, September 28, 1882, 202.

87. Liverpool *HCMB, August 1882 to February 1883*, October 11, 1882, 263.

88. LMI, *Minutes, 51st Session*, November 7, 1889. Carter was on the subcommittee that considered the proposals.

89. *Liverpool Mercury*, October 18, 1882, 5.

90. NA, CA.CM/Health/7, Borough of Nottingham, *Health Committee Minute Book* [hereafter cited as Nottingham *HCMB*], *December 22, 1876 to September 6, 1878*, December 14, 1877.

91. Ibid., January 11, 1878; NA, CA.CM/Health/9, Nottingham *HCMB, August 30, 1880 to November 24, 1882*, May 16, 1881.

92. Nottingham *HCMB, December 22, 1876 to September 6, 1878*, January 11, 1878; NA, Open Shelves, Borough of Nottingham, Reports Presented to the Council, 1884–85, *Report of the Town Clerk*, No. 55, July 22, 1885, 391–400.

93. Nottingham *HCMB, August 30, 1880 to November 24, 1882*, March 18 and 25, 1881.

94. Ibid., May 16, 1881. Seaton later revealed that the medical profession accorded neither him nor the health committee the respect they deserved when responding to what had been a "courteous and conciliatory" approach on their part. Nottingham *RHC, 1882*, 5.

95. Nottingham *HCMB, August 30, 1880 to November 24, 1882*, July 15, 1881. Seaton's account of the doctors' response was printed six months later in Nottingham *RHC, 1882*, 8.

96. "Nottingham Town Council," *Nottingham and Midland Counties Daily Express*, February 7, 1882.

97. NA, Open Shelves, Borough of Nottingham, *Minutes of the Town Council, 1881–2*, May 1, 1882. As well as in the local press, reports of this protest were made in *British Medical Journal* 1117 (May 27, 1882): 798; and "Private Bills," *Journal of the Vigilance Association for the Defence of Personal Rights* 17 (May 15, 1882): 47–49.

98. Bell Taylor played a founding role in the NA. See McHugh, *Prostitution and Victorian Social Reform,* 55; and Walkowitz, *Prostitution and Victorian Society,* 91–92. According to the *BMJ,* Bell Taylor was "a great individualist, and all that interfered with the liberty of the individual met with his uncompromising and eloquent denunciation." "Charles Bell Taylor, M.D. and F.R.C.S. Edin," *British Medical Journal* 2521 (April 24, 1909): 1033–34.

99. Nottingham *RHC, 1882,* 5, 28.

100. "Nottingham Town Council," *Nottingham and Midland Counties Daily Express,* February 7, 1882.

101. NA, CATC 10/38/5, Borough of Nottingham, *Town Clerk Letters Received, 1882–4,* J. S. Slanger, April 18, 1883.

102. "Notification of Infectious Disease," *Nottingham Journal,* May 8, 1883.

103. Ibid. Cropper was chair and treasurer of Sneinton and District Liberal Club.

104. Hatherly, "Notification of Infectious Diseases."

105. NA, Open Shelves, Borough of Nottingham, *Minutes of the Town Council, 1882–3,* May 7, 1883.

106. J. O. Brookhouse, "The Compulsory Notification," *Nottingham Journal,* May 9, 1883.

107. Johnson's apology for missing the VADPR's annual meeting in February 1883 was reported in "Annual Meeting," *Journal of the Vigilance Association for the Defence of Personal Rights* 26 (March 15, 1883): 21–26. In a letter marked "private" and written in his own hand, Johnson admitted to Nottingham's MP that he and the MOH had a difference of opinion on notification. NA, CATC10/38/47, Borough of Nottingham, *Town Clerk Letters Sent, 1881–4,* Arnold Morley, March 9, 1883.

108. Borough of Nottingham, *Town Clerk Letters Received, 1882–4,* E. Seaton, November 22, 1883.

109. Hennock, *Fit and Proper Persons,* 114.

110. BAH, *Birmingham City Council Sanitary Committee Minute Book* [hereafter cited as Birmingham *SCMB*], *May 10, 1871–July 15, 1874,* May 27, 1874.

111. Ibid., December 24, 1873.

112. BAH, Birmingham City Council Health Committee, Alfred Hill, *Report on the Health of the City of Birmingham for the Year 1883,* 44; BAH, Birmingham *SCMB, 27 July 1874–4 October 1876,* May 26 and June 2, 1875.

113. BAH, Birmingham City Council Health Committee, Alfred Hill, *Report on the Health of the City of Birmingham for the Year 1877,* 15.

114. BAH, Birmingham City Council, *Health Committee Minute Book* [hereafter cited as Birmingham *HCMB*], *October 18, 1876–July 17, 1878,* June 5, 1878.

115. Liverpool *Evidence,* Huddersfield Deputation, Dr. Rhodes, q. 347.

116. Hennock, *Fit and Proper Persons,* 114–16.

117. BAH, Birmingham City Council Health Committee, Alfred Hill, *Report on the Health of the City of Birmingham for the Year 1885,* 47; BAH, Birmingham *HCMB, October 18, 1876–July 17, 1878,* June 5, 1878.

118. BAH, Birmingham *HCMB, 6 February 1884–8 June 1886,* March 26, 1884.

119. BAH, Birmingham City Council Health Committee, Alfred Hill, *Report on the Health of the City of Birmingham for the Year 1882,* 35–36.

120. Similar arguments were being made in Liverpool; see Carter, "Is the Compulsory Notification . . . Useful?," 508.

121. "Compulsory Notification—Opposition in the Country," *Journal of the Vigilance Association for the Defence of Personal Rights* 23 (December 15, 1882): 111–12; Martineau, "Compulsory Notification of Infectious Disease." The Martineau brothers were nephews of Harriet Martineau and belonged to the same Birmingham "social set" as the Chamberlains. Hennock, *Fit and Proper Persons,* 46n87. Like his father, Robert, in 1846, Thomas Martineau served as mayor of Birmingham (1884–86), and he was knighted in 1887. Frank was a proponent of self-improvement through education and was secretary of the Birmingham and Midland Institute and trustee of Mason Science College. For more on these educational institutions, see Rodrick, *Self-Help and Civic Culture.*

122. "Compulsory Notification—Opposition in the Country," *Journal of the Vigilance Association for the Defence of Personal Rights* 23 (December 15, 1882): 111. Richard Chamberlain was Joseph's brother and was Birmingham's mayor in 1879–80.

123. Hastings, "Inaugural Address," 90.

124. BAH, Birmingham City Council, *Health Sub-Committee Minute Book, 1899–1902,* November 12, 1889, and February 25, 1890; BAH, Birmingham City Council Health Committee, Alfred Hill, *Report on the Health of the City of Birmingham for the Year 1890,* 42.

125. Elmy, "Local Government Board." Elmy was secretary of the VADPR from 1872. Fielding, "Ignota, the Unknown Woman," 155; "Mrs. Wolstenholme-Elmy," *Manchester Guardian,* March 13, 1918.

126. "City Council—Compulsory Notification of Infectious Diseases," *Birmingham Daily Post,* December 18, 1889, 7.

127. Ibid. In *Self-Help and Civic Culture,* Rodrick notes that Chamberlain's gospel "held that civic participation was a moral duty" (22).

128. Swales, "Leicester Anti-vaccination Movement"; Charlton, "Fight against Vaccination"; Fraser, "Leicester and Smallpox."

129. Parliamentary Archives (hereafter cited as PA), Records of the House of Commons, Private Bill Office, *House of Commons Select Committee on Private Bills: Evidence 1879, Vol. 18. L2, Leicester Corporation Bill, 20 May 1879* (hereafter cited as *Evidence LCB*), 47. The city's fever hospital at Freake's Ground had been opened in the midst of the 1871 smallpox epidemic, but subsequently it admitted scarlet fever patients.

130. Ibid., 6–9.

131. Record Office for Leicestershire, Leicester and Rutland (hereafter cited as ROLLR), CM46/4, Borough of Leicester, *Minute Book of Special Ad Hoc Committee, January 12, 1875–November 4, 1886,* February 5, 1879. The doctors' memorial against notification was dated January 1, 1879, but its content had been decided on at a meeting of the Leicester Medical Society held on December 27, 1878. See Leicester Medical Society (hereafter cited as LMS), *Minute Book, V, 1867–93,* December 27, 1878; and "Registration of Infectious Disease," *Sanitary Record* 10 (1879): 212–13.

132. *Leicester Advertiser,* January 18, 1879, 6. Six physicians and thirty-nine surgeons were registered in the city, so the memorial accounted for about three-quarters of the city's registered practitioners. Wright, *Directory of Leicester.*

133. ROLLR, CM32/9, Borough of Leicester, *Sanitary Committee Minute Book* [hereafter cited as Leicester *SCMB*], *1879–80,* January 3, 1879.

134. Crane later admitted signing the memorial but claimed ignorance of its precise contents: "had he known what was actually intended he should have not signed,

and he will take steps to have his signature erased." Ibid., January 10, 1879. He resigned in January 1880 due to ill health.

135. ROLLR, CM1/16, Borough of Leicester, *Minutes of Council*, January 16, 1879.

136. LMS, *Minute Book, V, 1867–93*, January 31, 1879.

137. Borough of Leicester, *Minutes of Council*, January 16, 1879; Borough of Leicester, *Minute Book of Special Ad Hoc Committee, 12 January 1875–4 November 1886*, March 14, 1879.

138. ROLLR, CM1/17, Borough of Leicester, *Minutes of Council*, March 18, 1879.

139. LMS, *Minute Book, V, 1867–93*, October 7, 1879, and September 7, 1880; BMAPBC *MB, 1875–87*, 84–86.

140. Lancaster, *Radicalism, Cooperation and Socialism*, 82–84.

141. Editorial, "Dr Johnston's 'Fad,'" *Leicester Advertiser*, January 18, 1879.

142. LMS, *Minute Book, V, 1867–93*, January 13, 1882.

143. "Report of the Committee on Registration of Disease," *British Medical Journal* 659 (August 16, 1879): 256–57.

144. Hart chaired the BMAPBC for twenty-five years until 1897. Coupled with his long-term editorship of the *BMJ*, he was able to coordinate and influence medical opinion on a range of issues. See Bartrip, *Themselves Writ Large*, 125.

145. BMAPBC *MB, 1875–87*, February 18 and April 30, 1885.

146. Carter, "Is the Compulsory Notification . . . Useful?" See also the contributions of Dr. Whittle, Dr. Houghton, and Mr. G. Brown to the subsequent discussion.

147. Fitzpatrick, "Notification of Infectious Diseases." Two shillings and sixpence was the usual amount a local authority paid to the doctor for a notification certificate. This amount was also the typical basic fee a doctor would charge for a visit, excluding medicine, to patients with a house rental of less than £50 per annum in the late 1870s. Many low-paid workers were covered by Friendly Society contributions, and doctors were heavily reliant on fees from their wealthier patients, who expected to pay anything up to 10s. About half of all single-handed general practices had a gross annual income of between £400 and £799 in the late 1870s. On the complex nature of the medical market, see Digby, *Making a Medical Living*, chap. 5.

148. Dr. E. Haughton, discussion, of Carter, "Is the Compulsory Notification . . . Useful?," 509.

149. Livy, "Notification of Infectious Diseases," 292; BMAPBC *MB*, Ernest Hart, "Special Report by the Chairman of the Parliamentary Bills Committee on the Progress of Legislation with Regard to the Notification to Sanitary Authorities of the Occurrence of Cases of Infectious Diseases" (hereafter cited as Hart, "Special Report").

150. "'Clinical Instruction' Again," *Personal Rights Journal* 65, no. 1 (December 1886): 104.

151. "Infectious Diseases Notification Bill," *Journal of the Vigilance Association for the Defence of Personal Rights* 4 (April 15, 1881): 36; Elmy, "Local Government Board."

152. Macara, "Confidentiality—a Decrepit Concept?"

153. Sykes, "On Organisation," 159; see also Kearns, "Tuberculosis."

154. Sykes, "On Organisation"; Livy, "Notification of Infectious Diseases," 292. Claims were made that general practitioners already betrayed the confidence of patients by giving a medical certificate of cause of death; however, considering the chain of events that could happen to patients and their families after notification,

death certification and disease notification were hardly comparable, and the medical profession easily rebuffed such points.

155. Liverpool *Evidence*, Warrington Deputation, Dr. Sherratt, q. 165, and Blackburn Deputation, Dr. Garstang, q. 187.

156. Crook, "Sanitary Inspection"; Hamlin, "Sanitary Policing"; Kearns, "Private Property"; Otter, *Victorian Eye*, chap. 3.

157. "It is an open secret that the [1883 notification] Bill is intended to pave the way to a more drastic and despotic measure to follow, viz., a compulsory Isolation Bill which would certainly operate most oppressively on the lower class of the community." Liberty and Property Defence League, *Overlegislation in 1883*, 15–16.

158. PA *Evidence LCB*, 60.

159. Dr. E. Whittle, discussion of Carter, "Is the Compulsory Notification . . . Useful?," 509; Liverpool *Evidence*, Warrington Deputation, Dr. Sherratt, q. 139.

160. "Infectious Diseases Notification Bill," *Journal of the Vigilance Association for the Defence of Personal Rights* 26 (March 15, 1883): 28–29; "Compulsion," *Journal of the Vigilance Association for the Defence of Personal Rights* 11 (December 15, 1881): 95–96; Elmy, "Compulsory Notification of Infectious Disease"; Elmy, "Local Government Board," 76; "Nemo," "Medical and Administrative Despotism," 68.

161. Carter, "Notification of Infectious Diseases."

162. The breakdown of MOHs' other professional commitments was as follows: eight MOHs had private practice, seven were disallowed it, and in eight cases the MOH's position was not stated.

163. Carpenter, "Right of the State."

164. PA *Evidence LCB*, 54.

165. The diploma in Public Health became a requirement of MOH employment from 1888. On professional credentialing and employment of MOHs, see Porter, "Stratification and Its Discontents," 86–89, 91–92, 96.

166. Ibid., 99–100.

167. Hart, "Special Report."

168. Peterson, *Medical Profession in Mid-Victorian London*; Waddington, *Medical Profession.*

169. Hart, "Special Report."

170. Jordan and Sharp, *Josephine Butler*, 4:19.

171. "Anti-compulsion Society" was the title given to this association in a report appearing in the Vigilance Association's journal. There is no other evidence that it went by this title, and in the report on the deputation to Sir Charles Dilke, it is simply referred to as an "association." "Medical Profession and Compulsory Notification of Infectious Diseases," *Journal of the Vigilance Association for Defence of Personal Rights* 20 (August 15, 1882): 74–75.

172. Ibid.

173. "Notification of Infectious Diseases at Bath," *Lancet* 121 (1883): 1013–14. See also "British Medical Association and the Compulsory Notification of Infectious Diseases," *Journal of the Vigilance Association for the Defence of Personal Rights* 21 (September 15, 1882): 81–83.

174. Liverpool *Circular*, 16.

175. Hill, "Notification of Infectious Disease."

176. "Compulsory Notification of Infectious Diseases," *Sanitary Record*, n.s., 3 (1882): 334.

177. Digby, *Making a Medical Living*, 148–55.

178. Carter, "Some Results," 36.

179. *Liberal Review*, September 9, 1882, 11. See also Liverpool *Evidence*, Edinburgh Deputation, Dr. Littlejohn, q. 220; "A Mother," "Infectious Diseases Notification Bills," 40.

180. Hance, "Relation of the State," 20–21.

181. Baldwin, "Victorian State."

182. It is difficult to arrive at a reliable estimate of incidence because age-specific data were rarely published. Using notification and population figures from Nottingham in the late 1890s as a guide, somewhere between 5 and 10 percent of all city-dwelling children below the age of fifteen years suffered from any one of these diseases in any given year.

183. ROLLR, L614, Borough of Leicester, William Johnston, *Annual Report on the Health of Leicester, 1883*, 26.

## Chapter Three

1. Hardie, "Duty of Municipal Authorities." Hardie, a surgeon and medical officer to Crumpsall Workhouse in Manchester, was honorary secretary to the MSSA. For a recent interpretation of the activities of the MSSA, see Platt, *Shock Cities*.

2. Hardie, "Duty of Municipal Authorities," 11. Hardie's call for an isolation hospital was part of an ongoing campaign in Manchester. A large public meeting had taken place at Manchester Town Hall four years earlier, pressing the mayor to provide additional hospital accommodations: "Hospital Accommodation for Infectious Diseases," *Manchester Guardian*, July 24, 1868. A facility was opened in the grounds of the infirmary at Monsall, which was not fully given over to the corporation until 1896. See Pickstone, *Medicine and Industrial Society*, 130–31, 161–62.

3. HCPP, C. 408, C. 408-I (1871), XIX.1, 29, *Report of Royal Commission upon the Administration and Operation of the Contagious Diseases Acts*, evidence of J. S. Mill, q. 20,015.

4. Hardie, "Duty of Municipal Authorities," 12. Lord Derby had recently opened a new hospital in Bootle, near Liverpool, on land he had donated. Derby's speech at the opening ceremony of the hospital—approvingly quoted by Hardie—had lauded the benefits of sanitary reform and prevention of ill health. "Lord Derby on Sanitary Reform," *Times*, April 11, 1872. On Lord Derby see Steele, "Stanley, Edward Henry."

5. Sanitary Act, 1866, 29 & 30 Vic., c. 90 s. 26.

6. Sheard, "Reluctant Providers?"

7. Beier, *For Their Own Good*, 172–74.

8. Worboys, *Spreading Germs*; Pickstone, *Medicine and Industrial Society*; Wohl, *Endangered Lives*.

9. Sheard, "Reluctant Providers?"

10. There is no monograph-length study of isolation hospitals in a national British context. The classic *England's First State Hospitals* by Gwendoline Ayers still serves as

a baseline study, immensely rich in detail despite many gaps and a singular focus on London. Margaret Currie's *Fever Hospitals and Fever Nurses* is an important book on fever nursing. There are two Scottish studies of individual hospitals: Porter and Williams, *Epidemic Diseases in Aberdeen*; and Gray, *Edinburgh City Hospital*. Some aspects of isolation and hospitals are dealt with by Weindling, "From Isolation to Therapy"; Hardy, *Epidemic Streets*; and Eyler, "Scarlet Fever and Confinement" and *Sir Arthur Newsholme*.

11. Porter and Porter, "Enforcement of Health."

12. Cox, "Compulsion, Voluntarism, and Venereal Disease."

13. Barnes, *Great Stink of Paris*.

14. *Metropolitan Workhouse Infirmaries*; *Report of Dr. Edward Smith*. In general, the diseases that eventually accounted for the majority of admissions to isolation hospitals—scarlet fever and, increasingly from the late 1880s, diphtheria—were acknowledged to be infectious. For qualifications to this generalization see Worboys, *Spreading Germs*. Smallpox was exceptional because of the controversy about whether the disease could be carried in the air over long distances, a clear problem if the hospital was located amid a populous district. This possibility sparked allegations that smallpox hospitals acted as foci for infection, which some public health activists were prepared to admit. See Barrow, "Victorian 'Pest-Houses.'"

15. Murchison, *Treatise on the Continued Fevers*; Currie, *Fever Hospitals and Fever Nurses*, 13; Richardson, *English Hospitals*; Bynum, "Hospital, Disease and Community."

16. McHugh, *Prostitution and Victorian Social Reform*, 64–65.

17. Young, "Removal and Isolation," 52.

18. "A Mother," "Infectious Diseases Notification Bills," 40.

19. Bailin, *Sickroom in Victorian Fiction*, 11; see also Murphy, *Our Homes*, chap. 88. I discuss the sickroom in chapter 5.

20. Beier, *For Their Own Good*, chap. 4.

21. "Liberty," "Medicine in Parliament," 38.

22. Ibid., 39.

23. Hendrick, *Child Welfare*; Fenton, "Citizenship in Private Space." On the increasing separation of parents from children in middle-class homes, see Adams, *Architecture in the Family Way*, chap. 5.

24. Rose, *Powers of Freedom*, 106; see also Valverde, "Despotism and Ethical Liberal Government," and Clor, "Mill and Millians."

25. HCPP, C. 408, C. 408-I (1871), XIX.1, 29, *Report of Royal Commission upon the Administration and Operation of the Contagious Diseases Acts*, J. S. Mill, qq. 20,026, 20,028.

26. Ibid., J. S. Mill, q. 20,065.

27. Therapeutically speaking, and discounting the actual medical effectiveness of interventions, in theory at least the medical and nursing staff of isolation hospitals did little, if anything, more than could have been done at home. I am, of course, disregarding the provision of food and warmth as "therapy" here, though there is evidence from oral testimonies that the sustenance on offer in isolation hospitals could be pretty meager. See Beier, *For Their Own Good*, 196.

28. Thorne, "Use and Influence of Hospitals," iv.

29. The Poor Law infirmaries had 94,001 beds and outstripped all other types of institution combined. Currie, *Fever Hospitals and Fever Nurses*, 20. There were,

however, more isolation hospitals (755) than Poor Law infirmaries (700) and general hospitals (594). Figures from Richardson, *English Hospitals*, 139.

30. NA, CA.CM/Health/9, Nottingham *HCMB, August 30, 1880 to November 24, 1882*; NA, CA.CM/Health/6, Nottingham *HCMB, July 13, 1874 to December 15, 1876*; NA, CA/HE/2/1/1, Borough of Nottingham, Edward Seaton, *Sixth Annual Report of the Medical Officer of Health for 1878.*

31. NA, CA.CM/Health/7, Nottingham *HCMB, December 22, 1876 to September 6, 1878*, October 26 and November 2, 1877, and March 8 and April 4, 1878; NA, CA.CM/Health/8, Nottingham *HCMB, September 13, 1878 to August 27, 1880*, January 3, 10, 17, 24, 31 and March 2, 1879.

32. NA, CA.CM/Health/9, Nottingham *HCMB, 30 August 1880 to 24 November 1882*, October 7, 1881, 266.

33. NA, CA/HE/2/1/1, Borough of Nottingham, Edward Seaton, *Monthly Report of Medical Officer of Health for January 1880, with Annual Summary for 1879*, 6–7.

34. See the many health committee discussions in NA, CA.CM/Health/11, Nottingham *HCMB, November 20, 1884 to January 14, 1887*; NA, CA.CM/Health/12, Nottingham *HCMB, January 21, 1887 to February 15, 1889*; NA, CA.CM/Health/13, Nottingham *HCMB, February 22, 1889 to February 27, 1891*; NA, CA.CM/Health/14, Nottingham *HCMB, March 6, 1891 to December 23, 1892*; and NA, CA.CM/Health/15, Nottingham *HCMB, December 30, 1892 to August 3, 1894.*

35. Sheffield Local Studies Library (hereafter cited as SLSL), 352.4 SQ, H. Harvey Littlejohn, *Annual Report of the Medical Officer of Health for Sheffield* [hereafter cited as Littlejohn, *Annual Report*], *1891*, 53.

36. Ibid., *1892*, 34.

37. Kaye, "Scarlet Fever."

38. Not dealt with here were the mass invasions by a curious public of newly constructed isolation hospitals that took place before they began admitting patients. On Edinburgh see Gray, *Edinburgh City Hospital*, 135. On Oldham see Thorne, "Use and Influence of Hospitals," 217; and on Nottingham see NA, Nottingham *HCMB, March 6, 1891 to December 23, 1892*, May 8, 1891.

39. HCPP, C. 1066 (1874), XXXI.33, *Reports of the Medical Officer of the Privy Council and Local Government Board, New Series, no. II, Supplementary Report to the Local Government Board on some Recent Inquiries under the Public Health Act, 1858.* See also "Fever Hospitals," *Manchester Guardian*, November 11, 1874.

40. Littlejohn, *Annual Report, 1892*, 53.

41. "Meeting at Mile End," *Journal of the National Association for the Defence of Personal Rights* 35 (December 15, 1883): 119–20, Mr. W. Joiner on 119.

42. The charge for hospital admission in Warrington had been 15s.: Liverpool *Evidence*, Warrington Deputation, qq. 93–100, and Huddersfield Deputation, Dr. Rhodes, q. 356.

43. HCPP, C. 3314 (1882), XXIX.1, *Royal Commission to Inquire Respecting Small-Pox and Fever Hospitals in Metropolis. Report, Minutes of Evidence, Appendix*, 174–75 (hereafter cited as *RCSFH*), evidence of Mr. Thomas Eccleston Gibb, who was clerk both to the vestry and to the guardians of the poor in St. Pancras. In the latter capacity, Gibb himself had struck patients off the voter list. In Edinburgh, MOH Littlejohn compelled the parochial authorities to attend to any family whenever the household

head and main breadwinner was hospitalized due to an infectious disease, thus pauperizing that family. Liverpool *Evidence*, qq. 264–65.

44. Smallpox vaccinating stations located on Poor Law premises suffered from similar problems. See Mooney, "Most Flagrant Anomalies."

45. Calculated from Thorne, "Use and Influence of Hospitals," 174–78, 230.

46. Ibid., 30.

47. Ibid., 218, 230.

48. Littlejohn, *Annual Report, 1891*, 34.

49. Ibid., 49; see also Nottingham *HCMB, July 13, 1874 to December 15, 1876*, April 16, 1875, 154.

50. That these deterrents operated is partly borne out by the evidence that in those towns where there was no infectious disease hospital to be removed to, the working-classes showed little compunction in calling for the MOH to make a domestic inspection. Liverpool *Evidence*, Blackburn Deputation, qq. 133–37.

51. BAH, Birmingham *HCMB, April 25, 1893–November 13, 1894*, 107.

52. Hawkley was due to be charged for willfully exposing other people to scarlet fever, though I have been unable to locate a report of any subsequent case in the court records or newspapers.

53. Thorne, "Use and Influence of Hospitals," 28. In addition to distributing a questionnaire to all English and Welsh sanitary authorities, Thorne visited a total of eighty-two authorities and sixty-seven hospitals. See also Manchester City Council Archives and Local History, 614.0942.S8, John Tatham, *Annual Report on the Health of Salford for the Year 1885.*

54. Porter and Porter, "Politics of Prevention"; Durbach, *Bodily Matters.*

55. "Nottingham Resolution," *Nottingham Daily Express*, March 3, 1891, 6.

56. C. J. Welton, "The Infectious Diseases Question," *Nottingham Daily Express*, April 16, 1891.

57. ROLLR, CM32/8, Leicester *SCMB, 1879–80*, March 7, 1879, 377–86.

58. "An Englishman," "The Proposed Compulsory Registration of Infectious Diseases," *Leicester Chronicle and Leicestershire Mercury*, January 18, 1879. It was unusual for local authorities to hospitalize someone suffering from whooping cough, and I have come across no evidence that this ever was the case in Leicester.

59. "Nottingham Resolution," *Nottingham Daily Express*, March 3, 1891; *RCSFH*, evidence of John Syer Bristowe and Mr. Alfred Godrich, district medical officer in Brompton.

60. Thomas Burnie, "The Nottingham Hospital for Infectious Disease," *Nottingham Daily Express*, April 6, 1891. Burnie's profession is listed in the city directory.

61. Thorne, "Use and Influence of Hospitals," 27.

62. BAH, Birmingham *HCMB, March 26, 1884–June 8, 1886*, 76; and *June 22, 1886–March 26, 1889*, September 25, 1888, 375, letter from Mrs. Lyons.

63. Littlejohn, *Annual Report, 1891*, 34.

64. By countenancing disclosure to employers within one week of adopting infectious disease notification, the health committee was demonstrating its intention to trespass yet further on the confidentiality of the physician-patient relationship, the fear of which had compelled many doctors to oppose notification legislation, both in Leicester and elsewhere.

65. "Memorial from the 'Rights and Liberties' Defence League," *Nottingham Daily Express,* April 7, 1891; Yeatman, "Slanders." The town clerk disputed this version of events in "Hospital," *Nottingham Daily Express,* May 5, 1891, with a rejoinder from Charles Bell Taylor, "The Corporation and the Liberty of the Subject," *Nottingham Daily Express,* May 7, 1891. See also "Veritas," "Letter," *Nottingham Daily Express,* March 30, 1891.

66. These examples come from Aldwinckle, "Isolation in Fever Hospitals"; and Freeman, *Planning of Fever Hospitals.*

67. Cameron, "On the Importance of Isolating"; Parker, "Isolation and Scarlet Fever"; "Discussion on Disinfection and Isolation: With Special Reference to the Control of Epidemics," *British Medical Journal* 1496 (August 31, 1889): 452–59.

68. NA, CA/HE/2/1/1, Borough of Nottingham, B. Arthur Whitelegge, *Annual Report of the Medical Officer of Health for 1888,* 38.

69. Aldwinckle, "Isolation in Fever Hospitals," 503.

70. Pollard, "Fever Hospitals of Europe," 207.

71. Seaton, "Clinical Instruction at Fever Hospitals," 501; "Diagnosis of Notifiable Diseases," *British Medical Journal* 2202 (1903): 622–24.

72. NA, Open Shelves, Borough of Nottingham, Philip Boobbyer, *Annual Health Report for 1899,* 52. The term used in the reports for "discharged" was "recovered"; this was common in hospital reports of the period.

73. BAH, Birmingham City Council, *Health Sub-Committee Minute Book,* November 24, 1905.

74. "Planning of Hospitals for Infectious Disease," *Sanitary Journal: A Journal of Hygiene and Public Health,* n.s., 17 (March 18, 1893): 23–24.

75. Reprinted as appendix A in HCPP, C. 6342 (1912–13), XXXVI.1, *Fortieth Annual Report of the Local Government Board, 1910–11: Supplement in Continuation of the Report of the Medical Officer of the Board for 1910–11, Containing a Report on Isolation Hospitals by H. Franklin Parsons, M.D., with an Introduction by the Medical Officer of the Board* (hereafter cited as Parsons, *Report on Isolation Hospitals*).

76. Freeman, *Planning of Fever Hospitals,* 78–79.

77. Parsons, *Report on Isolation Hospitals,* 30.

78. Ibid.; Goodall, "Account of the Isolation Chambers."

79. Developments in cubicle design at the London Fever Hospital, where funding delayed the opening of an isolation block until 1915, are discussed in Newsom Kerr, "Fevered Metropolis," 182–85. For the New York Children's Hospital see Kisacky, "Restructuring Isolation."

80. Parsons, *Report on Isolation Hospitals,* appendix B.

81. Ibid., 33.

82. London Metropolitan Archive (hereafter cited as LMA), LMA/MAB.2410, Hospitals Department, Isolation Accommodation, Frederic H. Thomson, *Report on the Working of the Cubicle System and the 'Box' Or Room System of Isolation at that [North-eastern] Hospital* (hereafter cited as Thomson, *Cubicle System*).

83. Ibid., 3; Parsons, *Report on Isolation Hospitals,* 36–37.

84. LMA, LMA/MAB.2485, Hospitals Department, Isolation Accommodation, 1908, *Report by Dr. F. Foord Caiger, Medical Superintendent, South-western Hospital, on the Working of the Cubicle Wards at that Hospital* (hereafter cited as Foord Caiger, *Cubicle Wards*), 2.

85. Parsons, *Report on Isolation Hospitals,* 131.

86. Ibid.

87. Thomson, *Cubicle System,* 2; Foord Caiger, *Cubicle Wards,* 2.

88. Crookshank, "Control of Scarlet Fever," 479; Rundle and Burton, "Bed Isolation of Cases."

89. Rosenberg, *Care of Strangers,* 35, 286–87.

90. In 1881 Sheffield's health committee proposed appointing a nonresident medical officer to its newly opened hospital. Of course, this was cheaper than having a resident medical officer, but it was also thought of as a viable step because the committee assumed "it will be impossible for friends, visitors or charitable persons to visit the patients." Sheffield Archives (hereafter cited as SA), Sheffield Town Council, *Minutes, 1882–3,* June 7, 1882, 344.

91. Thorne, "Use and Influence of Hospitals," 27; see also Nottingham *HCMB, December 22, 1876 to September 6, 1878,* April 4, 1878, 332.

92. *RCSFH,* evidence of William Gayton, qq. 2,680–81.

93. Thorne, "Use and Influence of Hospitals," 257.

94. Ibid., 83.

95. Ibid., 92.

96. Eyler, *Sir Arthur Newsholme,* 111.

97. Thorne, "Use and Influence of Hospitals," 92.

98. Ibid., 150, 217.

99. *RCSFH,* evidence of Deputy Surgeon General John Ashton Bostock (a manager of the MAB), q. 1,260.

100. Thorne, "Use and Influence of Hospitals," 176.

101. Currie, *Fever Hospitals and Fever Nurses,* 81, testimony of Sarah England (Hicks).

102. Thorne, "Use and Influence of Hospitals," 51.

103. Currie, *Fever Hospitals and Fever Nurses,* 63.

104. Anderson, *Fever Hospital,* 33.

105. Gray, *Edinburgh City Hospital,* 158; *RCSFH,* evidence of John Ashton Bostock, q. 1,260.

106. Thorne, "Use and Influence of Hospitals," 27, 51; Gray, *Edinburgh City Hospital,* 158; Porter and Williams, *Epidemic Diseases in Aberdeen,* 48.

107. Currie, *Fever Hospitals and Fever Nurses,* 81, testimony of Sarah England (Hicks).

108. Exceptions to visiting rules commonly were made in the case of erysipelas and enteric fever wards.

109. *RCSFH,* evidence of Rotherhithe MOH Dr. Benjamin Browning, q. 4,219. It is difficult to judge the accuracy of what must have been hearsay evidence. See Barrow, "Victorian 'Pest-Houses.'"

110. Thorne, "Use and Influence of Hospitals," 27, 51, 294; Porter and Williams, *Epidemic Diseases in Aberdeen,* 48.

111. Thorne, "Use and Influence of Hospitals," 134.

112. *RCSFH,* q. 2,057.

113. Thorne, "Use and Influence of Hospitals," 134.

114. Ibid., 27.

115. Ibid., 294.

116. Ibid., 51, 294.

117. Beier, *For Their Own Good*, 196.

118. Thorne, "Use and Influence of Hospitals," 51, 89.

119. Porter and Williams, *Epidemic Diseases in Aberdeen*, 48.

120. Currie, *Fever Hospitals and Fever Nurses*, 86, testimony of Jean Bell (Hall).

121. Ibid., 99, testimony of Olive Dodd (Cowley), Dunstable and District Joint Isolation Hospital, 1942–44.

122. Thorne, "Use and Influence of Hospitals," 150, 209, 294; *RCSFH*, 90.

123. Thorne, "Use and Influence of Hospitals," 8.

124. Gray, *Edinburgh City Hospital*, 149.

125. SA, Sheffield Town Council, *Minutes, 1882–3*, 344. The health committee in Sheffield also argued that a telephone would reduce the time and inconvenience that the MOH incurred when seeking out cases to induce them to come to the hospital.

126. Thorne, "Use and Influence of Hospitals," 176.

127. *RCSFH*, 315.

128. Eyler, *Sir Arthur Newsholme*. The utility of hospital quarantine for smallpox was sometimes used to argue that all infections could benefit from sequestration.

129. Biddle's objection to dual notification reflected the long-held opinions of the British Medical Association, which had formed a committee to consider the question of sickness registration as early as 1862. This Registration of Disease Committee originally had eighteen members, including William Farr of the GRO and his successor, William Ogle, and was chaired by Arthur Ransome. The committee consistently supported the implementation of infectious disease notification so long as the householder was responsible for reporting the case. See Ransome, "Scientific and Practical Objects"; and Mooney, "Public Health versus Private Practice."

130. Biddle, "Dual Notification," "Notification of Infectious Disease," and "Notification of Infectious Diseases."

131. For more on Humphries see Szreter, *Fertility*, 79n10.

132. "Dual Notification and the Death Rate," *British Medical Journal* 1747 (June 23, 1894): 1377.

133. Newsholme, "Notification and Registration of Sickness."

134. Kaye, "Scarlet Fever."

135. Millard, "Hospital Isolation of Scarlet Fever" and "Influence of Hospital Isolation." A Ministry of Health report later broadly endorsed Millard's findings.

136. Rose, *Powers of Freedom*; Joyce, *Rule of Freedom*; Mehta, "Liberal Strategies of Exclusion." These studies were invigorated by the writings of Michel Foucault; see Foucault, *Discipline and Punish*; and Faubion, *Michel Foucault: Power*.

137. Rose, *Powers of Freedom*, 72.

138. Bashford and Strange, "Isolation and Exclusion," 3; see also Dean, "Liberal Government and Authoritarianism."

139. Bashford and Strange, "Isolation and Exclusion," 3.

140. Barrow, "Victorian 'Pest-Houses,'" 134. Barrow does not name the historians he has in mind. "Isolation hospital" was a commonly used term by the late nineteenth century.

141. Rose, *Powers of Freedom*, 242.

## Chapter Four

1. Johnson, "Educational Policy"; Goldstrom, *Social Content of Education*; McCann, *Popular Education and Socialization*; Stannard, "Ideology, Education, and Social Structure."

2. Hurt, *Elementary Schooling*; Roberts, *Character in the Mind.*

3. J. MacKenzie, *Imperialism and Popular Culture*; Horn, "English Elementary Education."

4. Searle, *Quest for National Efficiency*, 60–67, 208–12.

5. Heathorn, *For Home, Country, and Race*, 142.

6. Ibid., 145.

7. Davin, "Child Labour"; Hall, "Victorian Domestic Ideology."

8. Tosh, *Man's Place*, chaps. 7 and 8; Gomersall and Campling, *Working-Class Girls*, 91–92; Davidoff et al., *Family Story*, chap. 4.

9. Heathorn, *For Home, Country, and Race*, 154–55, 163; Moscucci, *Science of Woman.*

10. Dyhouse, "Towards a 'Feminine' Curriculum"; Dyhouse, *Girls Growing Up.*

11. McDermid, *Victoria's Daughters*, 58–61.

12. Heathorn, *For Home, Country, and Race*, 166. Britain's public elementary schools required boys to take drawing from 1890.

13. Ravenhill, "Hygiene and Household Economics," quote from 91 and 106. Ravenhill became the first female fellow of the Sanitary Institute in 1904 and made reports for the institute as well as the Board of Education.

14. Kerr, *Annual Report . . . 1903*, 40.

15. Steedman, *Childhood, Culture, and Class*, 46, 203–4. McMillan and Kerr moved from Bradford to London at the same time. Kerr's departure was prompted by the abolition of the Bradford School Board by the 1902 Education Act.

16. Davidoff et al., *Family Story*, 56.

17. Ravenhill, "Hygiene and Household Economics," 75–76.

18. Ibid., 80–81.

19. For international comparisons of the impact of schools on infectious disease see Meckel, *Classrooms and Clinics*, 44–45.

20. Hirst, "Public Health"; Woodward, "School Medical Officer"; Lewis, *Edwin Chadwick.*

21. Hirst, "Public Health"; Woodward, "School Medical Officer," 125–26; Silver and Silver, *Education of the Poor*, 91–98. On the United States see Meckel, *Classrooms and Clinics*, 20–22.

22. Beale Collins, "Isolation Hospitals," 603.

23. HCPP, C. 6461 (1890–91), *Twentieth Annual Report of the Local Government Board, 1890–91: Supplement Containing the Report of the Medical Officer for 1890*, George Buchanan, "Memorandum on the Circumstances under Which the Closing of Public Elementary Schools or the Exclusion therefrom of Particular Children May Be Required in Order to Prevent the Spread of Diseases (December 1890)" (hereafter cited as Buchanan, "Memorandum").

24. For an exploration of classroom or school closure in an English public school, see Richardson, *Typhoid in Uppingham.*

25. Meckel, *Classrooms and Clinics*, 43.

26. Hirst claims the acceptance of "contagionist theories," besides their having financial benefits, was responsible for shifting the focus onto excluding individual pupils, rather than blanket school or class closures. See Hirst, "Public Health," 115.

27. Dorothy Porter has argued that advancements in knowledge of disease etiology "revealed the interdependence of those social and biological conditions which furthered their propagation"; hence a "causal attack" against disease could be developed under the umbrella of "social efficiency." Porter, "Enemies of the Race," 171–72.

28. Meckel, *Classrooms and Clinics*, 133–39.

29. "Pell's Clause" of the 1876 Education Act allowed the dissolution of a board if it had not yet built a school. See Sutherland, *Policy-making*, 82. On London see Spalding, *London School Board.*

30. Lewis, "Parents, Children, School Fees"; Martin, *Women and Schooling.*

31. Sutherland, *Policy-making*, 84.

32. Ibid., 350.

33. Whitbread, *Nursery-Infant School*, 68–69.

34. Teachers' salaries were sometimes linked to pupils' performance, a policy that was not abolished in London until 1883. See Hirst, "Public Health."

35. Robertson, "Children, Teachers and Society."

36. HCPP, C. 931 (1874), LI.241, Committee of Council on Education, *New Code of Regulations*, 6.

37. HCPP, C. 3152 (1882), L.511, Committee of Council on Education, *Minute, March 1882, Establishing New Code of Regulations*, 14. Interestingly, in 1876 the North West Association of Medical Officers of Health had memorialized the LGB suggesting that they should be granted this power. The LGB replied that "no hope could be held out for such legislation in the present session as had been asked for." See Manchester Medical Collection, John Rylands Library, University of Manchester, North West Association of Medical Officers of Health, *Minute Book, 1875–1894*, December 19, 1876, and March 27, 1877.

38. HCPP, C. 5663 (1889), LIX.31, Committee of Council on Education, *Code of Regulations, 1889*, 11; see also Buchanan, "Memorandum."

39. HCPP, C. 6923 (1893), LXVIII.1, Committee of Council on Education, *Code of Regulations with Schedules and Appendices*, 16.

40. Hirst, "Public Health," 115–16. Conflicts between public health and education authorities were replicated in the United States around the same time. Meckel, *Classrooms and Clinics*, 17–19.

41. BAH, Birmingham City Council, *Health Sub-committee Minute Book, 1899–1902*, 291.

42. SA, Sheffield Town Council, *Minutes, January 1880 to October 1880*, Health Committee, February 19, 1880, 169; "Sheffield Town Council—Dr Hime and the School Board," *Sheffield and Rotherham Independent*, August 9, 1883.

43. ROLLR, 22D57/74, Borough of Leicester, *Town Clerk Correspondence, Letters Out, May, 1880–December, 1880*, letter to Dr. Thomas Blunt, May 10, 1880. As Blunt pointed out, the local act required him to do nothing more than report the case. ROLLR, CM32/8, Leicester *SCMB, 1879–80*, letter from Dr. Thomas Blunt, May 14, 1880; also April 23 and 30, May 7, and July 2, 1880.

44. Buchanan, "Memorandum."

45. Leicester *SCMB, 1881–1882*, February 18, 1881; Kenwood and Taylor, "Means of Preventing," 591.

46. "School Notification of Measles," *Public Health* 10 (October 1897–September 1898): 23–24.

47. "Minutes of the Society of Medical Officers of Health," *Sanitary Record* 8 (January 25, 1878): 55.

48. ROLLR, L614, Borough of Leicester, William Johnston, *Annual Report on the Health and Sanitary Condition of the Borough of Leicester* [hereafter cited as Johnston, *Annual Report*], *1884*, 34.

49. Boyd, "School Notification of Infectious Disease," 98.

50. NA, CA/HE/2/1/1, Borough of Nottingham, Edward Seaton, *Sixth Annual Report of the Medical Officer of Health for 1878*, 27.

51. NA, CA.CM/Health/9, Nottingham *HCMB, August 30, 1880 to November 24, 1882*, September 16 and 23, 1881.

52. NA, CA.CM/Health/15, Nottingham *HCMB, December 30, 1892 to August 3, 1894*, June 29, 1894.

53. "Society of Medical Officers of Health," *Sanitary Record* 8 (April 26, 1878): 267.

54. NA, Open Shelves, Borough of Nottingham, Philip Boobbyer, *Annual Health Report for 1896*, 35. Boobbyer also reported that 230 adult members of these households continued working.

55. "School Notification of Measles," *Public Health* 10 (October 1897–September 1898): 23–24.

56. Newsholme, "Bearing of School Attendance."

57. Nottingham *HCMB, August 30, 1880 to November 24, 1882*, September 9, 1881.

58. Newsholme, "Bearing of School Attendance."

59. Rubinstein, "Socialization."

60. Some cases came to light when one GP found that attendance officers had encouraged children to attend school while convalescing from scarlet fever. "Infection from Schools," *Sanitary Record* 3 (June–December 1875): 310; Spear, "Public Elementary Schools," 34.

61. The situation was different in some US cities, where cadres of physicians were paid by local government to act as medical inspectors. Meckel, *Classrooms and Clinics*, 52–61.

62. Hime, "Schools and Scarlet Fever"; May, "School Closure for Measles," 453.

63. Boyd, "School Notification of Infectious Disease," 97; Newsholme, "Bearing of School Attendance."

64. SA, Sheffield Town Council, *Minutes, 1882–83*, July 12, 1883, 454–55.

65. BAH, Birmingham *HCMB, 10 November 1896–22 July 1898*, July 13, 1897, 161, 177.

66. BAH, Birmingham City Council, John Robertson, *Birmingham Medical Officer of Health Annual Report 1906*, 24.

67. Gilmour, "Measles and School Closure."

68. In 1898 Plumstead Vestry flatly refused MOH Davies access to inspect children in schools. "Proceedings of the Metropolitan Branch of the Incorporated Society of Medical Officers of Health," *Public Health* 10 (October 1897–September 1898): 78–79.

69. Kenwood and Taylor, "Means of Preventing."

70. Spear, "Public Elementary Schools," 35.

71. Boyd, "School Notification of Infectious Disease," 97.

72. BAH, Birmingham City Council, John Robertson, *Birmingham Medical Officer of Health Annual Report 1906*, 24. As early as 1878, Kensington Vestry paid to have the school board visitors' infectious disease registration form printed. "Epidemic Diseases and the London School Board Visitors," *Sanitary Record* 8 (March 1, 1878): 135.

73. Beier, *For Their Own Good*, 205.

74. SA, Sheffield Town Council, *Minutes, January 1880 to October 1880*, Health Committee, July 8, 1880, 345.

75. This was the same Dr. Alfred Crane who unwittingly signed the petition opposing the notification clauses in Leicester's local act (see chapter 2).

76. ROLLR, 19D59/VI/6, Borough of Leicester School Board, *General Minute Book, 1883–1888*, November 3, 1884.

77. "Medical Certificates and the School Board," *British Medical Journal* 1822 (November 30, 1895): 1375–76.

78. Newsholme, *School Hygiene*, tables on 118, 122. This book helped launch Newsholme's publishing career. At the time he was MOH in Clapham, London, and acted as an instructor and examiner of teachers for the London School Board.

79. Johnston, *Annual Report, 1884*, 32.

80. Watkins, "English Revolution," 196; Hirst, "Failure 'without Parallel,'" 282n8. Smith was employed with an annual salary of £400, but he also retained his other appointments such as a professorship at King's College Hospital, medical officer to the Bovril and London Milk Companies, and MOH and public analyst to Woolwich Borough Council. Hirst has suggested that Smith's appointment was not such an important landmark as it might appear, since many school boards already sought medical advice on the examination of candidates for teaching appointments and the inspection of children allegedly unfit to attend school.

81. "Infectious Disease Prevention and the London School Board," *Public Health* 3 (May 1890–September 1891): 309; "Periodical Examination of School Children for Diphtheria and Other Infectious Diseases," *Lancet* 153 (1899): 463; Biddle, "School Attendance and Diphtheria."

82. "Society of Medical Officers of Health," *British Medical Journal* 1517 (January 25, 1890): 182–83. Under Section 55 of the 1891 Public Health (London) Act, the MOH was required to send a notification to the headmaster.

83. London County Council, *Annual Report . . . 1896*, appendix II, 7. The LGB memorandum was noted in *Public Health* 3 (May 1890–September 1891): 343–45, and was reissued by in the LGB's annual report for 1896–97.

84. Wilkinson, "Beginnings," 218–21.

85. Hirst, "Failure 'without Parallel,'" 282. Smith came to the opinion that school attendance had little influence on the spread of diphtheria. He was criticized for this by Shirley Murphy in London County Council, *Annual Report . . . 1896*, appendix III; and in Newsholme, "Prevalence of Diphtheria."

86. On notification of measles see "Notification of Measles I"; "Notification of Measles II"; Armstrong, "Notification of Measles" and "Compulsory Notification"; Vallin, "Compulsory Notification of Measles"; Anderson, "Notification of Measles and

Whooping Cough" and "Notification of Measles"; Sykes, "Notification of Measles"; and Waldo and Walsh, "Murder by Measles." Measles is the most infectious of all the common fevers. Caused by a viral infection in the upper respiratory tract, it is communicated in person via droplet infection. Unlike scarlet fever, the virus does not appear to vary. It rarely occurs in children less than three months old, due to the transmission of maternal antibodies during the fetal stages of pregnancy, providing the mother has had the disease.

87. HCPP, C. 7906 (1895), LI.391, *Twenty-fourth Annual Report of the Local Government Board, 1894–95: Supplement Containing the Report of the Medical Officer for 1894–95*, Theodore Thomson, "Report by Dr Theodore Thomson upon Measles in England and Wales, and as to Measures That May Be and Which Have Been Adopted by Sanitary Authorities with a View to Obtaining Control of this Disease" (hereafter cited as Thomson, "Measles in England and Wales"), 137, 159. Seven urban and three rural sanitary districts had a system of compulsory notification in operation.

88. In London, St. George's Vestry health subcommittee estimated that the notification of measles would cost £210 per annum in doctors' fees alone, the employment of sanitary visitors would involve a further £1,000, while hospital accommodations would cost £1 7s. 6d. per week and disinfection about 6d. for every pound of rates paid. Under such circumstances, "the committee really could not recommend the vestry to take any further action in the matter." Wilkinson, "Beginnings," 227–28.

89. Smith, "Notification of Infectious Diseases."

90. ROLLR, L614, Borough of Leicester, Joseph Priestley, *Annual Report on the Health of Leicester, 1894*, 12.

91. Districts were forever adding and dropping measles from their notification schedules. In 1912 eighty-eight districts still used it; see Bannington, *English Public Health Administration*, 173.

92. Hardy, *Epidemic Streets*, 51. A school's list of pupils who had previously suffered from measles was particularly helpful in places where the disease was not on the notification schedule.

93. Thomson, "Measles in England and Wales," 143. In half the districts, information was systematically provided for the public elementary schools and more irregularly elsewhere.

94. Johnston, *Annual Report, 1884.*

95. BAH, Birmingham City Council, *Health Sub-committee Minute Book, 1899–1902*, 204.

96. Thomson, "Measles in England and Wales," 146.

97. HCPP, C. 8953 (1898), XL.1, *Twenty-seventh Annual Report of the Local Government Board, 1897–98: Supplement Containing the Report of the Medical Officer for 1897–98*, Theodore Thomson, "Report on Epidemic Measles in the Borough of Lancaster"; HCPP, C. 9445 (1899), XXXVIII.1, *Twenty-eighth Annual Report of the Local Government Board, 1898–99: Supplement Containing the Report of the Medical Officer for 1898–99*, Theodore Thomson, "Report upon Measles in the Borough of Burton-on-Trent."

98. NA, Open Shelves, Borough of Nottingham, Philip Boobbyer, *Annual Health Report for 1896*, 33.

99. Thomson, "Measles in England and Wales," 154.

100. London County Council, *Annual Report . . . 1901*, 28.

101. May, "School Closure for Measles."

102. "Control of Measles," *British Medical Journal* 2270 (July 2, 1904): 28–29.

103. Article 101* was removed in part because the Board of Education believed that the creation of new local education authorities in the 1902 Education Act lessened financial problems for individual schools; see Hirst, "Public Health."

104. Ibid.

105. Kerr, *Annual Report . . . 1903,* 9 and 14; see also Hirst, "Early School Medical Service," 72–73.

106. May, "School Closure for Measles," 453.

107. Armstrong, "Diphtheria." By 1896 antitoxin was used to treat diphtheria in more than 66 percent of the cases admitted to Metropolitan Asylums Board hospitals; between 1897 and 1904, this figure was around 80 percent. However, the quantity and immediacy of administering the serum are not known, and patients were often given the antitoxin without a diagnostic test. See Weindling, "From Isolation to Therapy," 134–35. Historians remain unsure about the legitimacy of ascribing all the credit for diphtheria's reduction to the antitoxin. At first, the antitoxin was difficult to obtain, doses were often small and weak, and subcutaneous injection was not the most effective method of administering it. In any case, the virulence of the disease may already have been declining by the time the antitoxin was introduced. See Hardy, *Epidemic Streets,* 102–9.

108. In 1907 Nottingham's laboratory examined no fewer than 1,728 diphtheria specimens. NA, Open Shelves, Borough of Nottingham, Philip Boobbyer, *Annual Health Report for 1907,* 99–100.

109. Kerr, *Annual Report . . . 1903,* 3.

110. Kerr, *Report of the LCC* (1905), 25.

111. Kerr, *Report of the LCC* (1904), 20, 22. Harry Hendrick has noted that "scientific" was "always an important adjective" in the development of social welfare policies. Hendrick, "Child Labour," 47.

112. Hammonds, *Childhood's Deadly Scourge.*

113. Kerr, *Annual Report . . . 1903,* 5.

114. Ibid., 6.

115. Kerr, *Report of the LCC* (1907), 45.

116. Figure calculated from Kerr, *Report of the LCC* (1905), 58.

117. Kerr, *Report of the LCC* (1908), 46.

118. Clearly "herd immunity" derives from veterinary science, but how and when it became popularized for human disease needs further research. The earliest reference to it that I have been able to find in writings from British epidemiology and public health came as a result of experiments with enteric disease on mice in the 1920s; see Topley and Wilson's "Spread of Bacterial Infection: The Problem of Herd-Immunity."

119. Kerr, *Report of the LCC* (1905), 51–52.

120. Kerr, *Report of the LCC* (1908), 46.

121. Kerr, *Report of the LCC* (1904), 60.

122. Kerr, *Report of the LCC* (1908), 44.

123. Sykes, "Measles and Elementary Schools." Sykes, the influential MOH of St. Pancras, in London, believed that complete success in measles control would only be achieved by disallowing education for children five years old or less.

124. Kerr, *Report of the LCC* (1906), 29.

125. London County Council, *Annual Report of the Council 1912*, 3:155.

126. Newsholme and Kerr, *Newsholme's School Hygiene*, 248, 256.

127. HCPP, C. 5426 (1910), XXIII.175, Board of Education, *Annual Report for 1909 of the Chief Medical Officer of the Board of Education* (hereafter cited as BoE, *Annual Report* [1909]), 19–20.

128. HCPP, C. 4259 (1908), LXXXII.527, Board of Education, *Report of the Consultative Committee on the School Attendance of Children below the Age of Five*, 31.

129. Sykes, "Measles and Elementary Schools," 475; capitalization of "HOME" in the original.

130. Sykes, "Mothercraft."

131. Sykes, "Measles and Elementary Schools," 475. On debates about the crèche system in the early twentieth century, see Mooney and Tanner, "Infant Mortality, a Spatial Problem."

132. HCPP, C. 4259 (1908), LXXXII.527, Board of Education, *Report of the Consultative Committee on the School Attendance of Children below the Age of Five*, 31.

133. Ibid., 17.

134. Hendrick, *Child Welfare*, 112. Schemes for medical inspection could be found in France, Belgium, Germany, and a host of other European nations.

135. Harris, *Health of the Schoolchild*, 22–23; HCPP, C. 2175 (1904), XXXII.1, Interdepartmental Committee on Physical Deterioration, *Report*, vol. 1 and appendix.

136. Besides education legislation, Harris enumerates related legislative outcomes, such as the Open Spaces Act (1906), Notification of Births Act (1907), Public Health (Regulations as to Food) Act (1907), Public Health Amendment Act (1907), and Maternity and Child Welfare Act (1918).

137. Welshman, "Bringing Beauty and Brightness," 200; Harris, *Health of the Schoolchild*, 6.

138. Harris, *Health of the Schoolchild*, 39.

139. Hurt, *Elementary Schooling*, 142–43; Hirst, "Growth of Treatment"; Hirst, "Early School Medical Service," 73–79. The LCC had particular problems configuring treatment services, as detailed in Hirst, "Failure 'without Parallel.'"

140. Combining the roles of MOH and school medical officer was seen as a cost-cutting approach. MOHs were already incredibly busy, and it was thought they would be unable to cope with the anticipated workload of inspections. It was also feared that such close association with the local public health authority would undermine the distinctiveness and effectiveness of SMS as a preventive and treatment package.

141. Harris, *Health of the Schoolchild*, 101.

142. HCPP, C. 4986 (1910), XXIII.1, Board of Education, *Annual Report for 1908 of the Chief Medical Officer of the Board of Education* (hereafter cited as BoE, *Annual Report* [1908]), 17.

143. Board of Education Circular 576, "Memorandum on Medical Inspection of Children in Public Elementary Schools, under Section 13 of the Education (Administrative Provisions) Act, 1907." The board did not issue this as a Parliamentary Paper, but reprinted it in its *Annual Report* (1908), 141–50, quote on 141.

144. Hendrick, "Child Labour," 62.

145. HCPP, C. 5925 (1911), XVII.449, Board of Education, *Annual Report for 1910 of the Chief Medical Officer of the Board of Education* (hereafter cited as BoE, *Annual* Report [1910]), 101–3.

146. BoE, *Annual Report* (1909).

147. BoE, *Annual Report* (1910), 99.

148. ROLLR, L614, Borough of Leicester, William Johnston, *Annual Report on the Health of Leicester, 1883,* 26; and BAH, Birmingham City Council Health Committee, Alfred Hill, *Report on the Health of the City of Birmingham for the Year 1882,* 41.

149. BoE, *Annual Report* (1909), 80–87; BoE, *Annual Report* (1908), 94–96.

150. London County Council, *Annual Report of the Council 1912,* 3:121–22. On the long-term development of care committees, see Chaddock, "Voluntary Social Services." By 1929 there were 934 of them in London, engaging the services of 5,905 voluntary workers. This aspect of the SMS deserves more attention than I have been able to devote to it.

151. BoE, *Annual Report* (1909), 83.

152. London County Council, *Annual Report of the Council 1913,* 3:146. In practice, a care committee member was present at about 80 percent of inspections and 70 percent of reinspections.

153. Hendrick, "Child Labour," 62.

154. BoE, *Annual Report* (1909), 73–74; HCPP, C. 7184 (1914), XXV.401, Board of Education, *Annual Report for 1912 of the Chief Medical Officer of the Board of Education* (hereafter cited as BoE, *Annual Report* [1912]), 4–5.

155. The majority of legal proceedings related to children whose clothes or bodies were riddled with vermin. Brighton instigated 198 cases in 1913. The 1908 Children's Act gave local authorities the power to clean children and their clothing. Manchester used this law to clean 219 children in 1913. Given that the annual national number of inspections of head, clothes, and body ran into the hundreds of thousands, the scale of infractions was comparatively small. HCPP, C. 7730 (1914–16), XVIII.277, Board of Education, *Annual Report for 1913 of the Chief Medical Officer of the Board of Education,* 316. On truancy see Rubinstein, "Socialization," 245.

156. Hirst, "Early School Medical Service," 67.

157. HCPP, C. 6530 (1912–13), XXI.439, Board of Education, *Annual Report for 1911 of the Chief Medical Officer of the Board of Education* (hereafter cited as BoE, *Annual Report* [1911]), 102.

158. BoE, *Annual Report* (1908), 21.

159. BoE, *Annual Report* (1911), 103.

160. London County Council, *Annual Report of the Council 1913,* 3:149.

161. BoE, *Annual Report* (1908), 73.

162. BoE, *Annual Report* (1910), 89.

163. Calculated from London County Council, *Annual Report of the Council 1913,* 3:151.

164. On open-air schools see Bryder, "Wonderlands"; and Châtelet, "Breath of Fresh Air."

165. Bryder, *Below the Magic Mountain,* 36–45.

166. London County Council, *Annual Report of the Council 1913,* 3:156.

167. SLSL, 352.4 SQ, Harold Scurfield, *Annual Report of the Medical Officer of Health for Sheffield, 1909,* xiii.

168. BoE, *Annual Report* (1912), 88–89.

169. BoE, *Annual Report* (1911), 102.

170. Porter, "Enemies of the Race," 173.

171. J. Kerr, quoted in Crowley, *Needs, Objects, and Method*, 12. In the United States, these sorts of opinions were often shaped in the Progressive Era by attitudes toward the immigrant urban poor, race improvement, and eugenics. See Meckel, *Classrooms and Clinics*, 93–99; and Hammonds, *Childhood's Deadly Scourge*.

172. Harris, "Educational Reform," 97; see also Hirst, "Early School Medical Service."

173. Aaby et al., "Severe Measles." On malnutrition and respiratory complications see Hardy, *Epidemic Streets*, 36–37, 42–43.

## Chapter Five

1. As Clive Edwards points out, "Even though it might be a representation of respectability and stability in contrast to other spheres, concerns over the home, its possessions and their messages bred their own anxieties for people." Edwards, *Turning Houses into Homes*, 150.

2. Flanders, *Inside the Victorian Home*, chap. 10.

3. According to Thomson, ornamentation should be conspicuous by its absence from the sickroom: one large table fitted with drawers to hold the necessary articles (jars, a basin, and other items such as sponge, scissors, and linen), a small bedside table, a sofa or invalid chair, no more than two additional chairs, and a chest of drawers. Thomson himself was lenient with carpet because it prevented wooden floors from getting wet and it muffled noise. The breadth of Thomson's definition of "infectious" is striking and included typhus fever, plague, childbed (puerperal) fever, influenza, whooping cough, consumption in its latter stages, smallpox, chicken pox, measles, scarlet fever, and erysipelas. Contagious diseases communicated only by contact and inoculation were itch, sivvens, venereal diseases, yaws, hydrophobia, ringworm of the head, and Egyptian ophthalmia. Thomson, *Domestic Management of the Sick-Room*, 112–22. For background details on Thomson see Bartrip, "Thomson, Anthony Todd (1778–1849)."

4. Murray, *Modern Householder*, 688; Brinckman, *Care of the Sick*, chap. 3; Crookshank, *Manual of Home Nursing*, chap. 2.

5. Bailin, *Sickroom in Victorian Fiction*, 17–18; Adams, *Architecture in the Family Way*, chap. 3.

6. Thomson, *Domestic Management of the Sick-Room*, 395–401.

7. Cleere, "Victorian Dust Traps," 134.

8. Gunn and Vernon, "Introduction," 7–9.

9. Bashford, *Purity and Pollution*, 9; see also Poovey, *Making a Social Body*, chap. 6.

10. Behlmer, introduction to *Friends of the Family*; Davidoff and Hall, *Family Fortunes*; Helly and Reverby, *Gendered Domains*. See also Sheller and Urry, *Mobile Technologies of the City*; and Sheller and Urry, "Mobile Transformations."

11. Gilbert, *Citizen's Body*, chap. 2; Hamlin, *Public Health and Social Justice*.

12. Gilbert, *Citizen's Body*, 18–24; see also Corrigan and Sayer, *Great Arch*, 150–51.

13. Kearns, "Private Property," 190.

14. Hamlin, "Muddling in Bumbledom"; Hamlin, *Public Health and Social Justice*.

15. Gilbert, *Citizen's Body*, 55; Hall, McClelland, and Rendall, *Defining the Victorian Nation*; McClelland and Rose, "Citizenship and Empire"; Tosh, *Man's Place*.

16. McClelland, "England's Greatness, the Working Man," 90.

17. On "character" see Collini, *Public Moralists.*

18. Davis and Tanner, "Borough Franchise after 1867"; Hoppen, "Franchise."

19. From 1867 the vote extended to all rate-paying adult male occupiers and renters in lodgings worth £10 or more who had been resident there for a minimum of one year.

20. McClelland, "England's Greatness, the Working Man," 94–95; Biagini, *Liberty, Retrenchment, and Reform,* chap. 5. Incidentally, historians continue to dispute the extent to which working-class electoral participation unlocked the door to increased public health spending at the local level. See Aidt, Daunton, and Dutta, "Retrenchment Hypothesis."

21. Harris, "Civic Virtue and Social Darwinism," 74–75, quoted in McClelland, "England's Greatness, the Working Man," 98.

22. Godwin, *London Shadows,* viii; emphasis in original.

23. Tosh, *Man's Place,* 4. On the separation of work and home, see Davidoff and Hall, *Family Fortunes*; on the frequent overestimation of this separation, see Donald, "Tranquil Havens?"

24. Chase and Levenson, *Spectacle of Intimacy,* 12–13.

25. Flanders, introduction to *Inside the Victorian Home*; Adams, *Architecture in the Family Way,* 75; Bryden and Floyd, "Introduction," 2; see also Smiles, *Happy Homes.*

26. "Social Topics: Home," *Manchester Times,* March 11, 1876.

27. Muthesius, *English Terraced House*; Daunton, "Public Place and Private Space."

28. According to Victorian literary critics Karen Chase and Michael Levenson, domesticity was the "special moral mission of the middle class" and contained lessons that the poor and working classes invariably failed to assimilate. Chase and Levenson, *Spectacle of Intimacy,* 6. There is some room for dispute over this characterization of working-class obduracy. Historian Martin Daunton, for example, has argued that from around the 1870s the increasing domesticity of the working class was a response to an extension of employer control and the loss of autonomy in the workplace. Daunton, *House and Home,* chap. 11. Sociologists and geographers have made much the same point; see Marshall et al., *Social Class*; and Franklin, "Working-Class Privatism."

29. Chase and Levenson, *Spectacle of Intimacy,* 8.

30. Hepworth, "Privacy, Security and Respectability," 19.

31. Otter, *Victorian Eye,* 258. Much social policy in the later nineteenth century envisioned the ordering of internal domestic space according to middle-class norms. This was particularly true of the infant welfare movement, maternalism, and "scientific motherhood." See, for example, Kleinberg, "Gendered Space," 156; and Abramovitz, *Regulating the Lives of Women.*

32. SLSL, 352.4 SQ, Griffiths, *Annual Report of the Medical Officer of Health for Sheffield, 1875,* 22.

33. Bailin, *Sickroom in Victorian Fiction.*

34. Cohen, *Household Gods.*

35. For a recent study of disinfection in England, see Whyte, "Changing Approaches."

36. Coleman, *Yellow Fever in the North,* 140. Coleman provides a nuanced analysis of disinfection and "modified" quarantine in France (see chap. 4).

37. Baldwin, *Contagion and the State*, 141–42.

38. Ibid., 165–66. The only sustained analyses of municipal disinfection appear in histories of French public health. See Corbin, *The Foul and the Fragrant*; Barnes, *Great Stink of Paris.*

39. Worboys, *Spreading Germs*, 275.

40. Wohl, *Endangered Lives*; Smith, *People's Health*; Porter, *Health, Civilization, and the State.*

41. Hardy, *Epidemic Streets*; Eyler, *Sir Arthur Newsholme*; Niemi, *Public Health.*

42. Barnes, *Great Stink of Paris*, chap. 4.

43. These examples are from Letheby, "Right Use of Disinfectants (a)" and "Right Use of Disinfectants (b)." See also Twelvetrees, "Disinfection," pt. 2.

44. Letheby, "Right Use of Disinfectants (a)," 487.

45. Kearns, "Cholera," 111–12; Durey, *Return of the Plague*, 84–85, 95.

46. Cunningham Glen, *Law Relating to Public Health*, 160, 522, 529–30.

47. Kearns, "Cholera," 116.

48. On the mid-nineteenth-century transformation of "nuisance," see ibid.; Hamlin, "Public Sphere to Public Health"; and Hanley, "Parliament, Physicians, and Nuisances."

49. Durey, *Return of the Plague*, 162–64.

50. Cunningham Glen, *Law Relating to Public Health*, 264, 269–70.

51. HCPP, C. 161 (1861), XVI.339, *Third Report of the Medical Officer of the Privy Council, 1860*, 38.

52. On the terms "infective," "infectious," "contagion," and "miasmatic" in the 1860s, see Worboys, *Spreading Germs*, 33; and for zymotic disease theory see 34–42.

53. HCPP, C. 208 (1870), XXXVIII.591, *Twelfth Report of the Medical Officer of the Privy Council, 1869*, "Memorandum on Precautions to Be Taken against Scarlatina."

54. Ibid., 13.

55. Hardwicke, "Importance of Complete Disinfection," 454; Bond, "Importance of Complete Disinfection."

56. RSC *First Report*), evidence of John Simon, qq. 2,048–51.

57. HCPP, C. 208 (1870), XXXVIII.591, *Twelfth Report of the Medical Officer of the Privy Council, 1869*, 13.

58. Bond, "Importance of Complete Disinfection," 457–58.

59. Thorne, "Use and Influence of Hospitals," iv.

60. Cameron, "Disinfection."

61. Rideal, *Disinfection and Disinfectants*, 283–84.

62. Hardwicke, "Importance of Complete Disinfection."

63. Sanitary districts were created by the public health acts of 1873 and 1875 and were classed as urban (USDs) or rural (RSDs). Port sanitary authorities were separate. USDs were formed by either the municipal borough, the Improvement Commissioners District or in any Local Government District formed under the Public Health Act (1848), or Local Government Act (1858). RSDs followed the boundaries of existing Poor Law unions formed in 1837, minus the urban sanitary districts. In 1894 USDs and RSDs were replaced by urban and rural district councils. In 1892 there were more than 1,600 sanitary districts in England and Wales.

64. Cameron, "Disinfection," 537.

65. Messiter and Bailey, "Disinfection of Clothing by Heat."

66. An extensive sanitary survey was conducted by Dr. Frederick Barry in 1892–94, when it was feared cholera might hop across the English Channel. The survey was curtailed by Barry's untimely death, but he painted a similar picture of incompleteness where disinfection is concerned. HCPP, C. 7815 (1895), LII.1, *Reports and Papers on the Port and Riparian Sanitary Survey of England and Wales, 1893–94*; HCPP, C. 8215 (1896), XXXVII.667, *Twenty-fourth Annual Report of the Local Government Board, 1894–95: Supplement in Continuation of the Report of the Medical Officer for 1894–95: Inland Sanitary Survey, 1893–95.*

67. "Report of the Lancet Special Sanitary Commission on Disinfecting in London," *Lancet* 137 (January 3, 1891): 47–48.

68. Freeman, *Planning of Fever Hospitals.*

69. Cameron, "Disinfection."

70. Hardwicke, "Importance of Complete Disinfection," 454.

71. "Fees for Disinfection in Marylebone," *Lancet* 132 (September 15, 1888): 533. In the nine months to January 1878, Nottingham received £22 5s. in payments, which barely covered one-quarter of the operating costs of the hot-air disinfector. See NA, CA.CM/Health/7, Nottingham *HCMB, December 22, 1876 to September 6, 1878,* December 14, 1877; and NA, CA.CM/Health/9, Nottingham *HCMB, August 30, 1880 to November 24, 1882.*

72. Liverpool *Circular,* 27.

73. Beier, *For Their Own Good,* 186. Compare this resistance to the removal of property in England to Paris, where disinfection practices in the early 1890s were initially very unpopular. See Barnes, *Great Stink of Paris,* 146–51.

74. NA, CA/HE/2/1/1, Borough of Nottingham, Samuel George Johnson (town clerk) and Edward Seaton, *Report of the Health Committee to the 29th September 1884,* 7.

75. "Disinfection by Heat," *Daily News,* November 22, 1886.

76. Beier, *For Their Own Good,* 186.

77. Vincent, *Poor Citizens,* 11–12.

78. Beier, *For Their Own Good,* 186.

79. Taylor, *Sanitary Inspector's Handbook,* 227–28. In Nottingham, the manager of the disinfecting station maintained the disease notification ledgers. NA, CA/HE/2/1/1, Borough of Nottingham, Edward Seaton, *Annual Report of the Medical Officer of Health for 1882,* 15.

80. David Vincent notes how a visit to the pawnbroker "involved a profound loss of dignity. . . . It exposed to the public gaze both the precise state of personal possessions and the general fact that the household was too poor to subsist on cash income alone." Vincent, *Poor Citizens,* 12.

81. On the inseparability of science and the social, see Hacking, *Historical Ontology.*

82. "The examination of a substance for disinfectant capacity is an extremely complex matter. . . . No department of bacteriological enquiry is more encumbered with inconclusive researches than this investigation of disinfectants." Pearmain, Hewlett, and Moor, *Applied Bacteriology,* 373. In 1903 Samuel Rideal and J. T. Ainslie Walker developed the Rideal-Walker test that is still used today to assess the effectiveness of disinfectants. See Rideal and Walker, "Standardisation of Disinfectants."

83. Shann, "Disinfecting Property of Heat"; "Resolution on the Disinfecting Property of Heat," *Transactions of the National Association for the Promotion of Social Science,* 1857 (1864): 593.

84. Henry, "Experiments" and "Further Experiments." For background information on William Henry and the Mancunian scientific community in this period, see Kargon, *Science in Victorian Manchester*; and Thackray, "Natural Knowledge in Cultural Context." According to Thackray, Henry was "second only to Dalton in the Manchester scientific community." Some late-nineteenth-century experts on disinfection with heat referenced the eighteenth-century experiments by Needham and Spallanzani that sparked the controversy over spontaneous generation. See Rideal, *Disinfection and Disinfectants*, 19–20.

85. Henry, "Letter from Dr. Henry."

86. "Disinfection," *Medical Times and Gazette*, n.s., 14 (1857): 436–37.

87. Crace-Calvert, "Heat on Protoplasmic Life."

88. Kargon, *Science in Victorian Manchester*, 97–100, 121–23.

89. Roll-Hansen, "Experimental Method and Spontaneous Generation."

90. Letheby, "Right Use of Disinfectants (a)," 516.

91. For Letheby's activities in the arena of water analysis, see Hamlin, *Science of Impurity*. On dry-heat machines, see Lalor, "On Disinfection"; "Disinfection of Clothing and Bedding," *Medical Times and Gazette* 2 (December 10, 1881): 686–87.

92. "New Disinfecting Apparatus," *Medical Times and Gazette* 1 (1870): 323.

93. Letheby, "Right Use of Disinfectants (a)," 515.

94. Ransom, "Mode of Disinfecting by Heat" and "Disinfection by Heat." See also Asherson, "Ransom, William Henry (1823–1907)." Francois De Chaumont, professor of hygiene at the Army Medical School, and a Dr. Lake at the Southampton Infirmary also conducted experiments assessing the impact of heat on bedding. De Chaumont, "Effects of High Temperatures."

95. Koch, Gaffky, and Loeffler, "Versuche Über Die Verwerthbarkeit Heisser Wasserdämpfe Zu Desinfectionszwecken"; Koch and Wolffhülge, "Untersuchungen Über Die Desinfection Mit Heisser Luft." For the wider context of Koch's disinfection experiments, see Gradmann, *Laboratory Disease*, 13; Brock, *Robert Koch*, chap. 12; Koch and Carter, *Essays of Robert Koch*, xiv.

96. Priestley, "Disinfectors and Disinfectants, 1874–95," 19–20.

97. The information in the rest of this paragraph is taken from "Disinfecting by Steam," *Sanitary Record*, n.s., 3 (October 15, 1881): 158–60.

98. Napier, *Manual of Dyeing*.

99. HCPP, C. 4516 (1884–85), XXXIII.227, *Fourteenth Annual Report of the Local Government Board 1884–85: Supplement Containing the Report of the Medical Officer for 1884*, appendix B, no. 10, Franklin H. Parsons, "Report on Disinfection by Heat," 218–303; Parsons, *Extracts from the Annual Report*. Parsons's *BMJ* obituary extolled his work on disinfection as a "landmark" contribution to the field. "Henry Franklin Parsons, M.D. Lond., P.P.H.," *British Medical Journal* 2758 (November 8, 1913): 1263–64. The periodic reports of this American Public Health Association committee provide a valuable shorthand guide to international developments in disinfection. "Report of Committee on Disinfectants for 1886," *Public Health Papers and Reports* 12 (1886): 198–28.

100. See Whyte, "Changing Approaches," 82–91, for additional aspects of the debate about steam disinfection.

101. NA, CA/HE/2/1/1, Borough of Nottingham, B. Arthur Whitelegge, *Annual Report of the Medical Officer of Health for 1888*, 43.

102. HCPP, C. 4516 (1884–85), XXXIII.227, *Fourteenth Annual Report of the Local Government Board 1884–85: Supplement Containing the Report of the Medical Officer for 1884*, appendix B, no. 10, Franklin H. Parsons, "Report on Disinfection by Heat," 244, 249.

103. When St. Helen's local authority purchased a Goddard machine in 1893, it was eventually forced to hand over £100 to Lyons, on top of the £205 it had paid for the disinfector itself. The authority believed it had been duped by Goddard's, which kept silent about the patent dispute with Lyon. Whyte, "Changing Approaches," 131–32.

104. Aldwinckle, "Disinfecting Apparatus," 296.

105. Thresh, "Steam from Saline Solutions."

106. "Lancet Special Sanitary Commission on Disinfection, II," *Lancet* 147 (January 11, 1896): 120–24; Barwise, "Disinfection by Steam."

107. Mackenzie, "Methods of Disinfection," pt. 2, 596. Chloride of lime was also known as chlorinated lime and bleaching powder. All were names for a mixture containing chlorinated calcium and hypochlorate of calcium in varying proportions.

108. Barker, "On Deodorisation and Disinfection"; Bond, "Conditions of Efficient Disinfection"; Dougall, "Disinfection by Acids," pts. 1 and 2. Fumigation was less commonly termed "deodorisation" or "aerial disinfection."

109. "Disinfection no. I," *Lancet* 98 (September 23, 1871): 434–35; "Disinfection no. II," *Lancet* 98 (September 30, 1871): 472–73; "Disinfection no. III," *Lancet* 98 (October 14, 1871): 558–59.

110. Koch, "Ueber Desinfection." See also the summary in Young, *Notes on Disinfectants and Disinfection*, 193–97; and Brock, *Robert Koch*, 106.

111. Thorne, "Use and Influence of Hospitals."

112. Ransome's own accounts do not give the precise date. A publication from November 1893 implies the meeting occurred in February 1892, Delépine and Ransome, "Disinfection of Tuberculously-Infected Houses," 990. Elsewhere, Ransome recalled that it took place in 1891; see Ransome, *Campaign against Consumption*, 53.

113. Mohr, "Dreschfeld, Julius"; Worboys, "Delépine, Auguste Sheridan." Delépine became head of the laboratory in 1891 when Dreschfeld took over as the chair of medicine.

114. James Niven, Tatham's successor as Manchester's medical officer of health, pointed out that the "disinfection" performed in Manchester at the time "was taken to mean fumigation." See Niven, "Notification of Tuberculosis." Delépine and Ransome, "Disinfection of Tuberculously-Infected Houses." The research was supported by the Scientific Grants Committee of the British Medical Association.

115. Delépine and Ransome, "Disinfection of Tubercle-Infected Houses," 353. On the popularity of sulfur fumigation, see "Society of Medical Officers of Health: The Present Position of Disinfection," *Lancet* 137 (March 7, 1891): 548–49.

116. "Practical Disinfection of Rooms," *Lancet* 146 (November 9, 1895): 1180, which also explores why carbolic acid was favored in Britain, despite its dangerousness and the fact that corrosive sublimate (bichloride of mercury) was more popular in France, Germany, and Italy.

117. Koch, "Address on Bacteriological Research," 383.

118. Delépine and Ransome, "Disinfection of Tubercle-Infected Houses," 351.

119. Downes and Blunt, "Effect of Light upon Bacteria"; Downes, "Action of Sunlight on Micro-Organisms." Other scientists experimenting with sunlight and

bacteria included Émile Declaux, a close colleague of Pasteur, and the English botanist H. Marshall Ward, who worked on anthrax. See Ward, "Action of Light" and "Further Experiments."

120. Hockberger, "History of Ultraviolet Photobiology."

121. Koch, "Address on Bacteriological Research," 383.

122. Stirland, "Auguste Sheridan Delépine, 1855–1921," 110–11; Worboys, *Spreading Germs*, 262–63.

123. On Koch's innovative use of silk thread, see Brock, *Robert Koch*, 107. Linen and cotton threads were widely used, as was muslin gauze. See Novy, *Laboratory Work in Bacteriology*, 518–27, on the testing of disinfectants.

124. Delépine, "Some Experiments," 530.

125. Russell, "On Disinfection," 403.

126. Beier, *For Their Own Good*, 185. For an American example see Novy and Waite, "Disinfection of Rooms."

127. Mackenzie, "Methods of Disinfection," pt. 2.

128. Delépine, "Some Experiments," 529–30.

129. Speake, "Infectious Milk."

130. Slater and Rideal, "On Formaldehyde as an Antiseptic"; Kenwood and Taylor, "Disinfection of Rooms"; Kanthack, "Use of Formalin Lamps"; "Formaldehyde Disinfection by Means of Lamps," *Lancet* 146 (September 21, 1895): 747. For experimental results see Delépine, "Some Experiments." The Alformant Lamp heated dry polymerized formalin tablets to produce active formic aldehyde. "Formalin and the Alformant Lamp," *Sanitary Record* 20 (August 20, 1897): 198–99.

131. Rideal, *Disinfection and Disinfectants*. The book ran to three editions between 1895 and 1903. Initially Rideal advocated that formalin spray should continue to be supplemented with vaporization: Rideal, "Formaldehyde Disinfection."

132. For a description of the use of formalin spray in Lancaster on the eve of World War I, see Beier, *For Their Own Good*, 169–70. See also Whyte, "Changing Approaches," 167–68, for Mackenzie's trials of the effects of formalin spray on wallpaper.

133. Mackenzie, "Methods of Disinfection," pt. 2, 594; Barnes, *Great Stink of Paris*, 141–60. Barnes does not consider contemporary debates about the relative efficacy of sprays. See Defries, "Disinfection of Rooms"; and Kenwood and Taylor, "Disinfection of Rooms," for the British discussion about the Parisian scheme and experiments in France. Defries and Sons of Houndsditch, London, manufactured spray disinfectors that were similar to those used in Paris (the "Equifex Spray Disinfector"). Crewe's MOH claimed to be the first British user; see "Disinfection: Object Lesson from Crewe," *Sanitary Record* 19 (January 1, 1897): 14.

134. Disinfectors were cautioned to change out of their daily clothing and don overalls. This clothing also helped protect them when they first rubbed walls down with breadcrumbs that were then collected and burned. This was a preliminary process sometimes used to absorb infectious debris and remove surface dirt: Mackenzie, "Methods of Disinfection," pt. 2, 595; Pearmain, Hewlett, and Moor, *Applied Bacteriology*, 386. In Manchester, walls were rubbed with dough as well as breadcrumbs, though only when disinfection could not be carried out by the municipal authority. See Whyte, "Changing Approaches," 113–14, 167–68. This procedure was based on Esmarch, "Der Keimgehalt Der Wände Und Ihre Desinfection." According

to Niven, "On the Notification of Phthisis," 19, almost 1,600 Mancunian householders disinfected their homes using this method in the year ending March 30, 1901. The use of dough and bread fell into abeyance during the war when flour became scarce. Niven, *Observations*, 99–100.

135. Mackenzie, "Methods of Disinfection," pt. 2, 601.

136. Pearmain, Hewlett, and Moor, *Applied Bacteriology*, 385.

137. Mackenzie, "Simple and Portable Spray Pump."

138. Thresh, "Portable Spraying Disinfecting Apparatus"; "Portable Spraying Apparatus for Disinfection," *Lancet* 159 (June 21, 1902): 1779.

139. "Spray Apparatus for Disinfecting with Formic Aldehyde," *Lancet* 160 (July 12, 1902): 83.

140. Robertson, "New Form of Spray Apparatus."

141. The permissive Infectious Disease (Prevention) Act of 1890 required that "from time to time" local authorities should provide temporary shelter or accommodations for householders who had to vacate their property in the event of disinfection. See Parkes, *Infectious Diseases*, 34–35.

142. Beier, *For Their Own Good*, 185–86. Sulfur fumigation was still being used in "a few places" on the eve of World War I. Hewat, "Disinfection of Tubercle-Infected Houses," 151. See also Pearmain, Hewlett, and Moor, *Applied Bacteriology*, 373; and Rideal, *Disinfection and Disinfectants*, 7. On fumigation's continuing—and, to most, baffling—use, see "Disinfection Processes," *Public Health* 9 (October 1896–September 1897): 287; Poyntz Wright, "Equifex Spray Disinfector"; and Spottiswoode Cameron, "Disinfectants," 399–400.

143. Parsons, "Discussion on Isolation and Disinfection," 455; Reid, *Practical Sanitation*, 212; Taylor, *Sanitary Inspector's Handbook*, 212–14; Whitelegge and Newman, *Hygiene and Public Health*, 538–42; Newsholme, *Hygiene*, 325–26; Parkes and Kenwood, *Hygiene and Public Health*, 617–24.

144. Mackenzie, "Methods of Disinfection," pt. 1, 445; Beier, *For Their Own Good*, 186.

145. Caldwell Smith, "Discussion on Isolation and Disinfection," 455; see also Mackenzie, "Methods of Disinfection," pt. 1, 445.

146. Baldwin, *Contagion and the State*, 525–26.

147. Beier, *For Their Own Good*, 203–4.

## Chapter Six

1. Mendelsohn, "'Like All That Lives,'" 14–15.

2. Worboys, "Before McKeown," 149.

3. Ibid., 163.

4. After several years of vacillation and following an international survey, the 1907 International Congress in Vienna adopted a resolution recommending compulsory notification of pulmonary tuberculosis. Voluntary notification had been advocated at the 1901 Tuberculosis Congress in London. Bulstrode, "State Section." An international committee was set up in 1906 to report to the congress the following year. Raw, "International Congress against Tuberculosis" and "Compulsory Notification of Tuberculosis." Raw was a member of an English delegation in 1907 that opposed

compulsory notification, as did the French. They were defeated by the Germans, Austrians, and Norwegians (notification was already compulsory in Norway), see "International Conference on Tuberculosis (from Our Vienna Correspondent)," *Lancet* 170 (November 9, 1907): 1348–49. There was also disagreement over the stage at which to notify a case.

5. Caldwell Smith, "Discussion on Isolation and Disinfection," 455; Murray, *Modern Householder.*

6. Though used in multiple medical contexts, "preventive therapy" is today most commonly associated with tuberculosis. The term describes a combination of measures including isoniazid drug treatment to thwart the development of active disease, infection control, and intensified case finding.

7. Warren Crowe stated in 1906 that the "day in which public institutions will afford services to all consumptives is far off." Crowe, *Consumption*, 3. See also Beier, *For Their Own Good*, 179–81, 192.

8. Eyler, *Sir Arthur Newsholme*, chap. 6; Bryder, *Below the Magic Mountain*, 42.

9. Niven, *Observations*, 97.

10. "Oldham Medical Society," *Lancet* 142 (November 18, 1893): 1255–57; "Notification of Phthisis," *British Medical Journal* 1716 (November 18, 1893): 1101; Eyler, *Sir Arthur Newsholme*, 151. The Medical Society in Oldham tried unsuccessfully to have phthisis voluntarily notified to the sanitary authority in 1893 when Niven was MOH there.

11. Niven, "On the Notification of Phthisis," 266. The appointment of two assistant medical officers dealt with the increased number of home visits. Niven had long been interested in the possibilities of phthisis notification, and while he was MOH in Oldham he had replicated the popular educational work of Arthur Ransome and the MSSA in the 1890s. Niven, "Notification of Tuberculosis," pt. 2, 1198. Local Government Board inspector H. Timbrell Bulstrode asserted that Manchester's scheme was not fully up and running until 1901, which may indeed have been the case. HCPP, C. 3657, 1907, XXVII.1, *Supplement to the Annual Report of the Medical Officer of Health to the Local Government Board 1905–06*, H. Timbrell Bulstrode, "On Sanatoria for Consumption and Other Aspects of the Tuberculosis Question" (hereafter cited as Bulstrode, "On Sanatoria").

12. "Voluntary Notification of Phthisis," *Tuberculosis* 1, no. 4 (1900): 130.

13. On Bolton see Robertson, "Terrible Scourge of Consumption."

14. Background to the history of respiratory tuberculosis notification in Britain can be found in Bulstrode, "On Sanatoria"; Bryder, *Below the Magic Mountain*, 41–43; and Eyler, *Sir Arthur Newsholme*, chaps. 6 and 9. The National Campaign for the Prevention of Consumption made a survey of local authorities in 1900. Out of sixty-two responses, thirty districts were distributing leaflets about the prevention of consumption, twenty-five provided disinfecting services free of charge, and nine carried out bacteriological examinations. "Report of Answers Received from Corporations and Medical Officers of Health to Circular Letter Issued," *Tuberculosis* 1, no. 5 (October 1900): 226–27.

15. Institutional isolation was not the primary goal of compulsory tuberculosis notification schemes in other parts of the world. In the United States toward the end of the 1890s, such schemes were "intended as a far-reaching program of sanitary inspection and monitoring of all cases." Fairchild et al., *Searching Eyes*, 41.

Compulsory tuberculosis reporting began in Michigan in 1893, in Baltimore in 1896, and in New York City in 1897. It was rejected in Philadelphia in 1894. See "Discussion on Registration of Tuberculosis." For more on the history of tuberculosis reporting in the United States, see esp. Fox, "Social Policy and City Politics." Other works on the social history of tuberculosis in the United States deal with the issue in somewhat less detail; see Teller, *Tuberculosis Movement*, 21–24, 71–73; Feldberg, *Disease and Class*, 83–84; and Rothman, *Living in the Shadow*, 187–90.

16. Ransome, *Campaign against Consumption*, 89. The association was a private organization whose membership included public appointees such as PLMOs and MOHs.

17. Niven, "On Municipal Administrative Measures," 186.

18. As with many other members of the medical and public health professions, Ransome's ideas about tubercular infection were undergoing refinement in this period. Before latching on to the dried-sputum hypothesis, he based his ideas on a layered spatiality. "Tubercular diseases cling especially to certain localities" within cities, partially the result of damp subsoils; within these "phthisis nests," poorly ventilated homes intensified the localized threat. Ransome, "Some Evidence Respecting Tubercular Infective Areas," reprinted in Ransome, *Campaign against Consumption*, 176–89. In an article originally published in the October 1892 issue of the *Medical Chronicle*, Ransome remained committed to an environmental component. Substituting the damp-soil argument with one that suggested there were parts of towns "where bacillus-laden dust is most likely to be met with," the "virus" (a slip of his pen?) nevertheless was "derived from the poisonous atmosphere of the home." Ibid., quotes on 152, 153.

19. Ibid., 89.

20. "Proceedings of the North-Western Branch of the Incorporated Society of Medical Officers of Health," *Public Health* 4 (October 1891–September 1892): 322–25. Ransome was not himself an MOH, but was an associate of the branch.

21. "Proceedings of the Incorporated Society of Medical Officers of Health," *Public Health* 5 (October 1892–September 1893): 66–75.

22. Niven, "On the Prevention of Phthisis." On tubercular cattle, see Waddington, *Bovine Scourge*.

23. Niven, "On the Prevention of Phthisis," 202.

24. Parkes, "Prevention of Phthisis: A Critique." Ransome himself worried about sufferers being shunned and disowned by their own families and forced into destitution once they were known to be infectious. Worboys, *Spreading Germs*, 230. To be fair to Ransome, he had unsuccessfully attempted to insert a paragraph to the effect that consumptives were not a danger to the community if their houses were kept clean and ventilated and they destroyed their sputum. Ransome, "Prevention of Phthisis"; see also Paget, "Prevention of Phthisis." Ransome thought notification should be voluntary, and he championed the success of broad environmental sanitary measures in reducing tuberculosis mortality rates. Ransome, "Consumption, a 'Filth Disease,'" "Sanitation v. Tuberculosis," and "Crusade against Tuberculosis."

25. NA, Open Shelves, Borough of Nottingham, Philip Boobbyer, *Annual Health Report for 1896*, 53.

26. Russell and Chalmers, *Public Health Administration in Glasgow*, 546.

27. Parkes, "Prevention of Phthisis," 308–9.

28. "Provincial Meeting of the Incorporated Society of Medical Officers of Health at Newcastle, August 4th, 1893: The Prevention of Phthisis," *Public Health* 5 (October 1892–September 1893): 362.

29. "Over zealous inspectors have by their visits drawn public attention to the fact that a person is tuberculous and hence in the view of some persons highly dangerous." Bulstrode, "On Sanatoria," 586.

30. In "Changing Approaches" (109), Whyte recognizes that disinfection after tuberculosis required a more sensitive approach, but her research into local activities in northwest England suggests it was generally accepted by 1900.

31. "Prevention of Consumption," *Quarterly Medical Journal (Yorkshire and Adjacent Counties)* 8 (November 1899–August 1900): 143–49, quote on 146. This article, though published anonymously, was probably penned by John Robertson.

32. SLSL, 352.4 SQ, John Robertson, *Annual Report of the Medical Officer of Health for Sheffield, 1903,* 50; and Harold Scurfield, *Annual Report of the Medical Officer of Health for Sheffield, 1904,* 9–13.

33. Notification statistics confirmed the gender imbalance seen in the mortality data. In 1904, for example, there were 559 male cases and 279 females. In subsequent reports relatively little was made of the relationship between employment conditions and phthisis cases (although phthisis *mortality* by occupation remained a feature of the reports). See HCPP, C. 3496 (1907), XXXIV.1075, *Report of the Departmental Committee on Compensation for Industrial Diseases: Report; Minutes of Evidence, Appendices, and Index (Employers' Liability: Industrial Diseases Compensation), 1907,* 54–55.

34. SA, CA608 (19), *Sheffield Corporation Bill 1903, Correspondence, April 28, 1902 to December 5, 1902,* John Robertson to Henry Sayer, October 29, 1902.

35. As to compulsory notification, the agents informed the town clerk that "it should be well known that this is not allowed." SA, CA608 (85), *Sheffield Corporation Bill 1903: Compulsory Notification of Tuberculosis of the Lung, Correspondence* (hereafter cited as Sheffield *Correspondence*), Sayer to Robertson, February 20 and April 24, 1903.

36. SA, CA608 (6), *Report of the Local Government Board on the Sheffield Corporation Bill, 1903,* 6. As John Eyler notes, the LGB sent out a standard letter to local authorities seeking to add consumption to the list of notifiable diseases. Eyler, *Sir Arthur Newsholme,* 150.

37. SA, CA608 (6), *Report of the Local Government Board on the Sheffield Corporation Bill, 1903,* 5. The LGB did not object to voluntary notification, so long as the local authority paid a fee to the notifying practitioner.

38. Sheffield *Correspondence, April 28, 1902 to December 5, 1902,* Robertson to Sayer, April 16, 1903. This was a restatement of an opinion expressed in a report on tuberculosis four years earlier where Robertson argued "special" powers be formulated to differentiate tuberculosis from other infections. SA, CA/608 (73), John Robertson, *Special Report on the Prevalence of Tuberculosis and the Measures for Its Prevention,* May 11, 1899, 10.

39. Sayer to John Lithiby, Secretary of the Local Government Board, April 24, 1903; John Lithiby to Sayer, May 8, 1903; Sayer to Messrs Sherwood and Co., May 9, 1903; Sayer to Lithiby, May 11, 1903—all in Sheffield *Correspondence.*

40. Thomson was appointed in December 1887 in the midst of the smallpox epidemic in Sheffield that had prompted the Local Government Board to sponsor infectious disease notification legislation in the first place (see chapter 2). "Appointment

of Medical Officer of Health," *Sheffield and Rotherham Independent,* December 9, 1887. He took up his post in February 1888 and left in 1891 when he joined the medical department of the Local Government Board.

41. Sayer to Robertson, May 14 and May 16, 1903; Lithiby to Sayer, May 18, 1903—in Sheffield *Correspondence.*

42. SLSL, 352.4 SQ, John Robertson, *Annual Report of the Medical Officer of Health for Sheffield, 1903,* 49. It seems the committee members were under the impression that Hall was a medical officer of health. The promoters of the bill made it clear to the committee that he was not, but admitted Hall was "connected with the hospital." The statement that he was "in no way" associated with the city was, at best, misleading, especially since committee members were concerned that they had not heard any "independent" evidence. SA, CA608 (18), *Sheffield Corporation Bill 1903: Printed Minutes of Evidence to House of Commons Select Committee on the Sheffield Corporation Bill, Tuesday June 23rd, 1903* (hereafter cited as SCB *Evidence*), 46–47. Evidence given to this select committee was not printed routinely as a Parliamentary Paper, so it is fortunate that a copy is available in the Sheffield Archives.

43. On the very close links between Sheffield University's medical school and the city health department, see Sturdy, "Political Economy of Scientific Medicine," 131–32.

44. I say that Sheffield had a "strategy" for the hearings because the archives contain "proofs" of the evidence given by the corporation's three witnesses: Robertson, Hall, and Newsholme. It is unlikely that legal counsel did not at least vet these statements prior to the bill's hearing, if not coach the witnesses beforehand. SA, *Sheffield Corporation Bill 1903, Proof of Evidence*: CA608 (69), Dr. John Robertson; CA608 (70), Dr. Arthur Newsholme; and CA608 (71), Professor Arthur Hall.

45. SCB *Evidence,* Robertson, q. 176, Newsholme, q. 246.

46. Newsholme referred to the educational scheme he had developed in Brighton, which involved open-air sanatorium treatment. Admission was contingent on negotiations between the patient and Newsholme. The committee did not much pursue this potentially damaging evidence—damaging in that the scheme prevented the patient from working, even with the patient's agreement. The absence of a sanatorium in Sheffield may have helped here. Ibid., Hall, qq. 229–31, Newsholme, qq. 264–65. See also Eyler, *Sir Arthur Newsholme,* 154.

47. SLSL, 352.4 SQ, John Robertson, *Annual Report of the Medical Officer of Health for Sheffield, 1902,* 53. Obviously, the MOH annual report for 1902 was published late enough for the clause to be included in that year's report.

48. SCB *Evidence,* Robertson, q. 185.

49. Ibid., Robertson, q. 43; Hall, q. 212.

50. Ibid., Hall, q. 216.

51. Ibid., Robertson, q. 180.

52. SA, CA/608 (73), John Robertson, *Special Report on the Prevalence of Tuberculosis and the Measures for Its Prevention,* May 11, 1899, 10.

53. SCB *Evidence,* Hall, q. 219.

54. Ibid., Fitzgerald, q. 208.

55. Ibid., Thomson, qq. 200–204.

56. Ibid., Boyce, qq. 44–45.

57. Ibid., Thomson, q. 282.

58. HCPP, C. 5645 (1889), LXV.45, *Report on Epidemic of Smallpox at Sheffield, 1887–88, by Doctor Barry, with Introduction by Medical Officer of Local Government Board*, 8.

59. The smallpox epidemic in 1888 prompted the disinfection of 3,225 houses.

60. The trial period represented a precaution taken because no dissenting medical voices had been heard and opposition might be mobilized in the future. The clauses were renewed in 1910 for a further ten years, along with those that had been granted for Bolton, Burnley, and Oldham. HCPP, C. 159 (1910), III.123, *Bolton, Burnley, Oldham, and Sheffield (Local Government: Provisional Orders Confirmation)*.

61. SLSL, 352.4 SQ, Harold Scurfield, *Annual Report of the Medical Officer of Health for Sheffield, 1904*, 17.

62. Ibid., *1910*, xi. The data blew out of the water any theory about the positive relationship between alcohol consumption and tuberculosis, since the male patients tended to drink more heavily than females. Domestic overcrowding meant that patients who had a bedroom and a bed to themselves were in the minority. Indeed, over two-thirds of sufferers shared their bed.

63. Gorsky, "Friendly Society Health Insurance."

64. SLSL, 352.4 SQ, Harold Scurfield, *Annual Report of the Medical Officer of Health for Sheffield, 1910*, xi.

65. Worboys, "Sanatorium Treatment," 53–54, 56–60, 64–65. These numbers are approximate rather than definitive, but they doubtless provide a reasonable indication of the level of provision and are probably a more accurate reflection than the available official figures.

66. Leslie, "State Insurance"; Howarth, "Sanatorium Benefit"; Thomson, "Insurance and Sanatorium Benefits"; Davies and Fitzgerald, "National Insurance"; Pearson, "Observations."

67. Hennock, *Origin of the Welfare State*, 265. For more on National Insurance and tuberculosis, see Bryder, *Below the Magic Mountain*, 36–41. For National Insurance more generally, see Digby, "Economic and Medical Significance" and *Making a Medical Living*, chap. 12.

68. "Paddington Dispensary for Tuberculosis: Some General Reflections," *Lancet* 175 (March 26, 1910): 867–68; Williamson, "Future."

69. Hennock, *Origin of the Welfare State*, 264–65.

70. Holden, "Danger" and "Domiciliary Treatment of Tuberculosis."

71. Cameron, "Home Treatment versus Sanatorium."

72. Jessel, "Bedroom of the Consumptive" and "Dispensary Supervision in Pulmonary Tuberculosis." For a counterargument see Wynne, "Dispensary Supervision in Pulmonary Tuberculosis."

73. Dixon, "Domiciliary Treatment"; Shrubsall, "Selection of Patients"; Clark, "Organisation of Scientific Methods." For a spectrum of opinion across the early decades of the twentieth century, see "Discussion on the Consumptive at the Home," *Journal of the Royal Sanitary Institute* 27, no. 6 (1906): 277–89; and "Care of the Advanced Consumptive," *British Journal of Tuberculosis* 13, no. 2 (April 1919): 49–71. Any sort of reliable comparison of dispensary/home versus sanatorium treatment only began to appear in the 1920s. See Lissant Cox, "Sanatorium Treatment Contrasted."

74. Condrau, "Urban Tuberculosis Patients."

75. It is important to recognize the contingent meaning of terms such as cured, healed, improved, or relieved in almost any historical context relating to institutions providing health care, but for sanatoria in particular. Ibid., 189–90, 200, 205. Graduated labor was a feature of the British model of sanatorium treatment, whereas in Germany prolonged periods of rest were emphasized.

76. Chowry-Muthu, "Sanatorium Treatment of Consumption"; Bryder, *Below the Magic Mountain*, 41–43; Condrau, "Urban Tuberculosis Patients," 190.

77. Worboys, "Sanatorium Treatment," 58–59. Many pertinent examples of campaigns centered on motherhood and physical degeneration can be found in Pennybacker, *Vision for London, 1889–1914*, 315.

78. Condrau, "Urban Tuberculosis Patients," 204–5.

79. Craddock, "Engendered/Endangered," 340; Craddock, *City of Plagues*.

80. The control of dairies and meat supply is beyond the scope of this chapter. For a summary of the various positions taken on tuberculosis control, see Worboys, "Before McKeown."

81. Oldham's campaign was funded by the local state. Manchester's was underwritten by the MSSA. Niven, "On Municipal Administrative Measures"; Ransome, *Campaign against Consumption*, 53. The gendered rhetoric of these educational materials tends to be implicit (at least compared to the explicitly gendered discourses of materialism and physical degeneration).

82. Kearns, "Tuberculosis."

83. Niven, *Observations*, 98.

84. Rosenberg, "Health in the Home."

85. Some journal articles on home treatment appeared in the National Association for the Prevention of Consumption's short-lived journal *Tuberculosis*. These were directed mainly at officials responsible for advising patients: Paterson and Shrubsall, "Hints for the Consumptive" and "Home Treatment"; Cummins, "Notes on the Difficulties."

86. Although each of these manuals went through multiple editions, it is beyond the scope of this chapter to analyze in any detail the differences between the editions. On questions about the value of domiciliary treatment, see Thomson, "Problem of Tuberculosis."

87. Crowe, *Consumption*, 3. As Kenwood and Taylor noted in 1903, "We are running a little wild on the subject of sanatoria." Kenwood and Taylor, "Two Years' Experience." Crowe founded the Charterhouse Rheumatism Clinic in London in 1928 and eventually was invited to join the Empire Rheumatism Council. See Cantor, "Aches of Industry," 230.

88. Bardswell, *Advice to Consumptives*, 144. Bardswell was medical superintendent of the King Edward VII Sanatorium in Sussex.

89. Cummins, "Notes on the Difficulties," 190.

90. Thomson, *Consumption*, 75. When the first edition was published in 1911, Thomson was medical superintendent of the Liverpool Sanatorium at Frodsham. By the third edition in 1928 (when the title of his book changed from *Consumption* to *Tuberculosis*), he had acquired a diploma in Public Health from Liverpool University and had moved on to become county medical officer of health, school medical officer of health, and tuberculosis officer for Hertfordshire. He was a prolific writer of books on tuberculosis.

91. Ibid., 7, 13, 28.

92. Crowe included an appendix on breathing exercises to ensure the undamaged part of the lungs were put to good use. Crowe, *Consumption*, 31–32.

93. Ibid., 30.

94. Thomson, *Consumption*, 56.

95. On the contested popularization of thermometry, see Hess, "Standardizing Body Temperature"; and Musher, Dominguez, and Bar-Sela, "Edouard Seguin."

96. Bardswell, *Advice to Consumptives*, 63–64.

97. Holton, "Through One's Own Powers," 86. On other aspects of the sanatorium experience from the patient's point of view, see Bryder, *Below the Magic Mountain*, chap. 7.

98. Crowe, *Consumption*, 17; Thomson, *Consumption*, 39–42.

99. Bardswell, *Advice to Consumptives*, 63.

100. Thomson, *Consumption*, 44–45.

101. Crowe, *Consumption*, 24.

102. In the 1906 edition of Crowe's *Consumption* available in the Historical Collection of the Johns Hopkins Welch Medical Library, two of these unmarked blank charts were tucked inside the back cover of the book.

103. Hess and Mendelsohn, "Case and Series," 300. On documentary technologies in medicine, see Jacyna, "Medicine in Transformation, 1800–1849."

104. Crowe, *Consumption*, 6; Thomson, *Consumption*, 29.

105. Thomson, *Consumption*, 68.

106. Crowe, *Consumption*, 4.

107. This was the price of the first edition of *Consumption* in 1906. Bardswell's book cost 1s. 6d.; Thomson's, 2s.

108. Paterson and Shrubsall, "Home Treatment," 184.

109. Bardswell, *Advice to Consumptives*, 140.

110. Ibid., 74.

111. Thomson, *Consumption*, 28, 30, 31.

112. Bardswell, *Advice to Consumptives*, 140. In *Below the Magic Mountain* (223), Bryder relates how an ex-patient of Bardswell's complained that the opening of windows excited so much prejudice among neighbors to the extent that the patient had changed accommodations four times in the same town.

113. Crowe, *Consumption*, 7.

114. Thomson, *Consumption*, 11. Occupational stress and overwork were warned against, but the improbability of one's being able to change jobs to alleviate this was recognized.

115. Ibid., 12. Bacteriological discoveries about the presence of tubercle bacilli in dried sputum propelled the significance of dust and the push for ventilated premises to new heights. See Tomes, *Gospel of Germs*.

116. Crowe, *Consumption*, 13.

117. Thomson, *Consumption*, 46.

118. Holton, "Through One's Own Powers," 86.

119. Patients lucky enough to have a garden were encouraged to build a shelter. Thomson, *Consumption*, 37. Some councils and sanatoria lent out a shelter to patients when they had been discharged from the sanatorium. Bryder, *Below the Magic Mountain*, 224–26.

120. According to Newsholme, this was especially true for poor patients. Newsholme, "Four and a Half Years' Experience," 254–55. Postdischarge lapses were common, and public health officers bemoaned how consumptives failed to comply with their verbal and printed instructions.

121. Crowe, *Consumption*, 4.

122. Thomson, *Consumption*, 23.

123. Ibid., 55.

124. Ibid., 26.

125. Hunt, *Governing Morals*, 157.

126. Bardswell, *Advice to Consumptives*, 136.

127. "Amusements for Tuberculosis Patients," *British Journal of Tuberculosis* 1, no. 1 (January 1907): 100.

128. Ibid. The mass production of plasticine began at a factory in Birmingham in 1900. On plasticine see Harbutt, *Harbutt's Plastic Method*.

129. Cohen, *Household Gods*, xii. It was a contradiction that such expressions of individuality were purchased at the cost of conforming to notions and standards of taste shaped outside domestic space. Forty, *Objects of Desire*, 94; see also Edwards, *Turning Houses into Homes*, 148–49.

130. It is worth stressing at this point that well into the twentieth century the nurturing of moral character remained a fundamental aspect of tuberculosis treatment.

131. Bartrip, *Mirror of Medicine*.

132. Nevett, "Advertising and Editorial Integrity," 154–59.

133. "Preparations and Appliances," *British Journal of Tuberculosis* 1, no. 1 (January 1907): 92–101.

134. "Foot-Rests," *British Journal of Tuberculosis* 6, no. 1 (January 1912): 63–64.

135. "Preparations and Appliances," *British Journal of Tuberculosis* 1, no. 1 (January 1907): 92–101; "Sanitary Scraper and Mat," *British Journal of Tuberculosis* 3, no. 1 (January 1909): 75. *Baby's World* was founded in 1910 and rejected advertisements when the products did not live up to the claims made for them. See Gurjeva, "Child Health," 108.

136. Some people also used networks of mail-order agents, partly because their origins lay in the culture of working-class savings clubs. See Coopey and Porter, "Agency Mail Order in Britain," and Coopey, O'Connell, and Porter, *Mail Order Retailing in Britain*, esp. 13–38. On furnishing the home through mail order, see Edwards, *Turning Houses into Homes*, 170.

137. Daunton, *Royal Mail*, 57–64; Perry, *Victorian Post Office*, 226–27.

138. Coopey and Porter, "Agency Mail Order in Britain."

139. Benson, *Rise of Consumer Society*, 23–26.

140. Cohen, *Household Gods*, 30; see also Davidoff and Hall, *Family Fortunes*; and Logan, *Victorian Parlour*.

141. Edwards, *Turning Houses into Homes*, 152–54.

142. Adapting terms from Breward, *Hidden Consumer*, 160; and Ugolini, "Men, Masculinities, and Menswear Advertising," 81.

143. This phrase is borrowed from Cronin, "Rags and Refuse," 583.

144. The image accompanying the Presto image showed a 16°C scale. "Saranac Thermometer," *British Journal of Tuberculosis* 12, no. 2 (April 1918): 93–94.

145. "Bed-Screen and Shelter," *British Journal of Tuberculosis* 3, no. 1 (January 1909): 75–76. The screen was priced at 8s. 6d.

146. "New Form of Bath," *British Journal of Tuberculosis* 3, no. 1 (January 1909): 72–73.

147. "Portable Douche," *British Journal of Tuberculosis* 6, no. 3 (July 1912): 195–96.

148. The Perfection Sprayer was made by Newton, Chambers and Co., which already manufactured Izal and Izal hygienic and sanitary preparations. "Sprayer for Disinfectants," *British Journal of Tuberculosis* 3, no. 3 (July 1909): 220. The sprayer was relatively affordable. The three models cost 4s., 4s. 9d., and 7s. 6d. For examples of the hygienic movement in the United States, see Tomes, *Gospel of Germs.*

149. "Requisites for the Sanatorium and the Hygienic Home," *British Journal of Tuberculosis* 4, no. 1 (January 1910): 60–61; "Hot Air Boot-Dryer," *British Journal of Tuberculosis* 4, no. 2 (April 1910): 138–39.

150. "'Boreas' Sweeper," *British Journal of Tuberculosis* 3, no. 2 (April 1909): 150–51. The sweeper cost 39s. 6d.

151. "Kumfee," *British Journal of Tuberculosis* 4, no. 3 (July 1910): 211. The Kumfee retailed at 25s.

152. "Dumbnurse," *British Journal of Tuberculosis* 6, no. 3 (July 1912): 191–92. The Dumbnurse was priced at 15s.

153. *British Journal of Tuberculosis,* July 1918, 140.

154. *British Journal of Tuberculosis,* July 1920, 136–38.

155. White and Hunt, "Citizenship," 105.

156. "Appliances for the Patient," *British Journal of Tuberculosis* 4, no. 1 (January 1910): 57–60.

157. In his "Discussion on the Relation of Phthisis to Factory and Workshop Conditions," James Niven was one of the first to suggest that the common practice of spitting on the floors of public houses made them dangerous places for people's health.

158. Thomson, *Consumption,* 13.

## Conclusion

1. The "family" Mackenzie had in mind was resolutely nuclear, in which resided a powerful transformative dynamic: "Broadly, if there is no child, there is no family. . . . So long as there is a father, a mother and a child, so long will there be a family capable of creating a new society." Mackenzie, "The Family and the City," 119.

2. Ibid., 124.

3. Ibid., 129.

4. Ibid., 126–27.

5. Ibid., 129.

6. Beier, *For Their Own Good.* On tracheotomy see Hardy, "Tracheotomy versus Intubation."

7. Beier, *For Their Own Good*; Pooley, "All We Parents Want."

8. Mackenzie, "The Family and the City," 132.

9. Ibid., 134.

10. Ibid., 138.

11. Mackenzie, "Administrative Control," 164.

# *Bibliography*

## Archival Sources

Birmingham, City of, Archives and Heritage
British Medical Association Archives
Leicester Medical Society
Leicestershire, Leicester and Rutland Record Office
Liverpool, City of, Archives and Local History, Liverpool Central Library
Liverpool Medical Institution
London Metropolitan Archives
Manchester, City of, Archives and Local History, Manchester Central Library
Manchester, University of, Medical Collection, John Rylands Library
Nottinghamshire Archives
Parliament, Great Britain
- Hansard's Parliamentary Debates
- House of Commons Parliamentary Papers
- Parliamentary Archives, Records of the House of Commons: Private Bill Office

Sheffield, City of, Archives, Sheffield Local Studies Library

## Published Sources


Aaby, Peter, Coovadia Hooson, Jetta Bukh, Ida Maria Lisse, Arjon J. Smits, Anne Wesley, and Photini Kiepiela. "Severe Measles: A Reappraisal of the Role of Nutrition, Overcrowding and Virus Dose." *Medical Hypotheses* 18 (1985): 93–112.

Abramovitz, Mimi. *Regulating the Lives of Women: Social Welfare Policy from Colonial Times to the Present.* Boston: South End Press, 1988.

Adams, Annmarie. *Architecture in the Family Way: Doctors, Houses, and Women, 1870–1900.* Montreal: McGill-Queen's University Press, 1996.

Aidt, Toke S., Martin Daunton, and Jayasri Dutta. "The Retrenchment Hypothesis and the Extension of the Franchise in England and Wales." *Economic Journal,* no. 120 (2010): 990–1020.

Aisenberg, Andrew R. *Contagion: Disease, Government, and the "Social Question" in Nineteenth-Century France.* Stanford, CA: Stanford University Press, 1999.

Alborn, Timothy L. "A Calculating Profession: Victorian Actuaries among the Statisticians." *Science in Context* 7, no. 3 (1994): 433–68.

———. *Regulated Lives: Life Insurance and British Society, 1800–1914.* Toronto: University of Toronto Press, 2009.

Aldwinckle, Thomas W. "Disinfecting Apparatus." *Public Health* 10 (October 1897–September 1898): 93–97.

———. "Isolation in Fever Hospitals." *Journal of the Royal Sanitary Institute* 27, no. 9 (September 1906): 502–9.

Ali, S. Harris, and Roger Keil. "Public Health and the Political Economy of Scale: Implications for Understanding the Response to the 2003 Severe Acute Respiratory Syndrome (SARS) Outbreak in Toronto." In *Leviathan Undone? Towards a Political Economy of Scale*, edited by Roger Keil and Rianne Mahon, 195–208. Vancouver: UBC Press, 2009.

Allan, Francis J. "The Early Days and the Early Work of the Society, with Special Reference to the Registration of Disease." *Public Health* 13 (October 1900–September 1901): 71–86.

Allen, John. *Lost Geographies of Power.* RGS-IBG Book Series 79. Oxford: John Wiley and Sons, 2011.

Anderson, A. Jasper. "The Notification of Measles." *Public Health* 5 (October 1892–September 1893): 207–10.

———. "The Notification of Measles and Whooping Cough." *Public Health* 9 (October 1896–September 1897): 155–58.

Anderson, Amanda. *The Powers of Distance: Cosmopolitanism and the Cultivation of Detachment.* Princeton, NJ: Princeton University Press, 2001.

Anderson, William K. *Fever Hospital: A History of Fairfield Infectious Disease Hospital.* Melbourne: Melbourne University Press, 2002.

Armstrong, David. "Medical Surveillance of Normal Populations." In *Technologies of Modern Medicine: Proceedings of a Seminar Held at the Science Museum, London, March 1993*, edited by Ghislaine Lawrence, 73–87. London: Science Museum, 1994.

———. "Public Health Spaces and the Fabrication of Identity." *Sociology* 27, no. 3 (1993): 393–410.

———. "The Rise of Surveillance Medicine." *Sociology of Health and Illness* 17 (1995): 393–404.

Armstrong, H. E. "Compulsory Notification of Measles and Whooping Cough: Experience at Newcastle-upon-Tyne." *Public Health* 11 (October 1898–September 1899): 206–10.

———. "Diphtheria, Its Extent and Fatality in the Large Provincial Towns of England and Wales, and in the Hospitals of the Metropolitan Asylums Board, during the Years 1894–1904 Inclusive, in Relation to the Use of Antitoxic Serum in the Treatment of the Disease." *Public Health* 18 (October 1905–September 1906): 227–32.

———. "The Notification of Measles." *Public Health* 4 (October 1891–September 1892): 261–62.

Asherson, Geoffrey L. "Ransom, William Henry (1823–1907)." In *Oxford Dictionary of National Biography.* http://www.oxforddnb.com/view/article/35672.

Ayers, Gwendoline. *England's First State Hospitals: The Metropolitan Asylums Board.* London: Wellcome, 1971.

Bachelard, Gaston. *The Poetics of Space.* With a new foreword by John R. Stilgoe. Boston: Beacon Press, 1994.

Bailin, Miriam. *The Sickroom in Victorian Fiction: The Art of Being Ill.* Cambridge: Cambridge University Press, 1994.

Baldwin, Peter. *Contagion and the State in Europe, 1830–1930.* Cambridge: Cambridge University Press, 1999.

———. "The Victorian State in Comparative Perspective." In *Liberty and Authority in Victorian Britain,* edited by Peter Mandler, 51–70. Oxford: Oxford University Press, 2006.

Ballard, Edward. *Results of an Analysis of Records of Sickness Kept in Islington during the 12 Years 1857 to 1868 Inclusive.* London: HMSO, 1869.

Bannington, Bertram George. *English Public Health Administration.* London: P. S. King & Son, Ltd., 1915.

Bardswell, Noel Dean. *Advice to Consumptives: Home Treatment, After-Care and Prevention.* London: A. & C. Black, 1910.

Barker, T. H. "On Deodorisation and Disinfection." *British Medical Journal* 262 (January 6, 1866): 1–16.

Barnes, David S. *The Great Stink of Paris and the Nineteenth-Century Struggle against Filth and Germs.* Baltimore: Johns Hopkins University Press, 2006.

Barrow, Logie. "Victorian 'Pest-Houses' amid London's March of Bricks and Mortar." *Recherches Anglaises et Américaines* 36, no. 3 (2003): 127–37.

Bartrip, Peter W. J. *Mirror of Medicine: A History of the British Medical Journal.* Oxford: British Medical Journal and Clarendon Press, 1990.

———. *Themselves Writ Large: The British Medical Association 1832–1966.* London: British Medical Journal, 1996.

———. "Thomson, Anthony Todd (1778–1849)." In *Oxford Dictionary of National Biography.* http://www.oxforddnb.com/view/article/27293.

Barwise, Sidney. "Disinfection by Steam." *Public Health* 8 (October 1895–September 1896): 196–98.

Bashford, Alison. *Purity and Pollution: Gender, Embodiment and Victorian Medicine.* Basingstoke, UK: Macmillan, 1998.

Bashford, Alison, and Carolyn Strange. "Isolation and Exclusion in the Modern World: An Introductory Essay." In *Isolation: Places and Practices of Exclusion,* edited by Carolyn Strange and Alison Bashford, 1–19. London: Routledge, 2003.

Bayer, Ronald, and Amy L. Fairchild. "Public Health: Surveillance and Privacy." *Science* 290, no. 5498 (2000): 1898–99.

Beach, Abigail. "Potential for Participation: Health Centres and the Idea of Citizenship c. 1920–1940." In *Regenerating England,* edited by Christopher Lawrence and Anna-K. Mayer, 203–30. Clio Medica/The Wellcome Series in the History of Medicine. Amsterdam: Rodopi, 2000.

Beale Collins, H. "Isolation Hospitals." *Public Health* 21 (March–September 1908): 83–84.

Beckingham, David. "An Historical Geography of Liberty: Lancashire and the Inebriates Acts." *Journal of Historical Geography* 36, no. 4 (2010): 388–401.

Behlmer, George K. *Friends of the Family: The English Home and Its Guardians, 1850–1940.* Stanford, CA: Stanford University Press, 1998.

Beier, Lucinda McCray. *For Their Own Good: The Transformation of English Working-Class Health Culture, 1880–1970.* Columbus: Ohio State University Press, 2008.

Bell Taylor, Charles. "Notification of Infectious Diseases." *Nottingham Journal*, May 16, 1883.

Bellamy, Christine. *Administering Central-Local Relations, 1871–1919: The Local Government Board in Its Fiscal and Cultural Context.* Manchester: Manchester University Press, 1988.

Bellamy, Richard. *Liberalism and Modern Society: An Historical Argument.* Cambridge: Polity Press, 1992.

———. *Victorian Liberalism: Nineteenth-Century Political Thought and Practice.* London: Routledge, 1990.

Benson, John. *The Rise of Consumer Society in Britain, 1880–1980.* London: Longman, 1994.

Biagini, Eugenio F., ed. *Citizenship and Community: Liberals, Radicals, and Collective Identities in the British Isles, 1865–1931.* Cambridge: Cambridge University Press, 1996.

———. "Liberalism and Direct Democracy: John Stuart Mill and the Model of Ancient Athens." In Biagini, *Citizenship and Community*, 21–44.

———. *Liberty, Retrenchment, and Reform: Popular Liberalism in the Age of Gladstone, 1860–1880.* Cambridge: Cambridge University Press, 1992.

Biagini, Eugenio F., and Alastair J. Reid, eds. *Currents of Radicalism: Popular Radicalism, Organised Labour, and Party Politics in Britain, 1850–1914.* Cambridge: Cambridge University Press, 1991.

Biddle, Daniel. "Dual Notification and the Death Rate." *British Medical Journal* 1745 (June 9, 1894): 1276–77.

———. "Notification of Infectious Disease." *Times*, August 28, 1889.

———. "Notification of Infectious Diseases." *Lancet* 131 (June 23, 1888): 1269–70.

———. "School Attendance and Diphtheria." *Lancet* 144 (October 20, 1894): 942.

Biernacki, Richard, and Jennifer Jordan. "The Place of Space in the Study of the Social." In *The Social in Question: New Bearings in History and the Social Sciences*, edited by Patrick Joyce, 133–50. London: Routledge, 2002.

Bond, Francis T. "The Importance of Complete Disinfection, and the Best Means of Providing for It by Sanitary Authorities." *Transactions of the National Association for the Promotion of Social Science, 1878* (1879): 457–67.

———. "On the Conditions of Efficient Disinfection, and on Some New Forms of Disinfectant." *British Medical Journal* 738 (February 20, 1875): 239–41.

Boyd, John. "School Notification of Infectious Disease." *Public Health* 16 (October 1903–September 1904): 94–98.

Brand, Jeanne L. *Doctors and the State: The British Medical Profession and Government Action in Public Health, 1870–1912.* Baltimore: Johns Hopkins Press, 1965.

Breward, Christopher. *The Hidden Consumer: Masculinities, Fashion and City Life 1860–1914.* Manchester: Manchester University Press, 1999.

Brinckman, Arthur. *Notes on the Care of the Sick and Practical Advice to Those in Charge of the Dying and the Dead.* London: G. J. Palmer, 1879.

Bristow, Edward. "The Liberty and Property Defence League and Individualism." *Historical Journal* 18, no. 4 (1975): 761–89.

Brock, Thomas D. *Robert Koch, a Life in Medicine and Bacteriology.* Madison, WI: Science Tech Publishers, 1988.

Brunton, Deborah. *The Politics of Vaccination: Practice and Policy in England, Wales, Ireland, and Scotland, 1800–1874.* Rochester, NY: University of Rochester Press, 2008.

Bryden, Inga, and Janet Floyd, eds. *Domestic Space: Reading the Nineteenth-Century Interior.* Manchester: Manchester University Press, 1999.

———. "Introduction." In Bryden and Floyd, *Domestic Space,* 1–17.

Bryder, Linda. *Below the Magic Mountain: A Social History of Tuberculosis in Twentieth-Century Britain.* Oxford: Oxford University Press, 1988.

———. "'Wonderlands of Buttercup, Clover, and Daisies': Tuberculosis and the Open-Air School Movement in Britain, 1907–39." In *In the Name of the Child: Health and Welfare, 1880–1940,* edited by Roger Cooter, 72–95. London: Routledge, 1992.

Buchanan, George. "Citizenship in Sanitary Work." *Practitioner* 17 (1876): 384–400.

———. "Sanitary Work." *Times,* October 24, 1876.

Bullin, F., F. Hutchinson, and Edward Digby. "The Memorial of the Medical Officers of the City of London Unions." *Lancet* 52 (1848): 615–16.

Bulstrode, H. Timbrell. "The State Section of the Congress." *Tuberculosis* 1, no. 9 (October 1901): 406–13.

Butler, Josephine E. "A Vigilance Committee." In *Josephine Butler and the Prostitution Campaigns: Diseases of the Body Politic.* Vol. 3, *The Constitution Violated: The Parliamentary Campaign,* edited by Jane Jordan and Ingrid Sharp, 123–28. London: Routledge, 2003.

Bynum, William F. "Hospital, Disease and Community: The London Fever Hospital, 1801–1850." In *Healing and History: Essays for George Rosen,* edited by Charles E. Rosenberg, 97–115. Dawson, NY: Science History Publications, 1979.

Cadnam, Louisa. "How (Not) to Be Governed: Foucault, Critique, and the Political." *Environment and Planning D: Society and Space* 28, no. 3 (2010): 539–56.

Caldwell Smith, P. "A Discussion on Isolation and Disinfection: With Special Reference to the Control of Epidemics." *British Medical Journal* 1496 (August 31, 1889): 455–56.

Cameron, Charles A. "Disinfection." *Dublin Journal of Medical Science* 98, no. 6 (1894): 520–38.

Cameron, Donald L. "Home Treatment versus Sanatorium: From the Consumptive Patient's Point of View." *British Journal of Tuberculosis* 7, no. 2 (April 1913): 99–101.

Cameron, J. S. "On the Importance of Isolating Slight and Doubtful Cases of Scarlet Fever." *Lancet* 124 (June 9, 1884): 400–401.

Cantor, David. "The Aches of Industry: Philanthropy and Rheumatism in Inter-War Britain." In *Medicine and Charity before the Welfare State,* edited by Jonathan Barry and Colin Jones, 225–45. London: Routledge, 1991.

Carpenter, Alfred. "An Address on Domestic Health." *British Medical Journal* 1095 (December 24, 1881): 1007–9.

———. "The Right of the State to Enforce Notification and the Best Method of Doing It." *Sanitary Record,* n.s., 6 (1884): 50.

Carter, William. "Is the Compulsory Notification of Infectious Disease by Medical Men Practically Useful?" *British Medical Journal* 1133 (September 16, 1882): 507–13.

———. "Notification of Infectious Diseases." *British Medical Journal* 1105 (March 4, 1882): 318.

———. "Some Results of Recent Sanitary Legislation, with Suggestions as to Its Safe Extension." *Proceedings of the Literary and Philosophical Society of Liverpool* 41 (1886–87): 1–37.

Cassedy, James H. "Hygeia: A Mid-Victorian Dream of a City of Health." *Journal of the History of Medicine and Allied Sciences* 17, no. 2 (1962): 217–28.

Chaddock, Robert E. "Voluntary Social Services in London Schools." *Social Forces* 11, no. 3 (March 1933): 342–47.

Charlton, Christopher. "The Fight against Vaccination: The Leicester Demonstration of 1885." *Local Population Studies* 30 (1983): 60–66.

Chase, Karen, and Michael H. Levenson. *The Spectacle of Intimacy: A Public Life for the Victorian Family.* Princeton, NJ: Princeton University Press, 2000.

Châtelet, Anne-Marie. "A Breath of Fresh Air: Open-Air Schools in Europe." In *History, Space, and the Material Culture of Children,* edited by Marta Gutman and Ning de Coninck-Smith, 107–27. New Brunswick, NJ: Rutgers University Press, 2008.

Chowry-Muthu, D. J. "The Sanatorium Treatment of Consumption: Is It Worthwhile?" *British Medical Journal* 2322 (July 1, 1905): 46.

Clark, Hilda. "The Organisation of Scientific Methods for the Control of Tuberculosis." *Public Health* 26 (October 1912–September 1913): 332–37.

Clarke, John. "Programmatic Statements and Dull Empiricism." *Journal of Cultural Economy* 2, no. 1–2 (2009): 227–31.

Cleere, Eileen. "Victorian Dust Traps." In *Filth: Dirt, Disgust, and Modern Life,* edited by William A. Cohen and Ryan Johnson, 133–54. Minneapolis: University of Minnesota Press, 2005.

Clor, Harry M. "Mill and Millians on Liberty and Moral Character." *Review of Politics* 47, no. 1 (January 1985): 3–26.

Cohen, Deborah. *Household Gods: The British and Their Possessions.* New Haven, CT: Yale University Press, 2006.

Coleman, William. *Yellow Fever in the North: The Methods of Early Epidemiology.* Madison: University of Wisconsin Press, 1987.

Collini, Stefan. "The Idea of 'Character' in Victorian Political Thought." *Transactions of the Royal Historical Society* 35 (1985): 29–50.

———. "Liberalism and the Legacy of Mill." *Historical Journal* 20, no. 1 (1977): 237–54.

———. *Public Moralists: Political Thought and Intellectual Life in Britain, 1850–1930.* Oxford: Clarendon Press, 1991.

Condrau, Flurin. "Urban Tuberculosis Patients and Sanatorium Treatment in the Early Twentieth Century." In *Medicine, Charity and Mutual Aid: The Consumption of Health and Welfare in Britain, c. 1550–1950,* edited by Anne Borsay and Peter Shapely, 183–205. Aldershot, UK: Ashgate, 2007.

Coopey, Richard, Sean O'Connell, and Dilwyn Porter. *Mail Order Retailing in Britain: A Business and Social History.* Oxford: Oxford University Press, 2005.

Coopey, Richard, and Dilwyn Porter. "Agency Mail Order in Britain, c. 1900–2000: Spare-Time Agents and Their Customers." In *A Nation of Shopkeepers: Five Centuries of British Retailing,* edited by John Benson and Laura Ugolini, 226–48. London: I. B. Tauris, 2003.

Corbin, Alain. *The Foul and the Fragrant: Odor and the French Social Imagination.* Cambridge, MA: Harvard University Press, 1986.

Corrigan, Philip, and Derek Sayer. *The Great Arch: English State Formation as Cultural Revolution.* Oxford: Blackwell, 1985.

Cox, Pamela. "Compulsion, Voluntarism, and Venereal Disease: Governing Sexual Health in England after the Contagious Diseases Acts." *Journal of British Studies* 46, no. 1 (2007): 91–115.

Crace-Calvert, F. "Action of Heat on Protoplasmic Life." *Proceedings of the Royal Society of London* 19 (1870–71): 472–76.

Craddock, Susan. *City of Plagues: Disease, Poverty and Deviance in San Francisco.* Minneapolis: University of Minnesota Press, 2000.

———. "Engendered/Endangered: Women, Tuberculosis, and the Project of Citizenship." *Journal of Historical Geography* 27, no. 3 (2001): 338–54.

Crawford, E. Margaret. *Counting the People: A Survey of the Irish Censuses, 1813–1911.* Dublin: Four Courts, 2003.

Cronin, Anne M. "Rags and Refuse: The Newspaper, Empire, and Nineteenth Century Commodity Culture." *Cultural Studies* 20, no. 6 (2006): 574–98.

Crook, Tom. "Accommodating the Outcast: Common Lodging Houses and the Limits of Urban Governance in Victorian and Edwardian London." *Urban History* 35, no. 03 (2008): 414–36.

———. "Putting Matter in Its Right Place: Dirt, Time and Regeneration in Mid-Victorian Britain." *Journal of Victorian Culture* 13, no. 2 (2008): 200–222.

———. "Sanitary Inspection and the Public Sphere in Late Victorian and Edwardian Britain: A Case Study in Liberal Governance." *Social History* 32, no. 4 (2007): 369–93.

Crookshank, F. G. "An Address on the Control of Scarlet Fever." *Lancet* 175 (February 19, 1910): 477–80.

Crookshank, Harry. *Manual of Home Nursing and Hygiene: Including First Aid to Be Rendered in Cases of Accidents and Emergencies.* London: W. Whiteley, 1881.

Crowe, Henry Warren. *Consumption: Treatment at Home and Rules for Living.* Bristol, UK: John Wright & Sons; London: Simpkin, Marshall, Hamilton, Kent & Co., 1906.

Crowley, Ralph H. *The Needs, Objects, and Method of the Medical Inspection of Primary Schools.* London: J. & A. Churchill, 1907.

Crowther, M. A. *The Workhouse System, 1834–1929: The History of an English Social Institution.* Athens: University of Georgia Press, 1982.

Cummins, Miss C. E. "Notes on the Difficulties to Be Encountered in the Home Care of Phthisical Out-Patients." *Tuberculosis* 4, no. 4 (1907): 189–94.

Cunningham Glen, William. *The Law Relating to Public Health and Local Government: Including the Law Relating to the Removal of Nuisances Injurious to Health, the Prevention of Diseases, and Sewer Authorities, with Statutes and Cases.* 6th ed. London: Butterworths; Knight and Co., 1873.

Currie, Margaret R. *Fever Hospitals and Fever Nurses: A British Social History of Fever Nursing: A National Service.* London: Routledge, 2005.

Curtis, Bruce. "Surveying the Social: Techniques, Practices, Power." *Histoire Sociale* 35, no. 69 (2002): 83–108.

Daston, Lorraine J., ed. *Biographies of Scientific Objects.* Chicago: University of Chicago Press, 2000.

Daunton, Martin J. *House and Home in the Victorian City: Working Class Housing, 1850–1914.* Studies in Urban History. Vol. 7. London; Baltimore: E. Arnold, 1983.

———. "Public Place and Private Space: The Victorian City and the Working-Class Household." In *The Pursuit of Urban History,* edited by Derek Fraser and Anthony Sutcliffe, 212–233. London: E. Arnold, 1983.

———. *Royal Mail: The Post Office since 1840.* London: Athlone Press, 1985.

Davidoff, Leonore, Megan Doolittle, Janet Fink, and Katherine Holden. *The Family Story: Blood, Contract, and Intimacy, 1830–1960.* London: Longman, 1999.

Davidoff, Leonore, and Catherine Hall. *Family Fortunes: Men and Women of the English Middle Class, 1780–1850.* London: Hutchinson, 1987.

Davies, Sidney, and Marion Fitzgerald. "National Insurance and the Home Treatment of Consumptives." *British Journal of Tuberculosis* 6, no. 2 (April 1912): 93–102.

Davin, Anna. "Child Labour, the Working-Class Family, and Domestic Ideology in 19th Century Britain." *Development and Change* 13, no. 4 (1982): 633–52.

Davis, John, and Duncan Tanner. "The Borough Franchise after 1867." *Historical Research* 69, no. 170 (1996): 306–27.

Dean, Mitchell. "Liberal Government and Authoritarianism." *Economy and Society* 21, no. 1 (2002): 37–61.

———. "'A Social Structure of Many Souls': Moral Regulation, Government, and Self-Formation." *Canadian Journal of Sociology* 19, no. 2 (1994): 145–68.

De Chaumont, F. "Report on the Effects of High Temperatures upon Woollen and Other Fabrics." *Lancet* 106 (December 11, 1875): 830–31.

Defries, Wolf. "Disinfection of Rooms." *Public Health* 7 (October 1894–September 1895): 335–37.

De Haan, Ido. "Vigorous, Pure and Vulnerable: Child Health and Citizenship in the Netherlands since the End of the Nineteenth Century." In *Cultures of Child Health in Britain and the Netherlands in the Twentieth Century,* edited by Marijke Gijswijt-Hofstra and Hilary Marland, 31–60. Clio Medica/The Wellcome Series in the History of Medicine. Amsterdam: Rodopi, 2003.

Delépine, A. Sheridan. "Some Experiments on the Disinfection of Rooms by Gaseous Formaldehyde." *Journal of State Medicine* (1898): 527–42.

Delépine, A. Sheridan, and Arthur Ransome. "On the Disinfection of Tuberculously-Infected Houses: Being a Preliminary Report to the Scientific Grants Committee of the British Medical Association." *British Medical Journal* 1714 (November 4, 1893): 990–92.

———. "A Report on the Disinfection of Tubercle-Infected Houses." *British Medical Journal* 1781 (February 16, 1895): 349–55.

Deleuze, Gilles, and Félix Guattari. *What Is Philosophy?* New York: Columbia University Press, 1994.

Dennis, Richard. *Cities in Modernity: Representations and Productions of Metropolitan Space, 1840–1930.* Cambridge Studies in Historical Geography. Cambridge: Cambridge University Press, 2008.

Desrosières, Alain. *The Politics of Large Numbers: A History of Statistical Reasoning.* Cambridge, MA: Harvard University Press, 1998.

Dickens, Charles. "Registration of Sickness." *All the Year Round* 4 (1860): 227–28.

Digby, Anne. "The Economic and Medical Significance of the British National Insurance Act, 1911." In *Financing Medicine: The British Experience since 1750,* edited by Martin Gorsky and Sally Sheard, 182–98. Abingdon, UK: Routledge, 2006.

———. *Making a Medical Living: Doctors and Patients in the English Market for Medicine, 1720–1911.* Cambridge: Cambridge University Press, 1994.

"Discussion on the Advisability of the Registration of Tuberculosis." *Transactions of the College of Physicians of Philadelphia* 16 (January 12, 1894): 1–27.

Dixon, Godfrey B. "The Domiciliary Treatment of Tuberculous Patients." *British Journal of Tuberculosis* 9, no. 1 (January 1915): 19–22.

Donald, Moira. "Tranquil Havens? Critiquing the Idea of Home as the Middle-Class Sanctuary." In Bryden and Floyd, *Domestic Space,* 103–20.

Donzelot, Jacques. *The Policing of Families.* New York: Pantheon Books, 1979.

Dougall, John. "Disinfection by Acids," pt. 1. *British Medical Journal* 984 (November 8, 1879): 726–28.

———. "Disinfection by Acids," pt. 2. *British Medical Journal* 985 (November 15, 1879): 770–72.

Douglas, Mary. "The Idea of Home: A Kind of Space." *Social Research* 58, no. 1 (1991): 287–307.

Downes, Arthur. "On the Action of Sunlight on Micro-Organisms, &c., with a Demonstration of the Influence of Diffused Light." *Proceedings of the Royal Society of London* 40 (1886): 14–22.

Downes, Arthur, and Thomas P. Blunt. "Researches on the Effect of Light upon Bacteria and Other Organisms." *Proceedings of the Royal Society of London* 26 (1877): 488–500.

Driver, Felix. *Power and Pauperism: The Workhouse System, 1834–1884.* Cambridge: Cambridge University Press, 1993.

Dudfield, Reginald. "A Critical Examination of the Methods of Recording and Publishing Statistical Data Bearing on Public Health; with Suggestions for the Improvement of Such Methods." *Journal of the Royal Statistical Society* 68 (1905): 1–49.

Dudfield, Thomas Orme. *25th Annual Report on the Sanitary Condition of the Parish of St. Mary Abbots, Kensington, 1880.* 1881.

Durbach, Nadja. *Bodily Matters: The Anti-vaccination Movement in England, 1853–1907.* Durham, NC: Duke University Press, 2005.

Durey, Michael. *The Return of the Plague: British Society and the Cholera, 1831–2.* Dublin: Gill and Macmillan, 1979.

Dyck, Erika, and Christopher M. Fletcher, eds. *Locating Health: Historical and Anthropological Investigations of Health and Place.* London: Pickering & Chatto, 2011.

Dyhouse, Carol. *Girls Growing Up in Late Victorian and Edwardian England.* London: Routledge & Kegan Paul, 1981.

———. "Towards a 'Feminine' Curriculum for English Schoolgirls: The Demands of Ideology 1870–1963." *Women's Studies International Quarterly* 1, no. 4 (1978): 297–311.

Edmonds, Thomas Rowe. "On the Laws of Collective Vitality." *Lancet* 2 (1834–35): 5–8.

———. "Statistics of the London Hospital." *Lancet* 2 (1835–36): 778–83.

Edwards, Clive. *Turning Houses into Homes: A History of the Retailing and Consumption of Domestic Furnishings.* Aldershot, UK: Ashgate, 2005.

Elmy, E. C. W. "Compulsory Notification of Infectious Disease." *Journal of the Vigilance Association for the Defence of Personal Rights* 11 (November 15, 1881): 91–93.

———. "Legislation by Private Bills and Provisional Orders." *Journal of the Vigilance Association for the Defence of Personal Rights* 16 (April 15, 1882): 41–42.

———. "The Local Government Board and Compulsory Notification of Infectious Disease." *Journal of the Vigilance Association for the Defence of Personal Rights* 9 (September 15, 1881): 76–78.

Esmarch, E. "Der Keimgehalt Der Wände Und Ihre Desinfection." *Zeitschrift Für Hygiene* 2, no. 1 (1887): 491–520.

Eyler, John M. "Scarlet Fever and Confinement: The Edwardian Debate Over Isolation Hospitals." *Bulletin of the History of Medicine* 61 (1987): 1–24.

———. *Sir Arthur Newsholme and State Medicine, 1885–1935.* Cambridge: Cambridge University Press, 1997.

———. *Victorian Social Medicine: The Ideas and Methods of William Farr.* Baltimore: Johns Hopkins University Press, 1979.

Fairchild, Amy L., Ronald Bayer, and James Keith Colgrove, with Daniel Wolfe. *Searching Eyes: Privacy, the State, and Disease Surveillance in America.* Berkeley: University of California Press; New York: Milbank Memorial Fund, 2007.

Farnie, D. A. *The English Cotton Industry and the World Market, 1815–1896.* Oxford: Clarendon Press, 1979.

Farr, William. "General Sanitary Statistics." In *Report of the Proceedings of the Fourth Session of the International Statistical Congress, London, 16 July 1860,* edited by William Farr, R. Valpy, and J. T. Hammack, 45–59. London: HMSO, 1861.

Feldberg, Georgina D. *Disease and Class: Tuberculosis and the Shaping of Modern North American Society.* New Brunswick, NJ: Rutgers University Press, 1995.

Fenton, Laura. "Citizenship in Private Space." *Space and Culture* 8, no. 2 (May 2005): 180–92.

"Fidelis." "The Sanitary and Police Clauses and Mr Sclater-Booth's Proposed New Standing Order." *Journal of the Vigilance Association for the Defence of Personal Rights* 19 (July 15, 1882): 63–65.

Fielding, Muriel. "Ignota, the Unknown Woman: Elizabeth Clarke Wolstenholme Elmy, 1833–1918." In *Mary Wollstonecraft and 200 Years of Feminisms,* edited by Eileen Yeo, 152–55. London: Rivers Oram Press, 1997.

Fitzpatrick, Dr. "Notification of Infectious Diseases." *British Medical Journal* 1105 (March 4, 1882): 319.

Flanders, Judith. *Inside the Victorian Home: A Portrait of Domestic Life in Victorian England.* New York: W. W. Norton, 2004.

Flinn, Michael W. "Medical Services under the New Poor Law." In *The New Poor Law in the Nineteenth Century,* edited by Derek Fraser, 45–66. New York: St. Martin's Press, 1976.

Forty, Adrian. *Objects of Desire: Design and Society since 1750.* Paperback ed. New York: Thames and Hudson, 1992.

Foucault, Michel. *The Birth of Biopolitics: Lectures at the Collège De France, 1978–1979.* New York: Picador, 2008.

———. *Discipline and Punish: The Birth of the Prison.* Translated by Alan Sheridan. London: Allen Lane, 1977.

———. "Governmentality." In *The Foucault Effect: Studies in Governmentality*, edited by Graham Burchell, Colin Gordon, and Peter Miller, 87–104. London: Harvester Wheatsheaf, 1991.

———. *Security, Territory, Population: Lectures at the Collège De France, 1977–1978*, edited by Michel Senellart. Basingstoke, UK; New York: Palgrave Macmillan; République Française, 2007.

———. "The Subject and Power." In *Michel Foucault: Power*, edited by James D. Faubion, 326–48. Translated by Robert Hurley and others. New York: The New Press, 1994.

Fox, Cornelius B. "Why Should the Existing System of Registering Sickness Be Longer Perpetuated?" *Transactions of the National Association for the Promotion of Social Science* (1877): 562–69.

Fox, Daniel M. "Social Policy and City Politics: Tuberculosis Reporting in New York, 1889–1900." *Bulletin of the History of Medicine* 49 (1975): 169–95.

Frankel, Oz. *States of Inquiry: Social Investigations and Print Culture in Nineteenth-Century Britain and the United States.* Baltimore: Johns Hopkins University Press, 2006.

Franklin, A. "Working-Class Privatism: An Historical Case Study of Bedminster, Bristol." *Environment and Planning D: Society and Space* 7 (1989): 93–113.

Fraser, Stuart M. F. "Leicester and Smallpox: The Leicester Method." *Medical History* 24 (1980): 315–32.

Freeman, Albert C. *The Planning of Fever Hospitals and Disinfecting and Cleansing Stations.* London: Sanitary Publishing Company, 1909.

Froggatt, P. "Sir William Wilde and the 1851 Census of Ireland." *Medical History* 9 (1965): 302–27.

Gandy, Matthew. "The Bacteriological City and Its Discontents." *Historical Geography* 34 (2006): 14–25.

Gilbert, Pamela K. *The Citizen's Body: Desire, Health, and the Social in Victorian England.* Columbus: Ohio State University Press, 2007.

Gilmour, A. "Measles and School Closure." *Public Health* 25 (October 1911–September 1912): 448–53.

Godwin, George. *London Shadows: A Glance at the "Homes" of the Thousands.* 1854. Reprint, New York: Garland, 1985.

Goff, A., and J. H. Levy. *Politics and Disease.* Personal Rights. 3rd ser. London: P. S. King, Personal Rights Association, 1906.

Goldman, Lawrence. *Science, Reform and Politics in Victorian Britain: The Social Science Association, 1857–1886.* Cambridge: Cambridge University Press, 2002.

Goldstrom, J. M. *The Social Content of Education, 1808–1870; a Study of the Working Class School Reader in England and Ireland.* Shannon, IE: Irish University Press, 1972.

Gomersall, Meg, and Jo Campling. *Working-Class Girls in Nineteenth-Century England: Life, Work, and Schooling.* New York: St. Martin's Press, 1997.

Goodall, E. W. "An Account of the Isolation Chambers Recently Provided at the Eastern Hospital." *Public Health* 25 (October 1911–September 1912): 17–22.

Gorsky, Martin. "Friendly Society Health Insurance in Nineteenth-Century England." In *Financing Medicine: The British Experience since 1750*, edited by Martin Gorsky and Sally Sheard, 147–64. Abingdon, UK: Routledge, 2006.

Gradmann, Christoph. *Laboratory Disease: Robert Koch's Medical Bacteriology.* Translated by Elborg Forster. Baltimore: Johns Hopkins University Press, 2009.

Graham, Major George. "Remarks Submitted to the Consideration of the Royal Sanitary Commission by the Registrar-General of England and Wales." In *Thirty-first Annual Report of the Registrar-General of Births, Deaths and Marriages in England, 1868,* 285–91. London: HMSO, 1870.

Gray, James A. *The Edinburgh City Hospital.* East Lothian, UK: Tuckwell Press, 1999.

Green, David R. "Pauper Protests: Power and Resistance in Early Nineteenth-Century London Workhouses." *Social History* 31, no. 2 (May 2006): 137–59.

Griffin, Ben, Lucy Delap, and Abigail Wills. "Introduction: The Politics of Domestic Authority in Britain since 1800." In *The Politics of Domestic Authority in Britain since 1800,* edited by Lucy Delap, Ben Griffin, and Abigail Wills, 1–26. New York: Palgrave Macmillan, 2009.

Gunn, Simon. "From Hegemony to Governmentality: Changing Conceptions of Power in Social History." *Journal of Social History* 39, no. 3 (2006): 705–20.

Gunn, Simon, and James Vernon. "Introduction: What Was Liberal Modernity in Britain and Why was It Peculiar?" In *The Peculiarities of Liberal Modernity in Imperial Britain,* edited by Simon Gunn and James Vernon, 1–18. Berkeley: University of California Press, 2011.

Gurjeva, Lyubov G. "Child Health, Commerce and Family Values: The Domestic Production of the Middle Class in Late-Nineteenth and Early Twentieth Century Britain." In *Cultures of Child Health in Britain and the Netherlands in the Twentieth Century,* edited by Marijke Gijswijt-Hofstra and Hilary Marland, 103–25. Amsterdam: Rodopi, 2003.

Hacking, Ian. *Historical Ontology.* Cambridge, MA: Harvard University Press, 2002.

Hall, Catherine. "The Early Formation of Victorian Domestic Ideology." In *Fit Work for Women,* edited by Sandra Burman, 15–32. London: Palgrave Macmillan, 1979.

Hall, Catherine, Keith McClelland, and Jane Rendall. *Defining the Victorian Nation: Class, Race, Gender and the Reform Act of 1867.* Cambridge: Cambridge University Press, 2000.

Hall, Lesley A. "Venereal Diseases and Society in Britain, from the Contagious Diseases Acts to the National Health Service." In *Sex, Sin and Suffering: Venereal Disease and European Society since 1870,* edited by Roger Davidson and Lesley A. Hall, 120–36. London: Routledge, 2001.

Hamlin, Christopher. "Muddling in Bumbledom: On the Enormity of Large Sanitary Improvements in Four British Towns, 1855–85." *Victorian Studies* 32 (1988): 55–83.

———. *Public Health and Social Justice in the Age of Chadwick: Britain, 1800–1854.* Cambridge: Cambridge University Press, 1998.

———. "Public Sphere to Public Health: The Transformation of 'Nuisance.'" In *Medicine, Health and the Public Sphere in Britain, 1600–2000,* edited by Steve Sturdy, 189–204. London: Routledge, 2002.

———. "Sanitary Policing and the Local State, 1873–1874: A Statistical Study of English and Welsh Towns." *Social History of Medicine* 18 (2005): 39–61.

———. *A Science of Impurity: Water Analysis in Nineteenth Century Britain.* Berkeley: University of California Press, 1990.

Hammerton, A. James. *Cruelty and Companionship: Conflict in Nineteenth Century Married Life.* London: Routledge, 1992.

Hammonds, Evelynn Maxine. *Childhood's Deadly Scourge: The Campaign to Control Diphtheria in New York City, 1880–1930.* Baltimore: Johns Hopkins University Press, 1999.

Hance, Edward M. "On the Relation of the State to the Individual." *LSE Selected Pamphlets* (1885).

Hanley, James G. "Parliament, Physicians, and Nuisances: The Demedicalization of Nuisance Law, 1831–1855." *Bulletin of the History of Medicine* 80, no. 4 (2006): 702–32.

Hannah, Matthew G. *Governmentality and the Mastery of Territory in Nineteenth-Century America.* Cambridge: Cambridge University Press, 2000.

Harbutt, William. *Harbutt's Plastic Method and the Use of Plasticine in the Arts of Writing, Drawing & Modelling in Educational Work.* London: Chapman & Hall, 1897.

Hardie, James. "A Paper on the Duty of Municipal Authorities to Provide Hospital Accommodation for Cases of Infectious Diseases." *Manchester and Salford Sanitary Association Annual Report* (1872): appendix.

Hardwicke, William. "The Importance of Complete Disinfection, and the Best Means of Providing for It by Sanitary Authorities." *Transactions of the National Association for the Promotion of Social Science* (1878): 450–57.

Hardy, Anne. "Buchanan, Sir George (1827–1913)." In *Oxford Dictionary of National Biography.* http://www.oxforddnb.com/view/article/3839.

———. "Cholera, Quarantine and the English Preventive System, 1850–1895." *Medical History* 37, no. 3 (1993): 250–69.

———. *The Epidemic Streets: Infectious Disease and the Rise of Preventive Medicine, 1856–1900.* Oxford: Clarendon Press, 1993.

———. "Tracheotomy versus Intubation: Surgical Intervention in Diphtheria in Europe and the United States, 1825–1930." *Bulletin of the History of Medicine* 66, no. 4 (1992): 536–59.

Harling, Philip. "The Centrality of Locality: The Local State, Local Democracy, and Local Consciousness in Late-Victorian and Edwardian Britain." *Journal of Victorian Culture* 9, no. 2 (2004): 216–34.

———. "The Powers of the Victorian State." In *Liberty and Authority in Victorian Britain,* edited by Peter Mandler, 25–50. Oxford: Oxford University Press, 2006.

Harris, Bernard. "Educational Reform, Citizenship and the Origins of the School Medical Service." In *Cultures of Child Health in Britain and the Netherlands in the Twentieth Century,* edited by Marijke Gijswijt-Hofstra and Hilary Marland, 85–101. Clio Medica/The Wellcome Series in the History of Medicine. Amsterdam: Rodopi, 2003

———. *The Health of the Schoolchild: A History of the School Medical Service in England and Wales.* Buckingham, UK: Open University Press, 1995.

Harris, José. "Between Civic Virtue and Social Darwinism: The Concept of the Residuum." In *Retrieved Riches: Social Investigation in Britain, 1840–1914,* edited by David Englander and Rosemary O'Day, 67–87. Aldershot, UK: Ashgate, 1995.

Harvey, David. *Cosmopolitanism.* New York: Columbia University Press, 2009.

Hastings, George Woodyatt. "Inaugural Address." *Transactions of the Sanitary Institute of Great Britain* 10 (1888–89): 77–93.

Hatherly, Henry R. "Notification of Infectious Diseases." *Nottingham Journal*, May 11, 1883.

Hatton, John. *A Lecture on the Sanitary Condition of Chorlton-upon-Medlock.* Manchester, 1854.

Heathorn, Stephen J. *For Home, Country, and Race: Constructing Gender, Class, and Englishness in the Elementary School, 1880–1914.* Toronto: University of Toronto Press, 2000.

Helly, Dorothy O., and Susan Reverby, eds. *Gendered Domains: Rethinking Public and Private in Women's History; Essays from the Seventh Berkshire Conference on the History of Women.* Ithaca, NY: Cornell University Press, 1992.

Hendrick, Harry. "Child Labour, Medical Capital and the School Medical Service." In *In the Name of the Child: Health and Welfare, 1880–1940*, edited by Roger Cooter, 45–71. London: Routledge, 1992.

———. *Child Welfare: England, 1872–1989.* London: Routledge, 1994.

Hennock, E. P. *Fit and Proper Persons: Ideal and Reality in Nineteenth-Century Urban Government.* London: Edward Arnold, 1973.

———. *The Origin of the Welfare State in England and Germany, 1850–1914: Social Policies Compared.* Cambridge: Cambridge University Press, 2007.

Henry, William. "Experiments on the Disinfecting Powers of Increased Temperatures, with a View to the Suggestion of a Substitute for Quarantine." *Philosophical Magazine*, 2nd ser., 10, no. 59 (1832): 363–69.

———. "Further Experiments on the Disinfecting Powers of Increased Temperatures." *Philosophical Magazine*, 2nd ser., 11, no. 61 (1832): 22.

———. "Letter from Dr. Henry on a Modified Disinfecting Apparatus." *Philosophical Magazine*, 2nd ser., 11, no. 63 (1832): 205.

Hepworth, Mike. "Privacy, Security and Respectability: The Ideal Victorian Home." In *Ideal Homes? Social Change and Domestic Life*, edited by Tony Chapman and Jennifer Lorna Hockey, 17–29. London: Routledge, 1999.

Hess, Volker. "Standardizing Body Temperature: Quantification in Hospitals and Daily Life, 1850–1900." In *Body Counts: Medical Quantification in Historical and Sociological Perspective*, edited by Gérard Jorland, Annick Opinel, and George Weisz, 109–26. Montreal: McGill-Queen's University Press, 2005.

Hess, Volker, and J. A. Mendelsohn. "Case and Series: Medical Knowledge and Paper Technology, 1600–1900." *History of Science* 48, no. 3 (2010): 287–314.

Hewat, A. Middleton. "The Disinfection of Tubercle-Infected Houses." *British Journal of Tuberculosis* 8, no. 3 (July 1914): 147–51.

Hewitt, Martin. *The Emergence of Stability in the Industrial City: Manchester, 1832–67.* Aldershot, UK: Ashgate, 1996.

———. "The Travails of Domestic Visiting: Manchester, 1830–70." *Historical Research* 71 (1998): 196–227.

Higgs, Edward. "A Cuckoo in the Nest? The Origins of Civil Registration and State Medical Statistics in England and Wales." *Continuity and Change* 11 (1996): 115–34.

———. *Life, Death and Statistics: Civil Registration, Censuses and the Work of the General Register Office, 1836–1952.* Hatfield, UK: Local Population Studies, 2004.

Hill, Alfred. "The Notification of Infectious Disease: Its Importance and Its Difficulties." *Sanitary Record*, n.s., 6 (1884): 43.

Hime, T. W. "Schools and Scarlet Fever." *Lancet* 122 (1883): 301.

Hirst, J. David. "The Early School Medical Service in Wales: Public Care or Private Responsibility?" In *Medicine in Wales c. 1800–2000: Public Service or Private Commodity?*, edited by Anne Borsay, 65–85. Cardiff: University of Wales Press, 2003.

———. "A Failure 'without Parallel': The School Medical Service and the London County Council." *Medical History* 25 (1981): 281–300.

———. "The Growth of Treatment through the School Medical Service, 1908–18." *Medical History* 33 (1989): 318–42.

———. "Public Health and the Public Elementary Schools, 1870–1907." *History of Education* 20, no. 2 (1991): 107–18.

Hockberger, Philip E. "A History of Ultraviolet Photobiology for Humans, Animals and Microorganisms." *Photochemistry and Photobiology* 76, no. 6 (2002): 561–79.

Hodgkinson, Ruth G. *The Origins of the National Health Service: The Medical Services of the New Poor Law, 1834–1871.* Berkeley: University of California Press, 1967.

———. "Social Medicine and the Growth of Statistical Information." In *Medicine and Science in the 1860s*, edited by F. N. L. Poynter, 183–98. London: Wellcome Institute for the History of Medicine, 1968.

Holden, Oscar. "The Danger of the Domiciliary Treatment of Tuberculosis." *Medical Officer* 11 (1914): 99–101.

———. "The Domiciliary Treatment of Tuberculosis." *British Journal of Tuberculosis* 12, no. 2 (April 1918): 81–85.

Holton, Sandra Stanley. "To Live 'through One's Own Powers': British Medicine, Tuberculosis and 'Invalidism' in the Life of Alice Clark (1874–1934)." *Journal of Women's History* 11, no. 1 (1999): 75–96.

Hoppen, K. T. "The Franchise and Electoral Politics in England and Ireland, 1832–85." *History* 70 (1985): 202–17.

Horn, Pamela. "English Elementary Education and the Growth of the Imperial Ideal, 1880–1914." In *"Benefits Bestowed"? Education and British Imperialism*, edited by J. A. Mangan, 39–55. Manchester: Manchester University Press, 1988.

Howarth, William J. "Sanatorium Benefit for Tuberculous Patients, and National Insurance." *British Journal of Tuberculosis* 6, no. 4 (October 1912): 242–44.

Howell, Philip. *Geographies of Regulation: Policing Prostitution in Nineteenth-Century Britain and the Empire.* Cambridge: Cambridge University Press, 2009.

Huch, Ronald K. "The National Association for the Promotion of Social Science: Its Contribution to Victorian Health Reform, 1857–1886." *Albion* 17, no. 3 (1985): 279–99.

Huisman, Frank, and Harry Oosterhuis, eds. *Health and Citizenship.* London: Pickering & Chatto, 2013.

Hunt, Alan. *Governing Morals: A Social History of Moral Regulation.* Cambridge: Cambridge University Press, 1999.

Hurren, Elizabeth T. "Poor Law versus Public Health: Diphtheria, Sanitary Reform, and the 'Crusade' against Outdoor Relief, 1870–1900." *Social History of Medicine* 18 (2005): 399–418.

Hurt, J. S. *Elementary Schooling and the Working Classes, 1860–1918.* London: Routledge & Kegan Paul, 1979.

Jackson, Mark. "'Home Sweet Home': Historical Perspectives on Health and the Home." In *Health and the Modern Home*, edited by Mark Jackson, 1–17. New York: Routledge, 2007.

Jacyna, Stephen. "Medicine in Transformation, 1800–1849." In *The Western Medical Tradition, 1800 to 2000,* edited by William F. Bynum, Anne Hardy, Stephen Jacyna, Christopher Lawrence, and E. M. Tansey, 11–101. Cambridge: Cambridge University Press, 2006.

Jessel, George. "The Bedroom of the Consumptive." *British Journal of Tuberculosis* 10, no. 2 (April 1916): 75–79.

———. "Dispensary Supervision in Pulmonary Tuberculosis." *Lancet* 192 (December 28, 1918): 894–95.

Jessop, Bob, Neil Brenner, and Martin Jones. "Theorizing Sociospatial Relations." *Environment and Planning D: Society and Space* 26 (2008): 389–401.

Johnson, Richard. "Educational Policy and Social Control in Early Victorian England." *Past & Present* 49 (1970): 96–119.

Jones, Gareth Stedman. *Outcast London: A Study in the Relationship between Classes in Victorian Society.* 2nd ed. London: Penguin Books, 1984.

Jordan, Jane, and Ingrid Sharp, eds. *Josephine Butler and the Prostitution Campaigns: Diseases of the Body Politic.* Vol. 3, *The Constitution Violated: The Parliamentary Campaign.* London: Routledge, 2003.

———. *Josephine Butler and the Prostitution Campaigns: Diseases of the Body Politic.* Vol. 4, *Child Prostitution and the Age of Consent.* London: Routledge, 2003.

Joyce, Patrick. *The Rule of Freedom: Liberalism and the Modern City.* London: Verso, 2003.

———. *The State of Freedom: A Social History of the British State since 1800.* Cambridge: Cambridge University Press, 2013.

Kanthack, A. A. "The Use of Formalin Lamps for the Disinfection of Rooms (Alformant Lamps and Formogène Richard)." *Lancet* 152 (October 22, 1898): 1049–51.

Kargon, Robert Hugh. *Science in Victorian Manchester: Enterprise and Expertise.* Baltimore: Johns Hopkins University Press, 1977.

Kaye, James Robert. "Scarlet Fever: How Far Do Statistics Prove or Disprove the Utility of Hospital Isolation." *Public Health* 14 (October 1901–September 1902): 449–72.

Kearns, Gerry. "Cholera, Nuisances and Environmental Management in Islington, 1830–55." In *Living and Dying in London,* edited by William F. Bynum and Roy Porter, 94–125. London: Wellcome Institute for the History of Medicine, 1991.

———. "Private Property and Public Health Reform in England 1830–1870." *Social Science & Medicine* 26, no. 1 (1988): 187–99.

———. "Town Hall and Whitehall: Sanitary Intelligence in Liverpool, 1840–63." In *Body and City: Histories of Urban Public Health,* edited by Sally Sheard and Helen Power, 89–108. Aldershot, UK: Ashgate, 2000.

———. "Tuberculosis and the Medicalisation of British Society, 1880–1920." In *Coping with Sickness: Historical Aspects of Health Care in a European Perspective,* edited by John H. Woodward and Robert Jütte, 147–70. Sheffield, UK: European Association for the History of Medicine and Health Publications, 1995.

Kearns, Gerry, and Simon Reid-Henry. "Vital Geographies: Life, Luck, and the Human Condition." *Annals of the Association of American Geographers* 99, no. 3 (2009): 554–74.

Kenwood, Henry R., and Gerard C. Taylor. "Disinfection of Rooms by Formic Aldehyde Vapours." *Transactions of the Sanitary Institute of Great Britain* 18 (1897): 406–16.

———. "The Means of Preventing the Spread of Infection in Elementary Schools." *British Medical Journal* 2018 (September 2, 1899): 589–92.

———. "Two Years' Experience of the Voluntary Notification of Phthisis in the Metropolis—and Its Lessons." *Journal of the Sanitary Institute* 24 (1903): 261–65.

Kerr, James. *Annual Report of the Medical Officer of the London School Board, for the Year Ended 25 March 1903.* London, 1903.

———. *Report of the LCC Medical Officer (Education), for the Year Ended 25th March, 1904.* London, 1904.

———. *Report of the LCC Medical Officer (Education), for the Year Ended 31st March, 1905.* London, 1905.

———. *Report of the LCC Medical Officer (Education), for the Year Ended 31st March, 1906.* London, 1906.

———. *Report of the LCC Medical Officer (Education), for the Year Ended 31st March, 1907.* London, 1907.

———. *Report of the LCC Medical Officer (Education), for the 21 Months Ended 31st December, 1908.* London, n.d.

King, Nicholas B. "The Scale Politics of Emerging Diseases." *Osiris* 19, no. 1 (2004): 62.

Kisacky, Jeanne. "Restructuring Isolation: Hospital Architecture, Medicine and Disease Prevention." *Bulletin of the History of Medicine* 79 (2005): 1–49.

Kleinberg, S. J. "Gendered Space: Housing, Privacy and Domesticity in the Nineteenth-Century United States." In Bryden and Floyd, *Domestic Space*, 142–61.

Koch, Robert. "An Address on Bacteriological Research." *British Medical Journal* 1546 (August 16, 1890): 380–83.

———. "Ueber Desinfection." *Mittheilungen Aus Dem Kaiserlichen Gesundheitsamte* 1 (1881): 234–82.

Koch, Robert, and K. Codell Carter. *Essays of Robert Koch.* New York: Greenwood Press, 1987.

Koch, Robert, George Gaffky, and Friedrich Loeffler. "Versuche Über Die Verwerthbarkeit Heisser Wasserdämpfe Zu Desinfectionszwecken." *Mittheilungen Aus Dem Kaiserlichen Gesundheitsamte* 1 (1881).

Koch, Robert, and Gustav Wolffhülge. "Untersuchungen Über Die Desinfection Mit Heisser Luft." *Mittheilungen Aus Dem Kaiserlichen Gesundheitsamte* 1 (1881): 301–21.

Koven, Seth. *Slumming: Sexual and Social Politics in Victorian London.* Princeton, NJ: Princeton University Press, 2004.

Lalor, Joseph. "On Disinfection." *British Medical Journal* 580 (February 10, 1872): 153–54.

Lambert, Royston. *Sir John Simon and English Social Administration, 1816–1904.* London: MacGibbon & Kee, 1963.

———. "A Victorian National Health Service: State Vaccination 1855–71." *Historical Journal* 5 (1962): 1–18.

Lancaster, Bill. *Radicalism, Cooperation and Socialism: Leicester Working-Class Politics 1860–1906.* Leicester, UK: Leicester University Press, 1987.

Laxton, Paul. "Fighting for Public Health: Dr Duncan and His Adversaries, 1847–1863." In *Body and City: Histories of Urban Public Health*, edited by Sally Sheard and Helen Power, 59–88. Aldershot, UK: Ashgate, 2000.

Lefebvre, Henri. *The Production of Space.* Oxford: Blackwell, 1991.

Leigh, John. *Report on Infectious Disease in Manchester.* Presented to the Health Committee on December 19, 1870. Manchester, 1871.

Leslie, R. Murray. "State Insurance and the Machinery for the Detection and Treatment of Tuberculosis." *British Journal of Tuberculosis* 5, no. 4 (October 1911): 275–82.

Letheby, Henry. "On the Right Use of Disinfectants (a)." *Medical Times and Gazette* 2 (1873): 487–89.

———. "On the Right Use of Disinfectants (b)." *Medical Times and Gazette* 2 (1873): 514–17.

Lewis, James. *Suggestions for National Returns of Sickness.* London: C. P. Alvey, 1870.

Lewis, Jane. "Parents, Children, School Fees and the London School Board, 1870–1890." *History of Education* 11, no. 4 (1982): 291–312.

Lewis, R. A. *Edwin Chadwick and the Public Health Movement 1832–1854.* London: Longmans, Green, 1952.

"Liberty." "Medicine in Parliament and Common Sense Outside." *Journal of the Vigilance Association for the Defence of Personal Rights* 16 (April 15, 1882): 37–39.

Liberty and Property Defence League. *Overlegislation in 1883: Report on the Bills of the Session.* London, 1883.

———. *Overlegislation in 1884: Review of the Bills of the Session.* London, 1884.

———. *Self-Help v. State-Help: The Liberty and Property Defence League: Its Origin, Objects, and Inaugural Meeting.* London, 1882.

Lissant Cox, G. "Sanatorium Treatment Contrasted with Home Treatment: After-Histories of 4,067 Cases." *British Journal of Tuberculosis* 17, no. 1 (January 1923): 27–30.

Litsios, Socrates. "Charles Dickens and the Movement for Sanitary Reform." *Perspectives in Biology and Medicine* 46 (2003): 183–99.

"Liverpool: The Notification of Infectious Disease." *British Medical Journal* 1134 (September 23, 1882): 598.

Livingstone, David N. *Putting Science in Its Place: Geographies of Scientific Knowledge.* Chicago: University of Chicago Press, 2003.

Livy, John. "The Notification of Infectious Diseases." *British Medical Journal* 1128 (August 12, 1882): 291–92.

Logan, Thad. *The Victorian Parlour.* Cambridge: Cambridge University Press, 2001.

Longmate, Norman. *The Hungry Mills: The Story of the Lancashire Cotton Famine, 1861–5.* London: Temple Smith, 1978.

London County Council. *Annual Report of the Council 1912.* Vol. 3, *Public Health (Including the Report of the County Medical Officer of Health and the School Medical Officer, Main Drainage, Housing of the Working Classes).*

———. *Annual Report of the Council 1913.* Vol. 3, *Public Health (Including the Report of the County Medical Officer of Health and the School Medical Officer, Main Drainage, Housing of the Working Classes).*

———. *Annual Report of the Medical Officer of Health of the Administrative County of London, 1896.*

———. *Annual Report of the Medical Officer of Health of the Administrative County of London, 1901.*

Lowndes, Frederick W. "The Medical Profession in Liverpool, and the Notification of Infectious Diseases." *Sanitary Record*, n.s., 3 (1882): 323–24.

Macara, Alexander. "Confidentiality—a Decrepit Concept?" *Journal of the Royal Society of Medicine* 77 (1984): 577–84.

MacKenzie, John M. *Imperialism and Popular Culture*. London: Manchester University Press, 1986.

Mackenzie, W. Leslie. "Administrative Control of Pulmonary Phthisis in Scotland." *Lancet* 176 (July 16, 1910): 162–64.

———. "The Family and the City: Their Functional Relations." *Sociological Review* 1, no. 1 (1908): 118–38.

———. "Methods of Disinfection," pt. 1. *Public Health* 12, no. 6 (March 1900): 438–48.

———. "Methods of Disinfection," pt. 2. *Public Health* 12, no. 8 (May 1900): 593–611.

———. "A Simple and Portable Spray Pump for Disinfection." *British Medical Journal* 2126 (September 28, 1901): 898–900.

MacLeod, Roy M. "Law, Medicine and Public Opinion: The Resistance to Compulsory Health Legislation 1870–1907: Part I." *Public Law* (Summer 1967): 107–28.

———. "Law, Medicine and Public Opinion: The Resistance to Compulsory Health Legislation 1870–1907: Part II." *Public Law* (Fall 1967): 189–211.

Maglen, Krista. *The English System: Quarantine, Immigration and the Making of a Port Sanitary Zone*. Manchester: Manchester University Press, 2014.

Mahood, Linda. *The Magdalenes: Prostitution in the Nineteenth Century*. London: Routledge, 1990.

Manchester and Salford Sanitary Association. *Annual Report of the Committee of the Manchester and Salford Sanitary Association, Being a Summary of Their Proceedings for the Year 1864*. Manchester, 1865.

———. *Annual Report of the Committee of the Manchester and Salford Sanitary Association, Being a Summary of Their Proceedings for the Year 1869*. Manchester, 1870.

———. *Annual Report of the Committee of the Manchester and Salford Sanitary Association, Being a Summary of Their Proceedings for the Year 1880*. Manchester, 1881.

———. *Annual Report of the Manchester and Salford Sanitary Association, November 1853 to October 1854*. 1854.

———. *Annual Report of the Manchester and Salford Sanitary Association, November 1857–November 1858*. 1859.

———. *Report of the Committee of the Manchester and Salford Sanitary Association; Being a Summary of Their Proceedings for the Year 1859 and 1860*. Manchester, 1861.

———. *Report of the Committee of the Manchester and Salford Sanitary Association; Being a Summary of Their Proceedings for the Year 1861*. Manchester, 1862.

———. *Report of the Committee of the Manchester and Salford Sanitary Association; Being a Summary of Their Proceedings for the Year 1862*. Manchester, 1863.

Mandler, Peter, ed. *Liberty and Authority in Victorian Britain*. Oxford: Oxford University Press, 2006.

Marcus, Sharon. *Apartment Stories: City and Home in Nineteenth-Century Paris and London*. Berkeley: University of California Press, 1999.

Marks, Harry M. "'Until the Sun of Science . . . the True Apollo of Medicine has Risen': Collective Medical Investigation in Britain and America, 1880–1910." *Medical History* 50 (2006): 147–66.

Marshall, Gordon, David Rose, Gordon Newby, and Carolyn Vogler. *Social Class in Modern Britain.* London: Hutchinson, 1988.

Martin, Jane. *Women and the Politics of Schooling in Victorian and Edwardian England.* London: Leicester University Press, 1999.

Martineau, R. F. "Compulsory Notification of Infectious Disease." *Journal of the Vigilance Association for the Defence of Personal Rights* 6 (June 15, 1881): 55–56.

Massey, Doreen. *For Space.* London: Sage, 2005.

May, Francis H. "School Closure for Measles." *Public Health* 18 (October 1905–September 1906): 451–56.

McCann, Phillip, ed. *Popular Education and Socialization in the Nineteenth Century.* London: Methuen, 1977.

McClelland, Keith. "'England's Greatness, the Working Man.'" In *Defining the Victorian Nation: Class, Race, Gender and the Reform Act of 1867,* edited by Catherine Hall, Keith McClelland, and Jane Rendall, 71–118. Cambridge: Cambridge University Press, 2000.

McClelland, Keith, and Sonya Rose. "Citizenship and Empire, 1867–1928." In *At Home with the Empire: Metropolitan Culture and the Imperial World,* edited by Catherine Hall and Sonya Rose, 275–97. Cambridge: Cambridge University Press, 2006.

McDermid, Jane. *Victoria's Daughters.* Hoboken, NJ: Taylor and Francis, 2013.

McHugh, Paul. *Prostitution and Victorian Social Reform.* London: Croom Helm, 1980.

Meckel, Richard A. *Classrooms and Clinics: Urban Schools and the Protection and Promotion of Child Health, 1870–1930.* New Brunswick, NJ: Rutgers University Press, 2013.

"Medico-Meteorological Observations." *Association Medical Journal* 1, no. 40 (October 7, 1853): 891–92.

Mehta, Uday C. "Liberal Strategies of Exclusion." *Politics and Society* 18, no. 4 (1990): 427–54.

Mendelsohn, J. Andrew. "'Like All That Lives': Biology, Medicine and Bacteria in the Age of Pasteur and Koch." *History & Philosophy of the Life Sciences* 24, no. 1 (2002): 3–36.

Messiter, A. F., and Alfred Bailey. "The Disinfection of Clothing by Heat." *Lancet* 150 (December 4, 1897): 1482.

Mezei, Kathy, and Chiara Briganti. *The Domestic Space Reader.* Toronto: University of Toronto Press, 2012.

Millard, C. Killick. "The Hospital Isolation of Scarlet Fever: Some Points of Uncertainty." *Public Health* 14 (October 1901–September 1902): 285–94.

———. "The Influence of Hospital Isolation in Scarlet Fever: An Appeal to Statistics." *Public Health* 13 (October 1900–September 1901): 462–503.

Milroy, Gavin. "Suggestions for Utilising the Statistics of the Disease among the Poor." *Transactions of the Epidemiological Society of London* 1, no. 1 (1860–61): 69–75.

Mohr, Peter D. "Dreschfeld, Julius (1845–1907)." In *Oxford Dictionary of National Biography.* http://www.oxforddnb.com/view/article/32891.

Mooney, Graham. "Diagnostic Spaces: Workhouse, Hospital and Home in Mid-Victorian London." *Social Science History* (2009): 357–90.

———. "Public Health versus Private Practice: The Contested Development of Compulsory Notification of Infectious Disease in Late-Nineteenth-Century Britain." *Bulletin of the History of Medicine* 73, no. 2 (1999): 238–67.

———. "'A Tissue of the Most Flagrant Anomalies': Smallpox Vaccination and the Centralization of Sanitary Administration in Nineteenth-Century London." *Medical History* 41 (1997): 261–90.

Mooney, Graham, Bill Luckin, and Andrea Tanner. "Patient Pathways: Solving the Problem of Institutional Mortality in London during the Later Nineteenth Century." *Social History of Medicine* 12 (1999): 227–69.

Mooney, Graham, and Jonathan Reinarz. "Hospital and Asylum Visiting in Historical Perspective: Themes and Issues." In *Permeable Walls: Historical Perspectives on Hospital and Asylum Visiting*, edited by Graham Mooney and Jonathan Reinarz, 7–30. Clio Medica/The Wellcome Series in the History of Medicine. Amsterdam: Rodopi, 2009.

Mooney, Graham, and Andrea Tanner. "Infant Mortality, a Spatial Problem: Notting Dale Special Area in George Newman's London." In *Infant Mortality: A Continuing Social Problem*, edited by Eilidh Garrett, Chris Galley, Nicola Shelton, and Robert Woods, 169–90. Aldershot, UK: Ashgate, 2007.

Morris, Robert J. "Governance: Two Centuries of Urban Growth." In *Urban Governance: Britain and Beyond since 1750*, edited by Robert J. Morris and Richard H. Trainor, 1–14. Aldershot, UK: Ashgate, 2000.

Mort, Frank. *Dangerous Sexualities: Medico-Moral Politics in England since 1830.* London: Routledge & Kegan Paul, 1987.

Morus, Iwan Rhys. "Illuminating the Victorians." *History and Technology: An International Journal* 26, no. 2 (2010): 157–62.

Moscucci, Ornella. *The Science of Woman: Gynaecology and Gender in England, 1800–1929.* Cambridge: Cambridge University Press, 1990.

"A Mother." "Infectious Diseases Notification Bills." *Journal of Vigilance Association for Defence of Personal Rights* 16 (April 15, 1882): 39–40.

Murchison, Charles. *A Treatise on the Continued Fevers of Great Britain.* London: Parker, Son, and Bourn, 1862.

Murphy, Shirley Forster, ed. *Our Homes, and How to Make Them Healthy.* London: Cassell, 1883.

Murray, Ross. *The Modern Householder: A Manual of Domestic Economy in All Its Branches.* London: F. Warne; New York: Scribner, Welford, and Armstrong, 1872.

Musher, Daniel M., Edward A. Dominguez, and Ariel Bar-Sela. "Edouard Seguin and the Social Power of Thermometry." *New England Journal of Medicine* 316, no. 2 (1987): 115–17.

Muthesius, Stefan. *The English Terraced House.* New Haven, CT: Yale University Press, 1982.

Napier, James. *A Manual of Dyeing and Dyeing Receipts.* 3rd ed. London: Charles Griffin and Co., 1875.

"Nemo." "Medical and Administrative Despotism." *Journal of the Vigilance Association for the Defence of Personal Rights* 19 (July 15, 1882): 67–69.

Nevett, T. "Advertising and Editorial Integrity in the Nineteenth Century." In *The Press in English Society from the Seventeenth to Nineteenth Centuries*, edited by Michael Harris and Alan J. Lee, 154–64. Cranbury, NJ: Fairleigh Dickinson University Press, 1986.

Newsholme, Arthur. "The Bearing of School Attendance upon Infectious Disease." *Sanitary Record* 12 (September 15, 1890): 107.

———. "Four and a Half Years' Experience of the Voluntary Notification of Pulmonary Tuberculosis." *Journal of the Sanitary Institute* 24 (1903): 253–60.

———. *Hygiene: A Manual of Personal and Public Health.* London: George Gill, 1902.

———. "A National System of Notification and Registration of Sickness." *Journal of the Royal Statistical Society* 59, no. 1 (1896): 1–37.

———. "A National System of Notification of Sickness." *Public Health* 8 (October 1895–September 1896): 106–8.

———. "The Prevalence of Diphtheria, in London and Elsewhere, and Its Alleged Connection with the Elementary Schools." *Public Health* 8 (October 1895–September 1896): 338–40.

———. *School Hygiene: The Laws of Health in Relation to School Life.* London: Swan Sonnenschein, Lowrey & Co., 1887.

Newsholme, Arthur, and James Kerr. *Newsholme's School Hygiene: The Laws of Health in Relation to School Life.* New 14th ed. London: 1916.

Newsholme, Arthur, and T. H. C. Stevenson. "The Decline of Human Fertility in the United Kingdom and Other Countries as Shown by Corrected Birth-Rates." *Journal of the Royal Statistical Society* 69, no. 1 (1906): 34–87.

Newsom Kerr, Matthew L. "Fevered Metropolis: Epidemic Disease and Isolation in Victorian London." PhD diss., University of Southern California, 2007.

———. "'Perambulating Fever Nests of Our London Streets': Cabs, Omnibuses, Ambulances, and Other 'Pest-Vehicles' in the Victorian Metropolis." *Journal of British Studies* 49, no. 2 (April 2010): 283–310.

Niemi, Marjaana. *Public Health and Municipal Policy Making: Britain and Sweden, 1900–1940.* Aldershot, UK: Ashgate, 2006.

Niven, James. "A Discussion on the Relation of Phthisis to Factory and Workshop Conditions." *British Medical Journal* 2176 (September 13, 1902): 761–66.

———. "The Notification of Tuberculosis," pt. 1. *Lancet* 149 (April 17, 1897): 1116.

———. "The Notification of Tuberculosis," pt. 2. *Lancet* 149 (May 1, 1897): 1196–99.

———. *Observations on the History of Public Health Effort in Manchester.* Manchester: City of Manchester, 1923.

———. "On the Notification of Phthisis in Manchester." *Journal of the Sanitary Institute* 25, no. 3 (1903): 266–75.

———. "On Municipal Administrative Measures in Connection with Tuberculosis." *Tuberculosis* 1, no. 5 (October 1900): 185–96.

———. "On the Prevention of Phthisis." *Public Health* 5 (October 1892–September 1893): 195–202.

Noble, Daniel. *On Fluctuations in the Death Rate, with a Glance at the Causes, Having Especial Reference to the Supposed Influence of the Cotton Famine on Recent Mortality.* Manchester: Cave & Sever, 1863.

North, S. W. "Registration of Disease." *Sanitary Record* 8 (May 24, 1878): 321–22.

"Notification of Measles I." *Public Health* 9 (October 1896–September 1897): 301.

"Notification of Measles II." *Public Health* 10 (October 1897–September 1898): 124.

Novak, Steven J. "Professionalism and Bureaucracy: English Doctors and the Victorian Public Health Administration." *Journal of Social History* 6 (1973): 440–61.

Novy, Frederick G. *Laboratory Work in Bacteriology.* 2nd ed. Ann Arbor, MI: G. Wahr, 1899.

Novy, Frederick G., and H. H. Waite. "The Disinfection of Rooms." *Medical News* 72, no. 21 (May 21, 1898): 641–52.

Oddy, D. J. "Urban Famine in Nineteenth-Century Britain: The Effect of the Lancashire Cotton Famine on Working-Class Diet and Health." *Economic History Review* 36, no. 1 (1983): 68–86.

Ogborn, Miles. "Law and Discipline in Nineteenth-Century English State Formation: The Contagious Diseases Acts of 1864, 1866 and 1869." *Journal of Historical Sociology* 6 (1993): 28–55.

Osborne, Thomas, and Nikolas Rose. "Governing Cities: Notes on the Spatialisation of Virtue." *Environment and Planning D: Society and Space* 17 (1999): 737–60.

Otter, Christopher. *The Victorian Eye: A Political History of Light and Vision in Britain, 1800–1910.* Chicago: University of Chicago Press, 2008.

Paget, Charles. "The Prevention of Phthisis." *Public Health* 5 (October 1892–September 1893): 307–8.

———. *Wasted Records of Disease.* London: Edward Arnold, 1897.

Parker, R. W. "Isolation and Scarlet Fever." *British Medical Journal* 1410 (January 7, 1888): 42–43.

Parkes, Louis C. *Infectious Diseases: Notification and Prevention.* London: H. K. Lewis, 1894.

———. "The Prevention of Phthisis." *Public Health* 5 (October 1892–September 1893): 308–9.

———. "The Prevention of Phthisis: A Critique of Dr. Niven's Paper and of the Memorandum of the North-Western Branch." *Public Health* 5 (October 1892–September 1893): 246–47.

Parkes, Louis C., and Henry R. Kenwood. *Hygiene and Public Health.* Lewis's Practical Series. London: H. K. Lewis, 1901.

Parsons, H. Franklin. "A Discussion on Isolation and Disinfection, with Special Reference to the Control of Epidemics." *British Medical Journal* 1496 (August 31, 1889): 452–55.

———. *Extracts from the Annual Report of the Medical Officer of the Local Government Board for 1884: Disinfection by Heat.* London: Eyre and Spottiswoode, HMSO, 1886.

Paterson, M. S., and F. C. Shrubsall. "Hints for the Consumptive at Home." *Tuberculosis* 4, no. 3 (November 1906): 140–45.

———. "The Home Treatment of the Consumptive Invalid." *Tuberculosis* 4, no. 4 (February 1907): 178–84.

Pearmain, Thomas Hames, R. Tanner Hewlett, and Cresacre George Moor. *Applied Bacteriology: An Elementary Handbook for the Use of Students of Hygiene, Medical Officers of Health, and Analysts.* 3rd ed. London: Bailliere, Tindall and Cox, 1906.

Pearson, S. Vere. "Observations on the Working of 'Sanatorium Benefit.'" *British Journal of Tuberculosis* 8, no. 1 (January 1914): 8–15.

Pelling, Margaret. *Cholera, Fever and English Medicine, 1825–1865.* Oxford: Oxford University Press, 1978.

Pennybacker, Susan D. *A Vision for London, 1889–1914: Labour, Everyday Life and the LCC Experiment.* London: Routledge, 1995.

Perry, C. R. *The Victorian Post Office: The Growth of a Bureaucracy.* London: Royal Historical Society, 1992.

Peterson, M. Jeanne. *The Medical Profession in Mid-Victorian London.* Berkeley: University of California Press, 1978.

Philipson, George Hare. *On the Investigation of the Prevalent Diseases of the District by Means of Registration.* Newcastle-upon-Tyne: Northumberland and Durham Medical Society, 1863.

Pickstone, John V. *Medicine and Industrial Society: A History of Hospital Development in Manchester and Its Region, 1752–1946.* Manchester: Manchester University Press, 1985.

Platt, Harold L. "From Hygeia to the Garden City: Bodies, Houses, and the Rediscovery of the Slum in Manchester, 1875–1910." *Journal of Urban History* 33, no. 5 (2007): 756–72.

———. *Shock Cities: The Environmental Transformation and Reform of Manchester and Chicago.* Chicago: University of Chicago Press, 2005.

Pollard, Bailie James. "The Fever Hospitals of Europe." *The Sanitary Journal: A Journal of Hygiene and Public Health,* 3rd ser., 3 (June 1896): 198–209.

Pooley, Siân. "'All We Parents Want Is That Our Children's Health and Lives Should Be Regarded': Child Health and Parental Concern in England, c. 1860–1910." *Social History of Medicine* 23 (2010): 528–48.

Poovey, Mary. *A History of the Modern Fact: Problems of Knowledge in the Sciences of Wealth and Society.* Chicago: University of Chicago Press, 1998.

———. *Making a Social Body: British Cultural Formation, 1830–1864.* Chicago: University of Chicago Press, 1995.

Porter, Dorothy. "'Enemies of the Race': Biologism, Environmentalism, and Public Health in Victorian England." *Victorian Studies* 34 (1991): 159–78.

———. *Health, Civilization, and the State: A History of Public Health from Ancient to Modern Times.* London: Routledge, 1999.

———. "Stratification and Its Discontents: Professionalisation and Conflict in the British Public Health Service, 1848–1914." In *A History of Education in Public Health: Health That Mocks the Doctors' Rules,* edited by Elizabeth Fee and Roy M. Acheson. Oxford: Oxford University Press, 1991.

Porter, Dorothy, and Roy Porter. "The Enforcement of Health: The British Debate." In *AIDS: The Burdens of History,* edited by Elizabeth Fee and Daniel M. Fox, 97–120. Berkeley: University of California Press, 1988.

———. "The Politics of Prevention: Anti-vaccinationism and Public Health in Nineteenth-Century England." *Medical History* 32 (1988): 231–52.

Porter, Ian A., and Michael J. Williams. *Epidemic Diseases in Aberdeen and the History of the City Hospital.* Aberdeen History of Medicine Publications No. 2. Aberdeen, UK, 2001.

Porter, Roy. "Medical Futures." *Notes and Records of the Royal Society* 55 (2001): 309–23.

Powell, Richard C. "Geographies of Science: Histories, Localities, Practices, Futures." *Progress in Human Geography* 31, no. 3 (2007): 309–29.

Poyntz Wright, T. "On the Use of the 'Equifex Spray Disinfector,' for the Effective Disinfection of Rooms and Houses, as a Substitute for the Fumigation by Sulphurous Acid Gas." *Public Health* 9 (October 1896–September 1897): 63–65.

Prest, John M. *Liberty and Locality: Parliament, Permissive Legislation, and Ratepayers' Democracies in the Nineteenth Century.* Oxford: Clarendon Press, 1990.

Priestley, Joseph. "Disinfectors and Disinfectants, 1874–95: A Contrast." *Sanitary Record*, n.s., 17 (1895–96): 18–23.

Pugh, Martin. "The Limits of Liberalism: Liberals and Women's Suffrage, 1867–1914." In Biagini, *Citizenship and Community*, 45–65.

Ransom, W. H. "Disinfection by Heat." *British Medical Journal* 702 (June 13, 1874): 788–89.

———. "On the Mode of Disinfecting by Heat." *British Medical Journal* 662 (September 6, 1873): 274–75.

Ransome, Arthur. *Campaign against Consumption: A Collection of Papers Relating to Tuberculosis*. Cambridge: Cambridge University Press, 1915.

———. "Consumption, a 'Filth Disease.'" *Lancet* 151 (January 1, 1898): 14–17.

———. "The Crusade against Tuberculosis." *Lancet* 167 (June 16, 1906): 1714–15.

———. "On the Need for Combined Medical Observation." *British Medical Journal* 197 (October 8, 1864): 405–8.

———. "The Prevention of Phthisis." *Public Health* 5 (October 1892–September 1893): 284.

———. "Sanitation v. Tuberculosis." *Tuberculosis* 1, no. 3 (April 1900): 97–101.

———. "The Scientific and Practical Objects of the Registration of Disease." *British Medical Journal* 1133 (September 16, 1882): 505–7.

———. "Some Evidence Respecting Tubercular Infective Areas." *Transactions of the Epidemiological Society of London*, n.s., 6 (1886–87): 124–36.

Ravenhill, Alice. "Hygiene and Household Economics." In *The Nation's Need: Chapters on Education*, edited by Spenser Wilkinson, 75–106. Westminster: Archibald Constable & Co., 1903.

Raw, Nathan. "The Compulsory Notification of Tuberculosis." *Lancet* 170 (October 26, 1907): 1150–52.

———. "International Congress against Tuberculosis." *Tuberculosis* 4, no. 4 (1907): 185–88.

Reid, George. *Practical Sanitation: A Handbook for Sanitary Inspectors and Others Interested in Sanitation*. 13th ed. London: Charles Griffin and Co., 1906.

Reinarz, Jonathan, and Leonard Schwarz. *Medicine and the Workhouse*. Rochester, NY: University of Rochester Press, 2013.

Richardson, Benjamin Ward. *Hygeia: A City of Health*. London: Macmillan, 1876.

———. *A Ministry of Health and Other Addresses*. London: Chatto and Windus, 1879.

Richardson, Harriet. *English Hospitals 1660–1948: A Survey of Their Architecture and Design*. Swindon, UK: Royal Commission on the Historical Monuments of England, 1998.

Richardson, Nigel. *Typhoid in Uppingham: Analysis of a Victorian Town and School in Crisis, 1875–1877*. London: Pickering & Chatto, 2008.

Rideal, Samuel. *Disinfection and Disinfectants: Together with an Account of the Chemical Substances Used as Antiseptics and Preservatives*. London: Charles Griffin and Co., 1895.

———. "Formaldehyde Disinfection." *Public Health* 10 (October 1897–September 1898): 60–62.

Rideal, Samuel, and J. T. Ainslie Walker. "Standardisation of Disinfectants." *Journal of the Sanitary Institute* 24, no. 3 (January 1, 1903): 424–41.

Roberts, M. J. D. "Feminism and the State in Later Victorian England." *Historical Journal* 38, no. 1 (1995): 85–110.

Roberts, Nathan. "Character in the Mind: Citizenship, Education and Psychology in Britain, 1880–1914." *History of Education* 33, no. 2 (2004): 177–97.

Robertson, A. B. "Children, Teachers and Society: The Over-Pressure Controversy, 1880–1886." *British Journal of Educational Studies* 20, no. 3 (1972): 315–23.

Robertson, Stuart. "'The Terrible Scourge of Consumption Is amongst Us': The Guild of Help, Voluntarism and the Problem of Tuberculosis in Edwardian Bolton." In *Social Conditions, Status and Community, 1860–c. 1920*, edited by Keith Laybourn, 45–65. Stroud, UK: Sutton, 1997.

Robertson, William. "A New Form of Spray Apparatus." *Public Health* 15 (October 1902): 477–80.

Rockey, John. "From Vision to Reality: Victorian Ideal Cities and Model Towns in the Genesis of Ebenezer Howard's Garden City." *Town Planning Review* 54, no. 1 (January 1983): 83–105.

Rodrick, Anne B. *Self-Help and Civic Culture: Citizenship in Victorian Birmingham.* Aldershot, UK: Ashgate, 2004.

Rogers, Joseph. *Reminiscences of a Workhouse Medical Officer.* Edited, with a preface, by Prof. Thorold Rogers. London: T. Fisher Unwin, 1889.

Roll-Hansen, Nils. "Experimental Method and Spontaneous Generation: The Controversy between Pasteur and Pouchet, 1859–64." *Journal of the History of Medicine and Allied Sciences* 34, no. 3 (July 1, 1979): 273–92.

Rose, Nikolas. *Powers of Freedom: Reframing Political Thought.* Cambridge: Cambridge University Press, 1999.

Rosen, George. *A History of Public Health.* Expanded ed. Baltimore: Johns Hopkins University Press, 1993.

Rosenberg, Charles E. *The Care of Strangers: The Rise of America's Hospital System.* Baltimore: Johns Hopkins University Press, 1987.

———. "Health in the Home: A Tradition of Print and Practice." In *Right Living: An Anglo-American Tradition of Self-Help Medicine and Hygiene*, edited by Charles E. Rosenberg, 1–20. Baltimore: Johns Hopkins University Press, 2003.

Rosenkrantz, Barbara Gutmann. *Public Health and the State: Changing Views in Massachusetts, 1842–1936.* Cambridge, MA: Harvard University Press, 1972.

Rothman, Sheila M. *Living in the Shadow of Death: Tuberculosis and the Social Experience of Illness in America.* New York: Basic Books, 1994.

Rubinstein, David. "Socialization and the London School Board 1870–1904: Aims, Methods and Public Opinion." In *Popular Education and Socialization in the Nineteenth Century*, edited by Phillip McCann, 231–64. London: Methuen, 1977.

Rumsey, Henry W. *Essays and Papers on Some Fallacies of Statistics Concerning Life and Death, Health and Disease, with Suggestions towards an Improved System of Registration.* London: Smith, Elder and Co., 1875.

———. *Essays on State Medicine.* London: J. Churchill, 1856.

Rundle, C., and A. H. G. Burton. "The Bed Isolation of Cases of Infectious Disease." *Lancet* 179 (March 16, 1912): 720–21.

Russell, James Burn. "On Disinfection." *Glasgow Medical Journal* 22 (1884): 410–12.

Russell, James Burn, and Archibald Kerr Chalmers. *Public Health Administration in Glasgow: A Memorial Volume of the Writings of James Burn Russell.* Glasgow: J. Maclehose, 1905.

Russell, Rollo. "A Department of Health." *Nineteenth Century* 29, no. 170 (March 1, 1891): 615–23.

Rydz, D. L. *The Parliamentary Agents: A History.* London: Royal Historical Society, 1979.

Schweber, Libby. *Disciplining Statistics: Demography and Vital Statistics in France and England, 1830–1885.* Durham, NC: Duke University Press, 2006.

Scott, James C. *Seeing like a State: How Certain Schemes to Improve the Human Condition Have Failed.* New Haven, CT: Yale University Press, 1998.

Searle, G. R. *The Quest for National Efficiency: A Study in British Politics and Political Thought, 1899–1914.* Berkeley: University of California Press, 1971.

Seaton, Edward Cox. "Clinical Instruction at Fever Hospitals in Connection with the Operation of the Compulsory Notification Act." *British Medical Journal* 1548 (August 30, 1890): 501–2.

Shann, G. "On the Disinfecting Property of Heat." *Transactions of the National Association for the Promotion of Social Science, 1857* (1864): 558–63.

Sheard, Sally. "Reluctant Providers? The Politics and Ideology of Municipal Hospital Finance 1870–1914." In *Financing Medicine: The British Experience since 1750,* edited by Martin Gorsky and Sally Sheard, 112–29. Abingdon, UK: Routledge, 2006.

Sheller, Mimi, and John Urry. *Mobile Technologies of the City.* London: Routledge, 2006.

———. "Mobile Transformations of 'Public' and 'Private' Life." *Theory, Culture & Society* 20, no. 3 (2003): 107–25.

Shepherd, John A. *A History of the Liverpool Medical Institution.* Liverpool: Liverpool Medical Institution, 1979.

Shrubsall, F. C. "The Selection of Patients for Sanatorium Treatment." *Public Health* 26 (October 1912–September 1913): 230–36.

Sigsworth, E. Michael, and Michael Worboys. "The Public's View of Public Health in Mid-Victorian Britain." *Urban History* 21, no. 2 (1994): 237–50.

Sigsworth, E. Michael, and T. J. Wyke. "A Study of Victorian Prostitution and Venereal Disease." In *Suffer and Be Still: Women in the Victorian Age,* edited by Martha Vicinus, 77–99. Bloomington: Indiana University Press, 1972.

Silver, Pamela, and Harold Silver. *The Education of the Poor: The History of a National School 1824–1974.* London: Routledge & Kegan Paul, 1974.

Simon, John. *English Sanitary Institutions, Reviewed in Their Course of Development, and in Some of Their Political and Social Relations.* 2nd ed. London: Smith, Elder, 1897.

Slater, Charles, and Samuel Rideal. "On Formaldehyde as an Antiseptic." *Lancet* 143 (April 21, 1894): 1004–6.

*Slater's General and Classified Directory and Street Register of Manchester and Salford.* Manchester: Isaac Slater, 1863.

Smiles, Samuel. *Happy Homes and the Hearts That Make Them; or, Thrifty People and Why They Thrive.* Carefully revised, with additional matter, by Chas. A. Gaskell. Chicago: US Pub. House, 1883.

Smith, Edmund M. "The Notification of Infectious Diseases at Present Not Notifiable, and the Need for Medical Officers of Schools." *Quarterly Medical Journal (Yorkshire and Adjacent Counties)* 10 (1901–2): 203–8.

Smith, Francis B. "The Contagious Diseases Acts Reconsidered." *Social History of Medicine* 3 (1990): 197–215.

———. *The People's Health 1830 to 1910.* New York: Holmes & Meier, 1979.

Spalding, Thomas A. *The Work of the London School Board.* London: P. S. King and Son, 1900.

Speake, Stephen W. "Infectious Milk: Issues of Pathogenic Certainty within Ideational Regimes and Their Biopolitical Implications." *Studies in History and Philosophy of Science Part C: Studies in History and Philosophy of Biological and Biomedical Sciences* 42, no. 4 (2011): 530–41.

Spear, John. "Public Elementary Schools and the Spread of Infectious Disease." *Sanitary Record* 10 (January 17, 1879): 33–35.

Spottiswoode Cameron, J. "Disinfectants." *Transactions of the Sanitary Institute of Great Britain* 18 (1897): 397–402.

Stannard, Kevin P. "Ideology, Education, and Social Structure: Elementary Schooling in Mid-Victorian England." *History of Education* 19, no. 2 (1990): 105–22.

Steedman, Carolyn. *Childhood, Culture, and Class in Britain: Margaret McMillan, 1860–1931.* New Brunswick, NJ: Rutgers University Press, 1990.

Steele, David. "Stanley, Edward Henry, Fifteenth Earl of Derby (1826–1893)." In *Oxford Dictionary of National Biography.* http://www.oxforddnb.com/view/article/26266.

Stirland, R. M. "Auguste Sheridan Delépine, 1855–1921." In *Some Manchester Doctors: A Biographical Collection to Mark the 150th Anniversary of the Manchester Medical Society,* edited by Willis J. Elwood and A. Felicite Tuxford, 107–12. Manchester: Manchester University Press, 1984.

Sturdy, Steve. "The Political Economy of Scientific Medicine: Science, Education and the Transformation of Medical Practice in Sheffield, 1890–1922." *Medical History* 36 (1992): 125–59.

Sutherland, Gillian. *Policy-making in Elementary Education, 1870–1895.* Oxford: Oxford University Press, 1973.

Swales, J. D. "The Leicester Anti-vaccination Movement." *Lancet* 340 (October 24, 1992): 1019–21.

Sykes, John F. J. "Measles and Elementary Schools." *Public Health* 24 (October 1910–September 1911): 467–76.

———. "Mothercraft." *Journal of the Royal Sanitary Institute* 31 (1910): 573–88.

———. "Notification of Measles." *Public Health* 8 (October 1895–September 1896): 199.

———. "On Organisation and Administration of Infectious Diseases." *Sanitary Record,* n.s., 8 (1886): 159.

Szreter, Simon R. S. *Fertility, Class and Gender in Britain, 1860–1940.* Cambridge: Cambridge University Press, 1996.

———. "The GRO and the Public Health Movement in Britain, 1837–1914." *Social History of Medicine* 4 (1991): 435–63.

Tatham, John. "On the Compulsory Notification of Infectious Diseases." *Practitioner* 41 (1888): 472–80.

Taylor, Albert. *The Sanitary Inspector's Handbook.* 3rd ed. London: H. K. Lewis, 1901.

Teller, Michael E. *The Tuberculosis Movement: A Public Health Campaign in the Progressive Era.* New York: Greenwood Press, 1988.

Thacker, Stephen B. "Historical Development." In *Principles and Practice of Public Health Surveillance*, edited by Lisa M. Lee, Steven M. Teutsch, Stephen B. Thacker, and Michael E. St. Louis, 1–17. New York: Oxford University Press, 2010.

Thackray, Arnold. "Natural Knowledge in Cultural Context: The Manchester Mode." *American Historical Review* 79, no. 3 (1974): 672–709.

Thomson, Anthony Todd. *The Domestic Management of the Sick-Room: Necessary, in Aid of Medical Treatment, for the Cure of Diseases.* London: Longman, Orme, Brown, Green & Longmans, 1841.

Thomson, Henry Hyslop. "Insurance and Sanatorium Benefits." *British Journal of Tuberculosis* 6, no. 4 (October 1912): 248–49.

———. "The Problem of Tuberculosis." *Lancet* 190 (August 18, 1917): 251–53.

———. *Consumption, Its Prevention and Home Treatment: A Guide for the Use of Patients.* Oxford Medical Publications. London: Oxford University Press, 1911.

———. *Tuberculosis, Its Prevention and Home Treatment: A Guide for the Use of Patients.* Oxford Medical Publications. 3rd ed. London: Oxford University Press, 1928. Originally published as *Consumption, Its Prevention and Home Treatment: A Guide for the Use of Patients* (1911).

Thresh, John C. "Portable Spraying Disinfecting Apparatus." *Public Health* 14 (October 1901–September 1902): 625.

———. "Steam from Saline Solutions, with Special Reference to Its Disinfecting Powers." *Public Health* 9 (October 1896–September 1897): 131–34.

Tomes, Nancy. *The Gospel of Germs: Men, Women, and the Microbe in American Life.* Cambridge, MA: Harvard University Press, 1998.

Topley, W. W. C., and G. S. Wilson. "The Spread of Bacterial Infection: The Problem of Herd-Immunity." *Journal of Hygiene* 21, no. 3 (May 1923): 243–49.

Tosh, John. *A Man's Place: Masculinity and the Middle-Class Home in Victorian England.* New Haven, CT: Yale University Press, 1999.

Tuan, Yi-Fu. "A View of Geography." *Geographical Review* 81, no. 1 (1991): 99–107.

———. *Space and Place: The Perspective of Experience.* Minneapolis: University of Minnesota Press, 1977.

Twelvetrees, W. Noble. "Disinfection: Physical, Chemical, and Mechanical," pt. 2. *Sanitary Record*, n.s., 19 (1897): 505–7.

Ugolini, Laura. "Men, Masculinities, and Menswear Advertising, c. 1890–1914." In *A Nation of Shopkeepers: Five Centuries of British Retailing*, edited by John Benson and Laura Ugolini, 80–104. London: I. B. Tauris, 2003.

Vallin, E. "The Compulsory Notification of Measles and Infectious Pneumonia." *Public Health* 12 (October 1900–September 1901): 802–7.

Valverde, Mariana. "Despotism and Ethical Liberal Government." *Economy and Society* 25, no. 3 (1996): 357–72.

Vincent, David. *Poor Citizens: The State and the Poor in Twentieth-Century Britain.* London: Longman, 1991.

Waddington, Ivan. *The Medical Profession in the Industrial Revolution.* Dublin: Gill and Macmillan, 1984.

Waddington, Keir. *The Bovine Scourge: Meat, Tuberculosis and Public Health, 1850–1914.* Woodbridge, UK: Boydell Press, 2006.

Wahrman, Dror. *Imagining the Middle Class: The Political Representation of Class in Britain, c. 1780–1840.* Cambridge: Cambridge University Press, 1995.

Waldo, F. J., and David Walsh. "Murder by Measles." *Nineteenth Century* 39, no. 232 (June 1, 1896): 957–63.

Walkowitz, Judith R. *Prostitution and Victorian Society: Women, Class, and the State.* Cambridge: Cambridge University Press, 1980.

Wallis, Patrick. "Richardson, Sir Benjamin Ward (1828–1896)." In *Oxford Dictionary of National Biography.* http://www.oxforddnb.com/view/article/23544.

Ward, H. Marshall. "Experiments on the Action of Light on Bacillus Anthracis." *Proceedings of the Royal Society of London* 52 (1892): 393–400.

———. "Further Experiments on the Action of Light on Bacillus Anthracis." *Proceedings of the Royal Society of London* 53 (1893): 23–44.

Watkins, Dorothy. "The English Revolution in Social Medicine, 1889–1911." PhD diss., University of London, 1984.

Weindling, Paul. "From Isolation to Therapy: Children's Hospitals and Diphtheria in *Fin de Siècle* Paris, London and Berlin." In *In the Name of the Child: Health and Welfare, 1880–1940,* edited by Roger Cooter, 124–45. London: Routledge, 1992.

Welshman, John. "'Bringing Beauty and Brightness to the Back Streets': Health Education and Public Health in England and Wales, 1890–1940." *Health Education Journal* 56, no. 2 (1997): 199–209.

———. "Child Health, National Fitness, and Physical Education in Britain, 1900–1940." In *Cultures of Child Health in Britain and the Netherlands in the Twentieth Century,* edited by Marijke Gijswijt-Hofstra and Hilary Marland, 61–84. Clio Medica/The Wellcome Series in the History of Medicine. Amsterdam: Rodopi, 2003

Whitbread, Nanette. *The Evolution of the Nursery-Infant School.* Hoboken, NJ: Taylor and Francis, 2013.

White, Melanie, and Alan Hunt. "Citizenship: Care of the Self, Character and Personality." *Citizenship Studies* 4, no. 2 (July 1, 2000): 93–116.

Whitelegge, Arthur, and George Newman. *Hygiene and Public Health.* 12th ed. London: Cassell, 1911.

Whyte, Rebecca. "Changing Approaches to Disinfection in England, 1848–1914." PhD diss., University of Cambridge, 2012.

Wilkinson [now Hardy], Anne. "The Beginnings of Disease Control in London: The Work of the Medical Officers in Three Parishes, 1856–1900." PhD diss., University of Oxford, 1980.

Williamson, David J. "The Future of Dispensary and Domiciliary Management of Tuberculosis." *British Journal of Tuberculosis* 7, no. 1 (January 1913): 25–29.

Wohl, Anthony S. *Endangered Lives: Public Health in Victorian Britain.* Cambridge, MA: Harvard University Press, 1983.

Woods, Robert I. *The Demography of Victorian England and Wales.* Cambridge: Cambridge University Press, 2000.

Woodward, John H. "The School Medical Officer before the School Medical Service: England and Wales, 1850–1908." In *Coping with Sickness: Historical Aspects of Health Care in a European Perspective,* edited by John H. Woodward and Robert Jütte, 121–46. Sheffield, UK: European Association for the History of Medicine and Health, 1995.

Worboys, Michael. "Before McKeown: Explaining the Decline of Tuberculosis in Britain, 1880–1930." In *Tuberculosis Then and Now: Perspectives on the History of an Infectious Disease*, edited by Flurin Condrau and Michael Worboys, 148–70. Montreal: McGill-Queen's University Press, 2010.

———. "Delépine, Auguste Sheridan (1855–1921)." In *Oxford Dictionary of National Biography*. http://www.oxforddnb.com/view/article/57113.

———. "Practice and the Science of Medicine in the Nineteenth Century." *Isis* 102, no. 1 (2011): 109–15.

———. "The Sanatorium Treatment for Consumption in Britain, 1890–1914." In *Medical Innovations in Historical Perspective*, edited by John Pickstone, 47–71. New York: St. Martin's Press, 1992.

———. *Spreading Germs: Disease Theories and Medical Practice in Britain, 1865–1900.* Cambridge: Cambridge University Press, 2000.

Wright, C. N. *Commercial and General Directory of Leicester and Six Miles Round.* 5th ed. Leicester, 1880.

Wynne, Fred E. "Dispensary Supervision in Pulmonary Tuberculosis." *Lancet* 192 (November 16, 1918): 680–81.

Yeatman, John Pym. "The Slanders Uttered in the Nottingham Town Council." *Nottingham Daily Express*, April 8, 1891.

Young, Albion G. *Notes on Disinfectants and Disinfection.* Augusta, ME: Kennebec Journal Print, 1898.

Young, Meredith. "The Removal and Isolation of Infectious Patients in Populous Districts." *Journal of the Sanitary Institute* 24, no. 1 (January 1, 1903): 41–70.1.

# *Index*

Page numbers in italics refer to illustrations and graphs. For abbreviations used in subentries, please see the Abbreviations list on page xiii; as well, please note that in subentries, "TB" refers to tuberculosis, and "notification" refers to infectious disease notification.


Aberdare Hospital (Wales), 86
Académie des Sciences (Paris), 136–37
Alcester Hospital, 86, 87, 89
American Public Health Association, 140
Anti-compulsion Society, 61
antivaccination movement, 3, 42, 45–46, 48, 56, 61, 78; in Leicester, 43, 57–58, 80
Army Medical Department: Farr's work with, 24–26
Association of Metropolitan Medical Officers of Health (later SMOH), 23, 30, 31, 137. *See also* Society of Medical Officers of Health
Association of Municipal Corporations, 47, 50
attendance officers (AOs), school board, 100, 101–2, 103, 112, 116, 119

bacteriology: and diphtheria, 82, 98, 103, 107, 110, 120; and disinfection, 19, 124–25, 136–37, 143–47, 219n82; vs efficacy of infectious disease surveillance, 5, 6–7, 8, 14, 19; Koch's work in, 124, 139, 143, 145, 154; and school medical policies, 96, 103, 107, 110, 119–20; as source of income for medical schools, 160
Bagthorpe Hospital (Nottingham), 74, 75, 79, 82, 91
Baldwin, Peter, 7, 19, 64, 124, 125, 143, 152–53
Ballard, Edward, 31, 38
Bardswell, Noel: *Advice for Consumptives*, 165, 166, 168, 171, 172, 178, 230n112
Barnes, David, 7, 19, 125
Barry, Frederick, 219n66
Barwise, Sidney, 116
Bell, Jean, 89
Benham and Sons (disinfecting apparatus manufacturer), 140
Birmingham, 8; disinfection in, 125, 129, *130*, 143–44, *148*; hospitalization in, 73, 75, *76*, 77–78, 79, 82, 91; monitoring of schoolchildren in, 102, 104, 105; notification in, 12, 43, 47, 54–57, 58, 63, 64; scarlet fever in, 12, 55, 75, *76*, 77–78, 82, 91; smallpox epidemic in, 75, 129; and splits within elite families over notification, 56–57
Bligh, Alexander, 51–52
Board of Education, 93, 99; on care committees, 116–17; and Code of Regulations, 99, 106, 213n103; on combining MOH and SMO roles, 115, 214n140; and MOH access to schools, 102; on need for separate TB registers, 118; on starting age for schoolchildren, 112; on school closure/pupil exclusion, 112; and system of following-up, 115–17, 118, 119
Bolton, 118, 156; notification in, 2, 47, 48, 52–53

Bond, Francis, 128
Boobbyer, Philip, 91, 105–6, 157–58
Boston: board of health in, 1
Boyce, Herbert E., 160
Boyd, John, 102
Bradford, Thomas: steam disinfecting apparatus of, 138, *139*, 140
Braley, Francis, 79
Brighton (Mass.): abbatoir in, 1
Brighton (UK), 14. *See also* Newsholme, Arthur
British Doloment Company, hospital flooring made by, 81
*British Journal of Tuberculosis* (*BJTB*), 156, 172–78
British Medical Association (BMA): and Collective Investigation, 29, 38; and establishment of RSC, 23; on MOH access to schools, 102; and notification, 48, 49, 51–52, 53, 55, 58–59, 61–62, 63; Parliamentary Bills Committee of, 49, 58–59, 61; and Poor Law data collection, 35
Buchanan, George: on citizenship and notification, 1–2, 3, 6, 47, 179, 180, 183n10; and dispute with MSSA, 33; and LGB, 183n2; on need for isolation hospitals, 75
Burke, William, 23, 29
Burnie, Thomas, 79
Butler, Josephine, 52

Caiger, Foord, 85
Caius, John: *Boke or Counseill against the Disease commonly called the Sweate or Sweating Sickness*, 125
Cameron, Sir Charles, 129
carbolic acid (disinfectant), 126, 136, 143, 147, 221n116
care committees, and continued monitoring of schoolchildren, 116–17, 118, 119
Carpenter, Alfred, 14–15, 60, 153, 176
Carter, William, 52, 56, 61, 62, 63
certificates: diseases named on, 9; in dual notification system, 47; GPs' refusal to issue, 52; patients named on, 65; payments to GPs for, 47, 51, 55, 199n147; requesting disinfection, 127–28; for schoolchildren, 102–3, 106
Chadwick, Edwin, 32, 96, 122, 188n45
Chamberlain Joseph, 47, 55, 56, 198nn121–22
Chamberlain, Richard, 56, 198nn121–22
chicken pox, 85, 102, 112
children: cleaning of, 117, 215n155; Henry's vaccination experiments on, 136; hospital deaths of, 78, 79, 89; hospitalization of, 78–79, 84, 86–87, 89, *92*, 179, 180–81; recommended minimum school age for, 98, 112–13, 213n123; resistance to hospitalization of, 71–72, 75, 77, 78–81, 86–87, 92, 128; TB in, 107, 115, 118–19. *See also* contact tracing of schoolchildren; measles, *and entry following;* schools, *and entries following*
Children's Act (1908), 215n155
chloride of lime (disinfectant), 121, 126, 127, 143, 148, 221n107
cholera, 14, 24, 28, 32; disinfection against, 126, 127, 135–36, 139, 140; hospitals for, 12; London outbreak of (1849), 30; notification of, 47
citizenship, and relationship to public health/sanitation, 1–4, 6, 47, 61–62, 64, 179–82, 183n10; antivaccination movement and, 3, 42, 57; cleanliness/disinfection and, 122–23, 126, 161, 181; in home/domestic sphere, 93, 122–23; isolation hospitals and, 4, 12, 42, 57, 71, 181; as national/wartime duty, 93; and responsibility to state vs individual freedoms, 2–4; and working class/poor, 3, 32–33, 42, 78, 93–94, 122–23, 217n20
City Hospital (Edinburgh), 87
class: and citizenship, 3, 32–33, 42, 78, 93–94, 122–23, 217n20; and disinfection of home, 122–24, 126–27, 132–33, 140, 143, 145, 146–47, 149, 153; and home as locus

of infectious risk, 11, 32–33, 62–63, 96; and hospitalization, 42, 62-63, 70, 71–81, 87, 89; and monitoring of schoolchildren, 93–94, 96, 103, 110–11, 114–19, 120; and motherhood, 33, 80, 110–14, 120; and notification, 11, 29–34, 47, 62–63; and private practice, 62–63; and TB home care/therapy, 231n120; and TB notification/education campaigns, 156–57
Collective Investigation (BMA initiative), 29, 38
Collie, Alexander, 88
Combination Collapsible Ventilator Company, "CC" hospital windows made by, 81
Common Lodging Houses Acts, 46, 126; (1851), 45
consumer goods, as promoted to tuberculosis patients, 156, 172–78; through journal "puff pieces," 173–74, 175; and mail-order system, 174. *See also entry below*
consumer goods, as promoted to tuberculosis patients (specific): "Beb" Bath, and similar devices, 176; "Dumbnurse," 176, *177*; "Kumfee," 176, *177*; plasticine, 172, *173*, 175, 178; "Presto Thermometer," 175
consumption. *See* tuberculosis
contact tracing of schoolchildren, 4, 5–6, 13, 16, 120, 181; class aspects of, 110–11, 114–19; as facilitated by pupil exclusion, 110; and measles notification, 104–7; and measles study in Woolwich, 107–12; and "mothercraft," 112–14; SMS involvement in, 98, 114–19, 120; and system of following-up, 114–19; and TB notification, 119. *See also* measles, *and entry following;* schools, *and entries following*
Contagious Diseases Acts (1864, 1866, 1869), 3, 5, 42, 45, 46; opposition to, 45, 52, 61, 63; repeal of, 45, 52, 56, 70; Royal Commission on, 72–73
Contagious Diseases (Animals) Act (1869), 157
Crace-Calvert, Frederick, 136–37
Crane, Alfred W., 57–58, 103
Cropper, Henry S., 54
Crowe, Henry Warren: *Consumption: Treatment at Home and Rules for Living,* 165–66, 168, 170–72, 178, 224n7; appendix on breathing exercises in, 230n92; blank pages for doctor's use in, 170, 230n102; chart of a normal man in, 168, *170*
croup, 28, 103

Davies, Sydney, 107, 210n68
Delépine, A. Sheridan, 144–47. *See also* Ransome, Arthur
Deptford Hospital, 88
Derby, Edward Henry Stanley, Earl of, 69, 201n4
Dickens, Charles, 29–30
Dilke, Sir Charles, 61
diphtheria: antitoxin for, 107, 213n107; bacteriological testing for, 82, 98, 103, 107, 110, 120; in children, 12, 64, 86, 96, 97, 98, 103, 104, 107, 110, 120, 211n85; cleanliness/disinfection and, 14, 103, 127; deaths from, 75, 104; first English cases of, 188n61; hospitalization for, 12, 75, *76*, 82, 86, 159, 202n14; notification of, 40, *76*, 97, 103
disinfection: in hospitals, 81, 87, 88, 128, 131, 136, 138–39, 149; of hospital visitors, 88; in lodging houses, 45, 126
disinfection of homes, 5–6, 13–14, 16, 21, 75, 121–53; bacteriology and, 19, 124–25, 136–37, 143–47, 219n82; child illness and, 103, 104–5, 115; against cholera, 126, 127, 135–36, 139, 140; class aspects of, 122–24, 126–27, 132–33, 140, 143, 145, 146–47, 149, 153; citizenship and, 122–23, 126, 161, 181; as concern of urban life, 126–29; and disinfection of clothes/bedding, 45, 121, 124,

disinfection of homes—*(cont'd)* 126, 127, 128, 129, 133–36, 138, 140, 154; domestic space/privacy and, 121–24, 126, 127–28, 133, 135, 153; early guidelines/procedures for, 125–29; ensuring acceptance of, 132–33, 135, 153; experiments in, 135–53; and hospital capacity, 124, 128, 129; and inventory/treatment of householders' items, 132–33, 135, 153; and laboratory as "domestic" space, 143–53; legislation enabling, 41, 127–28, 129, 131; machinery for, 136–43; methods/substances used in, 121, 125, 126, 127, 135–49, 152, 154; MOHs and, 129, 142, 144, 149; notification and, 40–41, 57, 104, 127–28, 131, 132, 143–44, *144*, 153; safety concerns of, 135, 143, 148–49, 221n116; scholarship on, 124–25; as self-regulated/easily managed, 132–43, 153; statistics on, 129, *130*, 131–32, 133, 134, 143–44, *144*; in TB cases, 140, 144–46, 153, 154–55, 157, 158, 161, 162, 182; varying local approaches to, 130–31. *See also entries below*

disinfection of homes, machinery for *(by name/type)*, 136–43; Bradford (steam), 138, *139*, 140; Equifex (spray), 149, *152*; Fraser (dry-heat), 137–38, *138*, 140; Goddard (steam), 140–41, 221n103; Henry (dry-heat), 136, *137*, 138; Lumley (spray-pump), 149; Lyon (steam), 139–41, *141*; Mackenzie (spray-pump), 149, *150–51*, 179; Ransom (dry-heat stove), 138–39; Reynolds and Branson (spray-pump), 149; Thresh (steam), 142, *142*

disinfection of homes, methods/substances used in: carbolic acid, 126, 136, 143, 147, 221n116; chloride of lime, 121, 126, 127, 143, 148, 221n107; dough/breadcrumbs, 149, 222n134; dry heat, 127, 136–39, 140; formalin spray, 147–49, 154; fumigation, 121, 125, 126, 127, 131, 143–47, 149, 152, 154, 157; soap/water wash, 121, 127; steam, 131, 139–42, 148, 154

Dodson, John, 48

Downes, Arthur, and Thomas Blunt, 145

Dreschfeld, Julius, 144

Druitt, Robert, 23

dry heat disinfection, 127, 136–39; by Fraser, 137–38, *138*, 140; by Henry, 136, *137*, 138; by Ransom, 138–39

dual notification, 47, 48, 49–50, 51–52, 53, 61, 207n129. *See also* householders, notification duty of

Duncan, William Henry, 30, 34, 188n45

dysentery, 28

Edmonds, Thomas Rowe, 24, 188n45

Education Acts: (1870), 96, 99; (1876), 96, 209n29; (1880), 96; (1893), 114; (1899), 114; (1902), 99, 106, 114, 208n15

Education Code (1905), 106–7

Elmy, Elizabeth Wolstenholme, 57, 194n60

*Endymion* (MAB smallpox hospital ship), 139

"English System." *See* infectious disease surveillance, "English System" of

enteric fever, 12, 40, 64, 75, 82, 103, 206n108, 213n118. *See also* typhoid fever

Equifex spray disinfector, 149, *152*

erysipelas, 23, 28, 206n108, 216n3

Farquharson, Robert, 48

Farr, William, 23, 29, 38; army medical statistics compiled by, 24–26; vs Graham, 24–28

Fazakerley Hospital (Liverpool), observation pavilion designs in, 83, *84*

Finance Act (1911), 119

Fitzgerald, Gerald, 161

formalin spray disinfection, 147–49, 154; by Equifex, 149, *152*; by Lumley, 149; by Mackenzie, 149, *150–51*, 179; by Reynolds and Branson, 149

Forwood, Arthur, 52, 58, 196n83

Foucault, Michel, 4

Fraser, George: dry-heat disinfecting apparatus of, 137–38, *138*, 140
Friendly Societies, 11, 26, 29; about, 185n55; membership in, 122, 162, 199n147
Fulham Smallpox Hospital, 87, 89
fumigation, 19, 88, 121, 126, 131, 143–47; discrediting of, 143; formalin spray vs, 147, 149; historical/classical allusions to, 125; Ransome-Delépine experiments with, 144–47, 154, 157; with sulfur, 127, 143, 145, 149, 152, 223n142

Garden Hospital (Nottingham), 74
Gayton, William, 86
General Board of Health, 31, 96
general practitioners (GPs), 11; certificates issued by, 9, 47, 51, 52, 55, 65, 102–3, 106, 199n147; as citizens, 61–62; and compulsory notification, 19, 22, 40–65, 80, 90; and disinfection of homes, 127–28; and hospitalization, 77, 79, 81, 90; and MOHs, 41–42, 59–62; and monitoring/certification of schoolchildren, 98, 100, 102–3, 104; and opposition to notification, 41–42, 47–48, 51–65; and sickness registration, 21–22, 24, 26, 27–29, 38; and TB home care/therapy, 163, 168, 170, 175, 176, 178; and TB notification, 156, 158–59, 161. *See also entry below;* British Medical Association; medical officers of health; private practice
general practitioners (GPs), notification issues for, 58–63; householders' responsibility, 42, 47, 48, 49–52, 53, 61–62, 207n129; income, 47, 51, 55, 199n147; patient autonomy/priority, 59; patient confidentiality, 3, 24, 41–42, 59, 64, 204n64; political resistance/intervention, 47–51, 54, 55, 58–59; professional competition/poaching, 55, 60–61; threat posed by MOH, 60–61
General Register Office (GRO), 23, 90; Farr-Graham disagreement within, 24–28; and Poor Law data collection, 30, 35, 36, 188n70
Goddard company (disinfecting apparatus manufacturer), 140–41, 221n103
Godwin, George, 122–23
Graham, George, 23, 27–28, 30
Griffiths, Francis, 124
Greenock (Scotland): notification in, 2

Hall, Arthur, 160–61, 227n42, 227n44
Hamilton, Robert, 51–52, 61
Hardie, James, 69, 72, 201nn1–2
Hart, Ernest, 58–59, 199n144
Hastings, George Woodyatt, 48, 49, 50–51, 56, 61
Hawkley, Henry, 77–78, 204n52
Henry, William, 135–36, 220n84; heat disinfecting apparatus of, 136, *137*, 138
"herd immunity": in schools, 13, 110, 213n118; against TB, 154
Heron, Joseph, 34, 190n107
Hill, Alfred, 54–55, 56
Hippocratic Oath, 59, 62, 64
Hobbes, Thomas, 4
Hobhouse, Leonard Trelawney, 179
Holden, Oscar, 163
home, as locus of disease prevention, control, and care, 11, 14–16, 36, 54; for children under five, 112–13, 213n123; and class aspects of notification/hospitalization, 32, 47, 62–63, 70, 71–81, 89; disinfection and, 13–14, 16, 21, 121–53; family's "fitness" to maintain, 122; and resistance to hospitalization of children, 71–72, 75, 77, 78–81, 86–87, 92, 128; self-regulated management of, 132–43, 153, 164–66; as subject to be taught in school, 94–95; in TB cases, 5, 14, 16, 119, 155–56, 163–78, 182; women's importance to, 15–16, 93–94, 112–14. *See also* sickroom; tuberculosis, home care/preventive therapy for

home, as locus of infectious risk, 11, 22; architectural aspects of, 121, 123, 147; class aspects of, 11, 32–33, 62–63, 96; in clothes and furnishings, 121, 124, 126, 128, 133, 135, 171; vs environment of isolation hospital, 36, 70–71, 78, 85–86, 91–92; to family members, 88, 159, 162, 172; and infectious disease in schoolchildren, 13, 16, 93–120; in measles cases, 104–12; normalcy of, 64; in sickroom, 121, 124, 127, 132, 216n3; in TB cases, 162
Homerton Smallpox Hospital, 86, 88
hospitalization. *See* isolation hospitals, *and entries following;* Metropolitan Asylums Board (MAB) hospitals; private hospitals; sanatoria
householders, notification duty of: citizenship and, 2, 61–62; in dual system, 47, 48, 49–50, 53, 61, 207n129; physicians' support for, 42, 51–52, 53, 63; and possible recourse to unqualified healers, 61
Howard, Ebenezer, 20–21
Huddersfield (Yorkshire): early notification legislation of, 2, 47, 51; hospitalization/hospital rules in, 77, 88
Humphries, Noel, 90
Hygeia (fictional utopian city), 20–21, 34, 179

Imperial Office of Hygiene (Germany), 139
industry, and resistance/vulnerability to disease: among brass workers, 24; in Manchester mills, 33; in Sheffield steel/cutlery factories, 159
infectious disease notification, 1–4, 5–10; arguments for/against physician involvement in, 3, 21, 22, 24–29; Buchanan on need for, 1–2, 3, 6, 47, 179, 180; in city environment, 19–22; class aspects of, 11, 29–34, 47, 62–63; and concept of sickness registration, 4, 11, 19–39, 47–48; dual system of, 47, 48, 49–50, 51–52, 53, 61, 207n129; early local implementation of, 2, 5, 7–8, 40–65, 100; by Hygeia's physicians, 21, 34; as later made compulsory nationwide, 2, 19, 41, 51, 155; and Poor Law data collection, 22, 29–39; RSC and, 21–29, 34, 35–36, 37–38; rural lack of, 41, 50; of TB, 14, 119, 153, 155, 156–62, 182; and socially deviant, 44–45, 46, 126. *See also entries below; entries for specific cities;* tuberculosis, notification of
infectious disease notification, early local implementation of, 2, 5, 7–8, 40–65, 100; "bastard laws" enabling, 7–8, 42, 49, 53; and disinfection, 40–41, 45, 57; and experience of legislation regulating the socially deviant, 43–47; in Huddersfield, 2, 47, 51; and issues of liberty vs compulsion, 41–43; as leading to national legislation, 47–51; in Leicester, 43, 57–58, 80; LGB's resistance to, 47–51; and need for hospital accommodations, 41, 47, 48, 53, 55; opposition to, 41–42, 47–48, 51–65; and opposition to enforced hospitalization, 42, 69–70. *See also specific cities and towns*
infectious disease notification, opposition to: and antivaccination movement, 3, 42, 43, 45–46, 48, 56, 57–58, 61, 78, 80; and experience of legislation regulating the socially deviant, 43–47; by GPs, 41–42, 47–48, 51–65; LGB and, 47–51; radical liberalism and, 42–43, 45, 56–59, 60; in TB cases, 155, 156–62
Infectious Disease (Notification) Act (1889), 19, 41, 42, 43, 50–51, 52, 56–57, 100, 155, 157, 162
Infectious Disease (Notification) Act (1899), 2, 19, 41, 51, 155
Infectious Disease (Notification) Acts, 104, 157, 159–60
Infectious Disease (Prevention) Act (1890), 78, 129, 223n141

infectious disease surveillance, "English System" of, 1–16; and bacteriology, 5, 6–7, 8, 14, 19; and disinfection, 5–6, 13–14, 16, 121–53; early local implementation of, 2, 5, 7–8, 40–65, 100; and family/domestic sphere, 14–16; "inspectability" of, 8–10, 44; intrusive nature of, 3–4, 5, 6–7, 38, 43, 59, 98, 180; in isolation hospitals, 5–6, 11–12, 16, 69–92; and monitoring of schoolchildren, 5–6, 13, 16, 93–120; and sickness registration vs Poor Law data collection, 4, 11, 19–39, 47–48, 71; spatial aspects of, 8–14; and TB notification/home care, 5, 14, 16, 154–78
influenza, 28, 216n3
insanity, 23, 26
"inspectability," 8–10, 44
isolation hospitals, 5–6, 11–12, 16, 69–92; citizenship and, 4, 12, 42, 57, 71, 181; class aspects of removal to, 42, 62–63, 70, 71–81, 87, 89; coerced attendance at, 70, 80–81; compulsory attendance at, 69–70, 71–72, 77–81; costs of, 12, 73, 74, 78; deaths in, vs deaths at home, 78, 91, *92*; disinfection in, 81, 87, 88, 128, 131, 136, 138–39, 149; and disinfection of homes, 124, 128, 129; existence of, as needed to enable notification, 41, 47, 48, 53, 55; forcible removal to, 4, 71, 77–78; legislation governing, 70; Mill on, 69, 72–73; as new/retrofitted buildings, 73–74; opposition/resistance to, 69, 74–75, 77, 78–81, 90–91, 128; pauperism/pauperization in, 70, 74, 77; potential for cross-infection in, 23–24, 70–71, 81–82, 85–90; and pressures of notification, 74, 81–82, 83; private rooms in, 77, 87; resistance to children's sequestration in, 71–72, 75, 77, 78–81, 86–87, 92, 128; rules for visitors (permeability management) in, 85–90; rural vs urban provision of, 70, 73, 74; scarlet fever cases in, 55, 69, 71, 74–75, *76*, 77–78, 79, 80, 82, 83, 85, 86, 87, 89, 90–91, *92*, 159, 198n129, 202n14; separation/observation in, 81–85; uncertain success of, 90–92. *See also entries below*
isolation hospitals, architecture/design of, 81–85; cubicle-style wards in, 84–85, 205n79; as new construction, 73, 74; pavilion-style wards in, 81, 82–84, *84*; as retrofitted buildings, 74; windows/floors in, 81
isolation hospitals, visitors to, 85–90; as allowed only when patient near death, 87, 88, 89; parents as, 86–87; patient updates published for, 89–90; as requiring proof of vaccination, 88; special clothing for/cleansing of, 87–88; "window appointments" for, 89
Isolation Hospitals Act (1893), 70, 71

Johnson, S. G., 54, 197n107
Johnston, William, 57, 58, 60, 64–65, 79

Kaye, James Robert, 75
Kerr, James, 95, 115; first report of, 107; on parental neglect, 110–11, 120; on "right living"/hygiene as school subject, 94–95; on school closure as admission of defeat, 107, 112; and Woolwich measles study, 107–12
Koch, Robert, 6, 124, 139, 143, 145, 154

Ladies National Association, 45, 50
Lancashire: cotton famine in, 33, 35, 37; disinfection apparatus in, 129, 132; sulfur fumigation in, 149. *See also* Liverpool; Manchester
*Lancet, The*, 36, 90; on disinfection, 137, 142, 145
Lawrence, Sir Trevor, 48
leaflet campaigns: in contact tracing, 102; against TB/phthisis, 156, 157, 161, 164
Leeds: disinfection in, 131, 149

Leicester, 8; antivaccination movement in, and approach to smallpox, 43, 57–58, 80; disinfection in, 129, 132; children's chronic disease register in, 118; hospitalization in, 73, 79, 80, 89; monitoring of schoolchildren in, 100, 102, 103, 105, 118; notification in, 43, 57–58, 60, 64–65, 80. *See also entry below*
Leicester, MOHs of: Crane, 57–58, 103; Johnston, 57, 58, 60, 64–65, 79; Millard, 91, 102; Priestley, 105, 139
Leicester Medical Society (LMS), 58
Leicestershire, 73, 129, 132
Leigh, John, 34, 39
Letheby, Henry, 136–37, 188n45
Liberty and Property Defence League, 49, 60
Lithiby, John, 160
Liverpool, 8; disinfection in, 129, 131; early Poor Law data collection in, 30, 34; hospitalization in, 71, 83, *84*; monitoring of schoolchildren in, 104, 118; notification in, 43, 51–52, 56, 58, 60–61, 62–63, 64; voluntary TB notification in, 156, 158
Liverpool Medical Institution (LMI), 51–52, 58, 195n78
Liverpool Sanatory Act (1846), 30
Livy, John, 48
Local Government Act (1858), 46, 218n63
Local Government Board (LGB): Buchanan and, 1, 47, 75, 183n2; and disinfection, 140, 161; establishment of, 188n70; and isolation hospitals, 41, 74, 78, 82–85; Mackenzie and, 149, 179, 182; and MOH appointments/salaries, 53–55; and notification, 47–51, 56, 61, 63, 226n40; and Poor Law relief, 35, 36; and school closure/pupil exclusion, 96, 112, 209n37; and TB notification, 158–62; and Thomson's measles control study, 104–6
lodging houses, 15, 44–45; disinfection of, 45, 126; legislation governing, 45, 46, 126
London, 8, 64; diphtheria antitoxin used in, 107; disinfection in, 125, 129, 136–37, 139–41, 143; hospitalization in, 71, 77, 82, 85, 87, 89, 165; MAB hospitals in, 36–37, 41, 77, 82, 85; monitoring of schoolchildren in, 93–120; notification in, 41, 50, 59, 100; Poor Law data collection in, 22, 30–31, 32, 35, 37; struggle against measles in, 97, 98, 106, 107–12, 118, 120. *See also entries below*
London County Council (LCC), 96, 116–17, 118–19
London Fever Hospital, 87, 205n79
London School Board (LSB), 94–95, 96, 99; as first board to appoint medical officer, 103–4; as informing MOHs of cases, 100, 101; and notified cases of infectious disease (1906–14), 96, 97; and school closures for measles, 98, 106, 112; and Woolwich measles study, 98, 107–12, 118. *See also* contact tracing of schoolchildren; Kerr, James; measles, *and entry following;* schools, *and entries following*
Lumley (L.) and Co. (spray-pump manufacturer), 149
Lyon, Washington: steam disinfector of, 139–41, *141*

Mackenzie, W. Leslie: disinfectant spray-pumps of, 149, *150–51*, 179; on citizenship and notification, 179–82
malnutrition, 115; measles and, 33, 120; TB and, 118–19
Manchester, 8; cleaning of schoolchildren in, 215n155; disinfection process/experiments in, 13, 129, 131, 135–37, 143, 144–47, 154, 157; and dual notification, 50; hospitalization in, 39, 71, 72, 77, 201n2; monitoring of schoolchildren in, 104, 112; Poor Law data collection/disease reporting in, 22, 29, 31, 32–34, 37; poverty and disease in, 33, 39; TB leaflet campaign in,

156, 161, 164; TB notification in, 156. *See also* Niven, James
Manchester and Salford Sanitary Association (MSSA), disease reporting system of, 22, 29, 31, 32–34, 37, 69; and need for working-class responsibility/self-help, 32–33, 156–57
Marshall, T. H., 183n10
Martineau, Robert Francis (Frank), 56–57, 198n121
Martineau, Thomas, 56, 198n121
Massachusetts State Board of Health, 1
May, Francis, 106
McLaren, Walter, 50, 195n70
McMillan, Margaret, 95
measles, 13, 28, 85, 216n3; about, 212n86; as contracted in home, 104–12; cost of dealing with, 212n88; London's struggle against, 97, 98, 106, 107–12, 118, 120; and malnutrition, 33, 120; in rural and urban sanitary districts, 104. *See also entry below*
measles in schools, 96–98, 101, 102, 104–13; attendance and, 104–7; closures for, 98, 105–6, 112; "combustible material" of children vulnerable to, 108, *109*, 120; as studied in Woolwich, 98, 107–12, 118; as tracked through Nellie's case, 110–11, *111*
Medical Acts: (1858), 61; (1886), 60–61
medical officers of health (MOHs): appointments of, 11; associations of, 1–2, 23, 30, 31, 47, 137, 156–57; and disinfection, 129, 142, 144, 149; and GPs, 41–42, 59–62; and hospitalization, 34, 46, 70, 71, 74–75, 78, 81–82, 91, 203n43; and monitoring of schoolchildren, 96, 98, 99–103, 105–8, 111, 112–13, 115, 214n140; and notification, 2, 8, 40–65; powers of, 45, 46, 59–60, 63–64, 78, 96, 158; and private practice, 52–53, 54–55, 60–61, 200n162; professional credentialing of, 60–61, 200n165; and sickness registration vs Poor Law data collection, 28–31, 34, 38–39; and TB notification, 156–62, 224nn10–11. *See also* Leicester, MOHs of; Nottingham, MOHs of; Sheffield, MOHs of; *specific MOHs by name*
Metropolis Local Management Act (1855), 143
Metropolitan Asylums Board (MAB) hospitals, 36–37, 41, 82; cubicle layouts in, 83, 85; in and pauperization of patients, 37, 77; and smallpox, 85, 86, 87–88, 139; and visitor rules/monitoring, 86, 87–88. *See also* workhouses, infirmaries of
Mill, John Stuart, 46, 69, 72–73, 193n31; *On Liberty*, 69
Millard, Killick, 91, 102
Milroy, Gavin, 34, 190n110
mothers: and children's hospitalization, 79, 80, 86–87, 88; consumptive, 157; as important to home/domestic sphere, 15–16, 93–94, 112–14; need for education of, 105, 112–14, 117, 120, 164; and vulnerability to disease, 75, 88; working-class, 33, 80, 110–11, 120. *See also* women
mumps, 112
Murphy, Shirley F., 157, 211n85

National Anti-contagious Diseases Acts Association, 45, 61
National Association for the Prevention of Consumption, 156, 163; journal of, 229n85
National Association for the Promotion of Social Science, 23, 193n44
National Insurance Act (1911): "sanatorium benefit" of, 119, 163, 165
Nellie I. (Woolwich schoolchild), as origin of measles cases, 110–11, *111*
New Poor Law. *See* Poor Law, New (1834), *and entries following*
Newcastle, 50, 157–58; hospitalization in, 71, 74; Poor Law data collection in, 22, 31, 33–34, 37

Newman, George, 112, 115
Newsholme, Arthur, 101, 112, 125, 157–58, 227n44, 227n46; as proponent of notification, 9, 39, 90, 160; *School Hygiene*, 103, 211n78; and voluntary TB notification, 156, 158
Nightingale, Florence, 187n36, 188n45
Niven, James: as Manchester MOH, 112, 156–58, 160, 221n114, 222n134, 232n157; as Oldham MOH, 156, 224nn10–11
North, S. W., 38
Northumberland and Durham Medical Society (NDMS), 31, 33–34, 190n102
notification. *See* infectious disease notification, *and entries following*
Notification of Births Act (1907), 116
Nottingham, 8; disinfection process/manufacture in, 129, *130*, 132, 133, 134, 138, 140–41; hospitalization in, 73, 74–75, *76*, 78, 79–80, 81–82, 83, 89, 91, *92*, 138–39; monitoring of schoolchildren in, 100–101, 105–6; and notification, 40, 42, 43, 48–49, 52–53, 54, 56, 58; scarlet fever notifications/hospitalizations in, 82, 83; and TB notification, 157–58. *See also entry below*
Nottingham, MOHs of: Boobbyer, 91, 105–6, 157–58; Seaton, 40, 52–54, 64, 74, 157, 196n94; Whitelegge, 81–82, 83
Nottinghamshire, 73, 129, 132
Nuisances Removal Acts (1845, 1846, 1855), 30, 46, 126

Oldham: disinfection in, 129, 143; hospital rules for parents in, 87; Niven as MOH of, 156, 224nn10–11; TB leaflet campaigns in, 156, 164, 229n81
open-air aspects of medical care/home therapy, 119, 164, 165, 175, 176, 227n46, 230n119
Otter, Chris, 21; on "inspectability," 8–10, 44
outdoor relief of infectious paupers, 31, 35, 37, 77; as risky/unsustainable, 11, 22, 36; Smith on, 35, 36, 71
Owens College Pathological Laboratory (Manchester), 144–47; experimental disinfection chamber at, 147, *148*

Paget, Charles, 28
Parkes, Louis, 157–58, 160
Parsons, Franklin, 149, 152; disinfection experiments by, 140; report on hospitals by, 85
Pasteur, Louis, 6, 137, 145
Pasteur Institute (Paris), hospital of, 84
pauperization of infectious patients, 37, 77, 203n43
paupers, infectious, 22, 34–39, 44; as admitted to hospitals, 74, 77; enumeration of, 29–34; home treatment of, 36; on outdoor relief, 11, 22, 31, 35, 36, 37, 39, 71, 77; and TB notification, 156. *See also* Poor Law, New (1834), *and entries following;* workhouses, *and entry following*
Pearmain, Thomas Hames, et al.: *Applied Bacteriology*, 148
phthisis, 156–59, 182; in Sheffield, 159–60, 162. *See also* tuberculosis
plague, 12, 135, 216n3
plasticine, as promoted for TB patients' amusement, 172, *173*, 175, 178
Poor Law, New (1834), 3; and workhouse medical care, 11, 12, 22, 31, 32, 34, 35, 36–37, 55, 77, 155, 163. *See also entries below;* workhouses, *and entry following*
Poor Law Board (PLB), 30, 35, 36, 71
Poor Law data collection, 22, 29–39; administrative problems/disputes arising from, 30–31, 33, 34, 35; financial aspects of, 22, 29, 32; by MSSA, 32–34; in Newcastle, 33–34; and numbers of infectious paupers, 22, 29–37; and outdoor relief conditions/need for hospital treatment of paupers, 11, 22, 35, 36, 37, 39, 71; Smith's study of, 35–39, 71
Poor Law medical officers (PLMOs), 29–36; and lodging houses, 45; of

MSSA, 32–34; Simon and, 30–31; workload of, 34–36
Poor Law unions (London), hospitals created by, 37. *See also* Metropolitan Asylums Board (MAB) hospitals; workhouses, *and entry following*
Priestley, Joseph, 105, 139
private hospitals, 12, 71, 115; as sanatoria, 163
private practice: attempts to gather statistics from, 27–29; class aspects of, 62–63; competition/poaching in, 55, 60–61; MOHs and, 52–53, 54–55, 60–61, 200n162; PLMOs in, 191n116; sanctity of, 42, 59
Privy Council, Medical Department of the, 23, 27, 126
prostitution, 3, 42, 44–45, 46
Public Health Act (1848), 218n63
Public Health Act (1872), 21, 55
Public Health Act (1875): and disinfection, 129; and evolution from sickness registration to notification, 21, 47–48, 54, 59–60; and isolation hospitals, 21, 41, 70, 71, 74; and lodging houses, 45; and notification of infectious schoolchildren, 100

Queen's Memorial Infectious Diseases Hospital (Australia), 87

Ransom, William, 138–39
Ransome, Arthur, 38, 48, 51–52; fumigation experiments by, 144–46, 154, 157; and MSSA disease registration system, 29, 32; and phthisis, 156–57
Ravenhill, Alice, 94, 95, 116, 208n13
Reform Act (1867), 3, 122
Reynolds and Branson (spray-pump manufacturer), 149
Richardson, Benjamin Ward, 21, 38; *Hygeia*, 20–21, 34, 179; sickness registration scheme developed by, 28–29, 33
Rideal, Samuel: *Disinfection and Disinfectants*, 147; and Rideal-Walker test for disinfectant efficacy, 219n82
Ritchie, Charles, 50
Robertson, John, 159–61, 162, 226n38
Royal Commission on the Contagious Diseases Acts, 72
Royal Commission on Small-Pox and Fever Hospitals, 88
Royal Sanitary Commission (RSC), 21–29, 46, 47, 180; and Poor Law data collection, 22, 29, 34, 35–36, 37–38; and rejection of physicians' information, 24–29
Rumsey, Henry Wyldbore, 21–22, 23, 34, 38, 186–87nn23–24, 188n45, 190n107
Russell, Alexander: *The Natural History of Aleppo*, 136
Russell, James, 158

sanatoria, 163–66; care in, as adapted to home, 14, 155–56, 163, 165–72, 175–76, 178, 182; costs/insurability of care in, 119, 162, 163, 165; funding of, 163; as housing only small minority of TB patients, 14, 119, 155, 163, 165; open-air aspect of, 119, 164, 227n46, 230n119; treatment regime in, 164, 166, 229n75
Sanderson, John Burdon, 90
Sanitary Act (1866), 41, 45, 46–47, 59–60, 70, 71; and disinfection, 127–28
sanitary districts, rural and urban, 218n63; disinfection in, 129, 130–31; measles control in, 104; Midlands hospitals in, 73
Sayer, Henry, 159–60
scarlet fever, 12, 28, 32, 140, 211n86, 216n3; in children, 40, 64, 79, 80, 86, 96–97, 100–101, 103, 104, 110, 210n60; deaths from, 10, 75, 91, *92*, 104, 138; diagnosis of, 82; in Hawkley case, 77–78, 204n52; hospitalization for, 55, 69, 71, 74–75, *76*, 77–78, 79, 80, 82, 83, 85, 86, 87, 89, 90–91, *92*, 159, 198n129, 202n14; notification for, 2, 40, 53, 54, 55, 80, 82, 83, 100–101, 103; Simon's memorandum on, 128

school boards, 99; and handling of infectious diseases, 99–107, 211n80. *See also* London School Board
School Medical Service (SMS), 98, 114–19, 120, 214n140
schools: administration/funding of, 99–104; in era of heightened national identity/imperialism, 93–94, 114; gender roles and, 93–94; medical officers of (SMOs), 115, 214n140; and reification of home/domestic sphere, 93–95, 112–14, 116, 118, 120; and "right living"/hygiene as teachable subject, 94–95. *See also entries below;* contact tracing of schoolchildren; measles, *and entry following*
schools, attendance at: administrative/financial aspects of, 99–104; debate over proper starting age for, 98, 112–13, 213n123; measles' effect on, 104–7; officers tasked with monitoring, 100, 101–2, 103, 112, 116, 119
schools, closure of, 103, 115, 120; as admission of defeat, 107, 112; vs exclusion of pupils, 96, 98, 99, 105, 107–8, 110–12; for measles, 98, 105–6, 112; as threat to school income, 99, 106–7, 108; Woolwich measles study and, 98, 107–12, 118
schools, infectious diseases at, 5–6, 13, 16, 93–120; and administrative/financial aspects of attendance, 99–104; attendance officers and, 100, 101–2, 103, 112, 116, 119; care committees and, 116–17, 118, 119; class aspects of dealing with, 93–94, 96, 103, 110–11, 114–19, 120; and cleaning of children, 117, 215n155; closures caused by, 96, 98, 99, 103, 105–8, 110, 111–12, 115, 120; and disinfection of homes, 103, 104–5, 115; GPs and, 98, 100, 102–3, 104; "herd immunity" to, 13, 110, 213n118; and measles notification, 104–7; and measles study in Woolwich, 98, 107–12, 118; and medical inspections, 96, 102, 114–19; and "mothercraft," 112–14; problems/lapses in dealing with, 100–103; and system of following-up, 114–19
Sclater-Booth, George, 47–48
Scurfield, Harold, 162
Seaton, Edward, 40, 52–54, 64, 74, 157, 196n94
Seguin, Édouard, 95
Select Committee on Police and Sanitary Regulations (SCPSR), 49–51, 52, 63, 64, 195n62
sequestration. *See* isolation hospitals; sanatoria
Sheffield, 75, 90; disinfection in, 124, 129, 161–62; and evolution from voluntary to compulsory TB notification, 14, 50, 119, 159–62, 165, 182; monitoring of schoolchildren in, 100, 102, 118, 119; phthisis in, 159–60, 162. *See also entry below*
Sheffield, MOHs of: 159–61, 162, 226n38; Scurfield, 162; Thomson, 160, 162
Sick Children's Hospital (Necker Hospital, Paris), 84
sickness registration, 4, 11, 19–39, 47–48; Dickens on, 29–30; Farr's army work and, 24–26; GPs and, 21–22, 24, 26, 27–29, 38; MOHs and, 28–31, 34, 38–39; vs Poor Law data collection, 22, 29–39, 71; Richardson's scheme of, 28–29, 33; RSC and, 24–29; significance of, 37–39. *See also* infectious disease notification; Poor Law data collection
sickroom: cleanliness/disinfection of, 121, 124, 127, 132; attempted laboratory replication of, 146–47; as opened by notification, 59–60; and parents' right to care for child, 71–72; removal of furnishings from, 121, 132, 216n3; setup of, as reducing living space, 124; as ultimate private domestic space, 124.

*See also* tuberculosis, home care/ preventive therapy for
Simon, John, 35, 153, 188n45; disinfection memoranda by, 126–27, 128, 136, 154; as London MOH, 30–31; RSC testimony by, 23, 27, 128
smallpox, 28, 140, 202n14, 216n3; in children, 64, 86, 96, 103; deaths from, 75, 104; disinfection against, 57, 74, 129, 136, 137, 228n59; epidemics of, 50, 53, 75, 129, 137, 198n129, 226n40, 228n59; hospitalization for, 12, 41, 74, 75, 85, 86, 87, 88, 89, 198n129, 202n14, 207n128; "Leicester method" of dealing with, 43, 57–58, 80; MAB hospital ship for, 139; notification of, 40, 43, 47, 53, 54, 55, 57, 61–62, 103. *See also entry below*
smallpox vaccination, compulsory: for infants, 3, 5, 14, 44, 45, 63, 78; legislation governing, 45–46, 63; Leicester's experience with, 43, 57–58, 80; notification and, 40; opposition to, 3, 42, 43, 45–46, 48, 56, 57–58, 61, 78, 80; proof of, as needed for hospital visitors, 88
smallpox vaccine lymph, as used in disinfection experiment, 136
Smith, Charles, 74
Smith, Edward, 35–39; on outdoor relief conditions/need for hospital treatment of paupers, 35, 36, 71; on workhouse conditions, 36. *See also* Poor Law data collection
Smith, W. R., 103–4, 211n80, 211n85
Society of Medical Officers of Health (SMOH): Buchanan's speech to, 1–2, 47; phthisis memorandum of, 156–57; and TB, 157
Solihull Rural Sanitary District (Warwickshire): isolation hospital with steam disinfector in, 131
sputum: and airborne transmission of TB, 157, 230n115; destruction/ disposal of, 159, 161, 164, 225n24; as mentioned in leaflet campaigns, 156, 164; as tested for TB, 107, 160–61; as used in fumigation experiments, 144–45
steam disinfection, 131, 139–42, 148, 154; by Bradford, 138, *139*, 140; by Goddard, 140–41, 221n103; by Lyon, 138–41, *141*; by Thresh, 142, *142*
sulfur fumigation, 127, 143, 145, 149, 152, 223n142. *See also* fumigation
Sykes, John F. J., 59, 112–13, 157, 213n123

Tait, Lawson, 56
Tatham, John, 50, 144
Taylor, Charles Bell, 48–49, 51, 56, 197n98; on "bastard laws" of local notification, 42, 49, 53
Temperance Movement, 3
Thomas, C. J., 107, 110
Thomson, Anthony Todd, 121, 216n3
Thomson, Henry Hyslop: *Consumption, Its Prevention and Home Treatment*, 165–71, 172, 178, 229n90; progress chart in, 166, 168, *169*; thermometer illustration in, 166, *167*
Thomson, Theodore, 84, 85, 104–6, 160–62
Thorne, Richard Thorne, 78, 79, 86, 90
Thresh, John, and company of, 149; steam disinfecting apparatus of, 142, *142*
tuberculosis, 154–78; compulsory notification of, 14, 119, 153, 154–55, 156–62, 182; disinfection/fumigation against, 140, 144–46, 153, 154–55; home care/preventive therapy for, 5, 14, 16, 119, 155–56, 163–72, 178, 182; leaflet campaigns against, 156, 157, 161, 164; and malnutrition, 118–19; sanatoria for, 163–66; among schoolchildren, 107, 115, 118–19; in Sheffield, 14, 119, 159–62; stigma of, 157–58; in US, 224n15; varying opinions on control of, 154–55; voluntary notification of, 156–59; women's vulnerability to, 159, 162. *See also entries below;* sanatoria; sputum

tuberculosis, home care/preventive therapy for, 5, 14, 16, 119, 155–56, 163–72, 182; as adaptation of sanatorium care, 14, 155–56, 163, 165–72, 175–76, 178, 182; class aspects of, 231n120; open-air aspects of, 165, 175, 176, 230n119; and promotion of consumer goods, 156, 172–78; self-help manuals on, 14, 165–71, 172, 178; and vulnerability of women, 162. *See also* consumer goods, as promoted to tuberculosis patients, *and entry following*; sickroom; *specific self-help manuals by author*
tuberculosis, notification of: as compulsory, 14, 119, 153, 154–55, 159–62, 182; disinfection and, 154–55, 157, 158, 161, 162, 182; early voluntary systems of, 156–59; educational efforts accompanying, 155, 156–57, 161, 162, 164–71, 172, 178; evolution of, in Sheffield, 14, 50, 119, 159–62, 165, 182; as leading to home-based care/preventive therapy, 155–62; opposition to, 155, 156–62; as welcomed by public, 160–61
typhoid fever, 40, 54, 64, 103, 127. *See also* enteric fever
typhus, 28, 33, 52, 54, 69, 103, 216n3

Vaccination Acts: (1853), 45–46, 63; (1867), 193n31. *See also* smallpox vaccination, compulsory
venereal disease, 12, 27, 44, 45, 72–73, 216n3
Vigilance Association for the Defence of Personal Rights (VADPR), 48, 54, 59, 61, 62, 63, 200n171; feminists in, 194n47; on isolation hospitals, 77
visitors to hospitals. *See* isolation hospitals, visitors to

Walker, J. T. Ainslie, 219n82
Warwickshire, 73, 131, 132, 312. *See also* Birmingham
Water Works and Improvement Act (Huddersfield, 1876), 2, 47, 51
Watson, Thomas, 36–37
Welton, C. J., 78, 79
West Lane Fever Hospital (Middlesbrough), 89
Whitelegge, Arthur, 81–82, 83
Whittle, Ewing, 61
whooping cough, 13, 28, 33, 64, 79, 104, 112, 204n58, 216n3
Windley, Thomas, 57, 58
women, 36, 57; gendered education of, 93–94; as important to home/domestic sphere, 15–16, 93–94, 112–14; on school boards, 99; and VADPR, 48, 194n47; and vulnerability to TB, 159, 162, 172. *See also* mothers
Woolwich (London), measles study in, 98, 107–12, 118
Worboys, Michael, 4, 5, 6, 7, 19, 124–25, 154, 163, 164
workhouses, 31, 34, 77, 155; disinfection of clothing in, 136; vs outdoor relief, 22; as sites of later hospitals, 55, 74. *See also entry below*
workhouses, infirmaries of, 11, 12, 31, 32, 77, 155; bed capacity of, 73; poor record-keeping in, 35; studies of, 36–37; TB morbidity in, 163. *See also* Metropolitan Asylums Board (MAB) hospitals
Working Men's National League, 52
Wunderlich, Carl, 168

Yorkshire, 38. *See also entry below;* Huddersfield
Yorkshire (West Riding), 75, 94; disinfection apparatus in, 129, 132. *See also* Sheffield
Young, Meredith, 71

www.ingramcontent.com/pod-product-compliance
Lightning Source LLC
LaVergne TN
LVHW091526200926
848483LV00002B/317

* 9 7 8 1 5 8 0 4 6 5 2 7 4 *